PROSTHETIC TREATMENT
OF THE EDENTULOUS PATIENT

PROSTHETIC TREATMENT OF THE EDENTULOUS PATIENT

R. M. BASKER, DDS, MGDSRCS, LDSRCS
Professor of Dental Prosthetics, University of Leeds;
Consultant in Restorative Dentistry, Leeds General Infirmary and
Associated Hospitals Trust; Examiner, MGDS of the Royal
College of Surgeons of England; formerly External Examiner, the
Universities of Birmingham, Bristol, Dundee, London,
Manchester, Newcastle-upon-Tyne, Sheffield and Wales

J. C. DAVENPORT, PhD, BDS, FDSRCS
Senior Lecturer in Dental Prosthetics, University of
Birmingham; Consultant Dental Surgeon,
South Birmingham Health Authority; External Examiner, the
Universities of Wales, Dublin and Leeds; formerly External
Examiner, University of Glasgow

H. R. TOMLIN, DDS, LDSRCS
Emeritus Professor of Dental Prosthetics, University of
Birmingham; formerly External Examiner, Queen's University
Belfast and the Universities of Edinburgh, London, Leeds and
Wales

THIRD EDITION

M
MACMILLAN

First edition 1976
Reprinted (with corrections) 1979, 1980, 1981, 1982
Second edition 1983
Third edition 1992

Published by
MACMILLAN EDUCATION LTD
Houndmills, Basingstoke, Hampshire RG21 2XS
and London
Companies and representatives
throughout the world

ISBN 0–333–56704–8
ISBN 0–333–56705–6

A catalogue record for this book is available from the
British Library.

Printed in Hong Kong

To our families

Contents

Preface to the First Edition

Over the years, the writings and researches of many prosthetists have hastened the swing from the mechanistic to the biological approach in complete-denture prosthetics. With this change in outlook there has been an increasing awareness of the tremendous variation that is found in edentulous patients: the variation in quality of the denture-bearing tissues and their response to function, the varying behaviour of the jaw mechanisms, the differing patterns of muscle function which act upon the dentures and, finally, the varying and often unexpected response of patients to the challenge of wearing complete dentures. Clinical techniques have been devised and modified to meet these variations.

Effective clinical procedures are built on a sound theoretical basis and in this text an attempt is made to present the theoretical background in the early chapters and to use this background to justify the clinical techniques which are subsequently described. In an effort to economise in an age of ever-rising costs, repetition has been avoided wherever possible and frequent references are made to other parts of the book where particular items are considered in greater detail.

Because of the varied response mentioned earlier, it is not sufficient for the clinician to possess only one basic technique of constructing complete dentures, no matter how sophisticated. Instead, it is of the utmost importance to develop a flexible approach when devising a treatment plan and to have available alternative methods of treatment appropriate to the needs of the individual patient. We have avoided presenting detailed descriptions of clinical techniques in the belief that once the background information is understood one can become proficient only by chairside tuition and clinical experience. Only practice makes perfect and the greater one's clinical experience, the more one will have learnt from successes and failures.

The background information on materials science, pre-prosthetic surgery and prosthetic laboratory techniques has not been included as these subjects are covered fully in well-established texts which are readily available to students.

The purpose of the bibliography at the end of each chapter is two-fold. First, to include references which may be related directly to clinical techniques described in the text, and second, to provide a selection of key sources which will enable the reader to commence a search of the literature on a particular topic of interest.

Inevitably, the replacement of lost tissues by complete dentures is a compromise; in spite of modern developments there remain limitations to this aspect of restorative dentistry and some patients continue to have difficulty in coming to terms with these limitations. Because of the understandable demands of the patients for good-looking, comfortable and efficient complete dentures, no matter what the problems in the mouth, complete-denture prosthetics remains a demanding and challenging aspect of a dentist's clinical life.

Birmingham, 1976   R.M.B.
                                                           J.C.D.
                                                           H.R.T.

Preface to the Third Edition

In preparing the third edition we have again attempted to preserve the principles which governed the structure of the book in the first instance. At the same time we have undertaken a thorough revision of the text bearing in mind the changes which have occurred during the last eight years – perhaps the most significant being the continuing fall in numbers of edentulous patients together with the transition to the completely artificial dentition being generally made somewhat later in life.

High levels of full clearances in previous years mean that there are still large numbers of people, indeed the majority of those over 65 years of age, with complete dentures. There will therefore remain a considerable need for replacement dentures for many years to come. However, those individuals requiring full clearances and complete dentures for the first time will be increasingly elderly and will become fewer in number. The consequence of this changing pattern is that, although there will be a gradual reduction in the volume of complete-denture prosthetics over the next 50 years, the work will become more demanding as it increasingly relates to the welfare of elderly patients.

In the new edition, we have introduced a specific section on the problems of elderly patients. Also included for the first time is a section on the prevention of cross-infection. Major alterations have been made to topics such as copy dentures, the treatment of mucosal lesions and the management of those people who suffer from the burning mouth syndrome. We have broadened the approach of the chapters dealing with patient assessment and muscular control of dentures. All other chapters have been revised thoroughly to take account of the changes in technique and the approach to treatment that have occurred since the second edition was published.

Leeds, Birmingham and Gresford, 1991

R.M.B.
J.C.D.
H.R.T.

Foreword to the First Edition

This addition to prosthetic literature must be widely and warmly welcomed. For a number of years there has been a shortage of British texts for students concerning the edentulous patient. The authors have, correctly, stressed the serious problems that more and more frequently present themselves now that life expectancy is on the increase and the average age of the edentulous is advancing. The dental profession is becoming aware of the particular geriatric situations it now has to face and this book will undoubtedly help in solving many prosthetic geriatric problems.

Emphasis has been placed more upon general principles than upon the minutiae of clinical or technical operative detail. Given a sound basic understanding of the principles to be observed in the treatment of the edentulous, chairside experience rapidly perfects each individual's manipulative skills.

Being not unfamiliar with the labours involved in producing textbooks one is conscious of the time and effort that has gone into the preparation of this book. It should achieve all the success that these efforts of one's former colleagues deserve.

Shalfleet, Isle of Wight, 1975   JOHN OSBORNE

Acknowledgements

We are most grateful to Professor R. J. Anderson, Dr O. J. Corrado and Dr C. J. Watson for checking sections of the latest edition and offering their constructive comments. For those sections of the book which have not required revision this time we should like to acknowledge the invaluable assistance of other colleagues for their contributions to the earlier editions.

We acknowledge with thanks the permission of the Editor of the *British Dental Journal* to reproduce Figures 3.3 and 7.10, and the permission of Munksgaard International Publishers Ltd to reproduce Figure 1.3 which is a modified version of an illustration that appeared in *Geriatric Dentistry* edited by Poul Holm-Pedersen and Harold Löe. We would also like to thank Mr J. P. Ralph and Dr C. J. Watson for allowing us to reproduce Figures 3.2 and 8.9 respectively.

Our grateful thanks are extended to all the members of the Medical and Dental Illustration Unit of the University of Leeds and the Photographic Department of the Dental School at the University of Birmingham for skilfully preparing the new illustrative material.

Finally, the support and contributions by our secretaries, Mrs Gill Bunney and Miss Alison Peacock, have been invaluable in bringing this project to fruition.

1 An Appraisal of the Complete-denture Situation

Perhaps the most fundamental question to ask in the first chapter of a book on complete dentures is 'What is the demand for such treatment?' Fortunately, more and more evidence has become available to provide an increasingly accurate answer and one which enables future trends to be determined with reasonable confidence. Particularly notable are the series of studies of adult dental health in the UK which have succeeded in painting a detailed picture over the last 20 years, a period during which major changes have occurred. The dental health of adults living in England and Wales has been studied on three occasions, in 1968, 1978 and 1988. Scotland and Northern Ireland were not included on the first occasion.

First, let us look at the proportion of edentulous adults in the UK in 1988 (Table 1.1). Overall, 21 per cent of all adults were edentulous and tooth loss was strongly correlated with age. Although within the younger age groups edentulousness varied little between different areas of the UK, from middle age onwards there were marked regional differences with total tooth loss occurring most frequently in northern England and Scotland, and least often in southern England.

An intriguing picture develops when one examines the proportion of edentulous adults in England and Wales over the 20-year period (Table 1.2 and Figure 1.1).

The result for any age group, other than the youngest, in 1988 is of course influenced by the amount of tooth loss recorded on the previous

Table 1.1

Age	Proportion edentulous (%)
16–24	–
25–34	1
35–44	4
45–54	17
55–64	37
65–74	57
75 and over	80

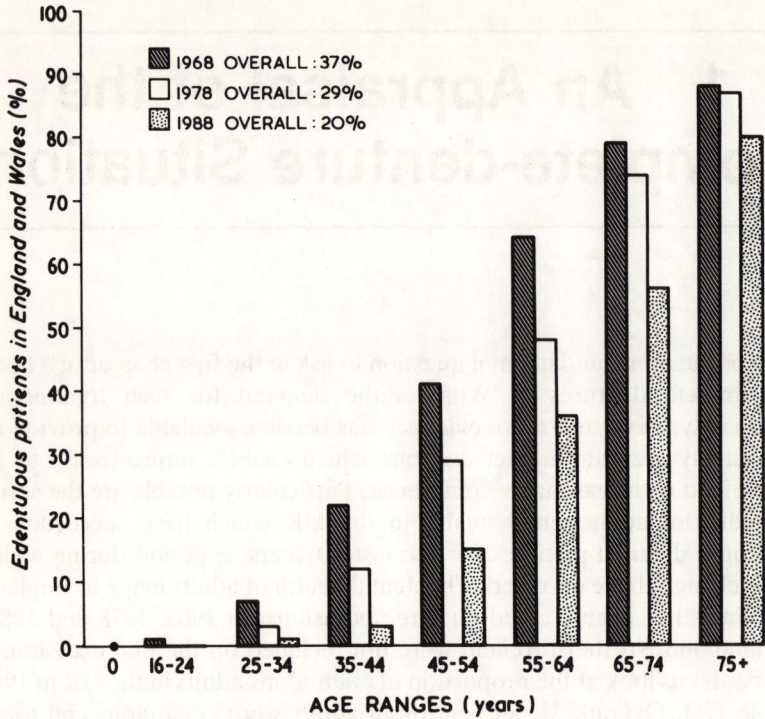

Figure 1.1　Relationship of total tooth loss to age

Table 1.2

Age	Proportion edentulous (%)		
	1968	1978	1988
16–24	1	–	–
25–34	7	3	1
35–44	22	12	3
45–54	41	29	15
55–64	64	48	36
65–74	79	74	56
75 and over	88	87	80
All ages	37	29	20

·occasions when that age cohort was either 10 or 20 years younger. For example, the major reduction in edentulousness of the age group 45–54 between 1978 and 1988 is due to the fact that the dental health of the 35–44 year olds in 1978 deteriorated very little over the subsequent 10 years. Of course, it takes a considerable time for the improvement to work its way

Table 1.3

Country	Report	Proportion of 65 and over edentulous (%)
Canada	Canadian Dept of National Health and Welfare, 1977	53
	Kandelman and Lepage, 1982	66
Denmark	Grabowski and Bertram, 1975	72
Norway	Rise and Heloe, 1978	68
USA	US Dept of Health, Education and Welfare, 1974	51

From MacEntee, 1985

through the whole population and thus one can say that the demand for complete dentures will be considerable in the foreseeable future. However, the trend will be for more and more of the prosthetic effort to be devoted to the older patients.

Similar trends are being reported in other industrialised countries. However, the magnitude of the problem does vary from country to country as can be seen from statistics reported in recent years (Table 1.3).

MAIN REASONS FOR TOOTH LOSS

Most teeth are extracted as a result of caries or periodontal disease. The former is the most common oral disease in the younger age groups, while periodontal disease increases in prevalence and severity with increasing age. A not inconsiderable number of teeth are lost in adults as a matter of convenience when a number of teeth have already been extracted by reason of caries or periodontal disease. Inevitably, the reasons for such massive tooth loss must be many and varied and are conveniently discussed under two headings, the attitude of the population towards dental health and the availability of treatment for the preservation of natural teeth.

The Attitude of the Population in the UK towards Dental Health

This can be gauged from the pattern of dental attendance, treatment preferred and attitudes towards complete dentures. It has been reported that approximately 50 per cent of the population in the UK attend the dentist only on an irregular basis. Even in the younger age group, who have benefited from the wider availability of dental treatment and from increasing dental health propaganda in recent years, over one-third seek treatment only when troubled by their teeth. Thus, it is perhaps not surprising that a similar proportion prefers a painful back tooth to be extracted rather than filled and is not at all upset by the possibility of having to wear complete dentures. As might be expected, those patients who attend for regular treatment are keener to save the natural teeth and are more likely to find the prospect of complete dentures upsetting.

With regard to the public attitude towards the prevention of dental disease, it is also regrettable to note that although it has been confirmed beyond all doubt that fluoridation of the water supply brings about a 50 per cent reduction in dental caries, only 10 per cent of the population of the UK benefit from this measure in spite of active campaigning by dental authorities over more than 30 years. Fortunately, 97 per cent of toothpaste sold in this country contains fluoride.

The Availability of Dental Treatment

The availability of treatment designed to preserve the teeth is related to ready access to a dental practice and, in any state-assisted health scheme, to the provision of sufficient funds and incentives for preventive dentistry to be practised. A recent introduction of a new contract for general dental practitioners in the UK, in which greater emphasis is placed on prevention and continuing care, may well improve dental health further. It has been estimated that a regular attender with natural teeth provides a work load approximately two-and-a-half times greater than the patient who seeks treatment only when troubled. Unless resources are increased to meet a stimulated demand, problems are created in areas where the dentist/patient ratio is already unfavourable. Steps are being taken to reduce this problem in the UK by the introduction of incentive schemes within the National Health Service to encourage dentists to set up practices in these areas.

FUTURE DEMAND FOR TREATMENT

What is the likelihood of the marked decline in edentulousness (Figure 1.1) accelerating further? With regard to the prevention of caries by water fluoridation, the easiest and most effective community measure, it is believed that even if such a measure could be introduced universally in the 1990s it would be well into the twenty-first century before the full effects were realised. The prevention of periodontal disease is even more of a problem as success depends primarily on the effort of the individual in maintaining a high level of oral hygiene. The control of existing peri-odontal disease requires treatment, occasionally surgical in nature, and a subsequent programme of efficient home care. Present evidence does not therefore indicate that widespread prevention and cure are around the corner.

THE LIMITATIONS OF COMPLETE DENTURES

Before discussing in some detail the problems of elderly patients, it is worth while considering the limitations of the conventional complete denture which, after all, is the common method of rehabilitating the edentulous patient. Although in recent years there has been enormous interest shown in implant dentures, the technique is extremely expensive and it would be unrealistic to believe that it could be regarded as routine treatment in the foreseeable future. It is of fundamental importance to remember that the extraction of teeth does not simply mean the loss of the visible crowns. With the loss of the roots, the surrounding alveolar bone resorbs to a great extent. Whereas it is relatively simple to provide an effective replacement for the crowns with a denture, it is frequently difficult, or even impossible, to make good all the lost alveolar bone; the more bone that is resorbed, the greater is the problem. Furthermore, it must be remembered that loss of bone is progressive throughout edentu-lous life and thus the problems are likely to worsen in elderly patients.

The limitations of complete dentures in restoring tissue loss, and thus supporting the lips and cheeks fully, contribute to an appearance of premature ageing in the edentulous patient (Figure 1.2). The facial muscles may lose some of their tone through the ageing process. In addition, it may be argued that loss of tone may also occur because the muscles are unable to function with the same degree of freedom because the underlying artificial support is only sitting on the mucosa and is not held rigidly to the rest of the facial skeleton. In fact, one can liken the difference in function to that of a person striding briskly along a path rather than moving gingerly over a sheet of ice.

Complete dentures certainly help in the control and breaking up of a bolus of food, but their chewing efficiency is considerably lower than that of natural teeth. Natural teeth are firmly attached to the surrounding bone whereas dentures are merely sitting on the mucosa and thus must be actively controlled by the patient. Furthermore, because the pain threshold of the denture-bearing mucosa is relatively easily exceeded, the biting force is necessarily lower. A correlation exists between biting force and chewing efficiency and it has been shown that the biting force of dentate patients can be five to six times more than that of complete-denture wearers. With increased resorption of bone, the dentures become less stable with consequent deterioration in masticatory performance. Al-though it has been shown that a higher intake of essential nutritional

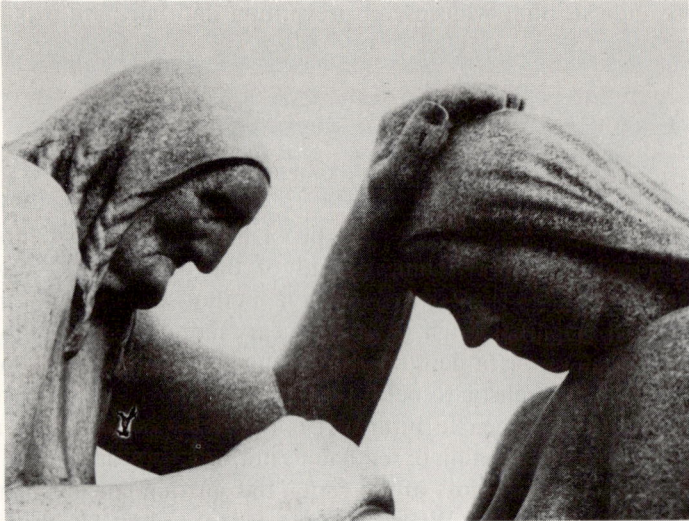

Figure 1.2   This sculpture of age and youth by Gustav Vigeland in Frogner Park, Oslo, illustrates the aged edentulous face well. Bone loss below the anterior nasal spine has occurred and is virtually impossible to replace with a complete upper denture

factors is associated with an efficient natural dentition, the wearing of complete dentures does not mean that nutrition will be deficient; modern food technology enables an adequate diet to be obtained in a form which is readily assimilated even by the most inefficient dentitions. Most important is the fact that the enjoyment of eating depends upon the ability to chew, thus making the most of the flavour of the food while it is in the mouth. Furthermore, the sense of touch within the oral cavity enables us to distinguish the textures of different foods, a process which heightens the enjoyment of a meal. Such pleasure in eating encourages people to maintain an interest in food. If complete dentures are painful or if their control becomes a problem, eating a meal becomes a chore. In addition, coverage of the palate by the upper denture prevents the full appreciation of the texture and temperature of the food. People with complete dentures are thus more likely to lose interest in eating and switch from such things as meat, fruit and salads to less demanding foods.

In spite of the limitations of dentures, the majority of patients manage well and are relatively happy to have a substitute for the real thing. There remain, however, a significant number of people who find complete dentures troublesome. Various reports quote figures of from 13 to 20 per cent of complete-denture wearers who find they have to leave one or both dentures out for all or a part of the day.

Occasionally, one meets patients whose attitude towards dental disease is that the easiest and most convenient approach is to have all the natural teeth extracted and replaced by complete dentures. Indeed, many years ago it used to be common practice in some areas for this treatment to be carried out for a bride-to-be in the belief that she would not saddle her new husband with major dental expenses in the future. Fortunately, this attitude is no longer prevalent. From the evidence presented, there surely could be no convincing argument for undertaking such a drastic step in early adulthood. Even though the first few years of edentulous life are most likely to be happy, it is impossible to prophesy whether each individual patient will maintain a satisfactory level of comfort and function, or will proceed to a state where denture problems reduce the quality of life.

THE ELDERLY EDENTULOUS PATIENT

Earlier in the chapter it was pointed out that the provision of complete dentures now, and even more so in the future, will be directed towards the elderly patient.

In recent years, a great deal has been written about the elderly patient. The purpose of this section of the book is to highlight some of the significant points which relate particularly to complete-denture treatment. For a more detailed presentation of the topic the reader is referred to the bibliography at the end of the chapter which cites textbooks and papers that we have used to compile this summary.

Demographic Changes

An elderly patient is usually defined as someone over the age of 65. However, it is current fashion to call those in the 60–74 age group the 'new elderly' and to describe those over 75 as 'old old'. Just how long these definitions will stand remains to be seen; one suspects that many people in the latter category would find the description faintly insulting.

Throughout the world the elderly population is growing rapidly. Figure 1.3 shows the proportion of the total population aged 60 and over living in selected regions. The figures were produced at the World Health Organisation (WHO) World Assembly on Aging in 1982. It can be seen that there is a big difference between areas which contain industrialised countries and those which are composed largely of less developed countries.

The distribution of elderly people in England and Wales is shown in Figure 1.4. The pattern of a gradual increase in the 'old old' and a slight

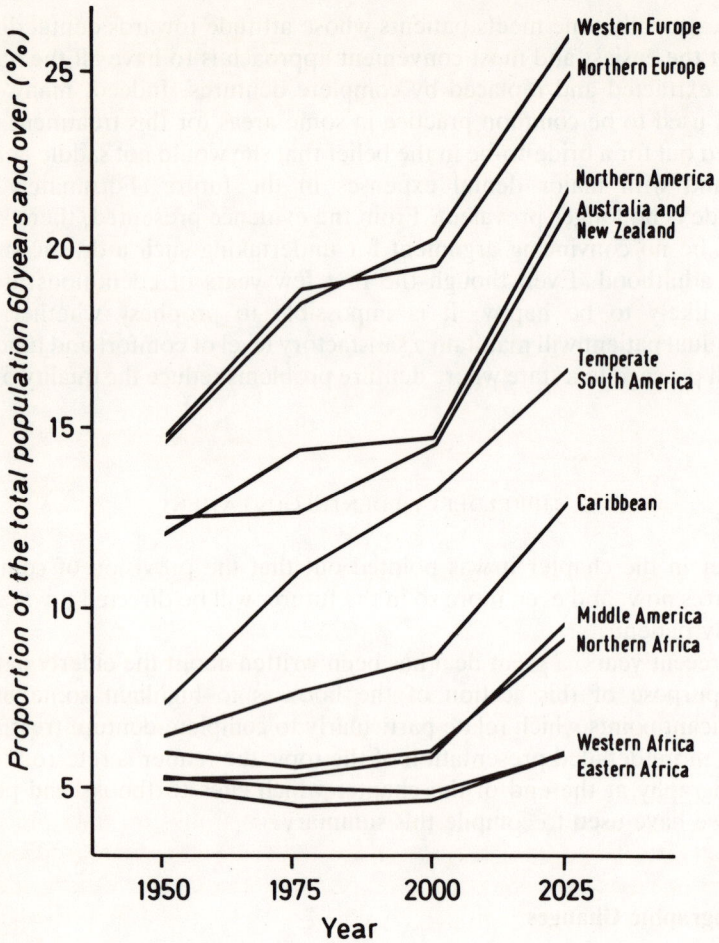

Figure 1.3　The growth of elderly populations in various regions of the world

reduction in the 65–74 age group is also mirrored in other industrialised countries. These trends are the result of the subtle balance between changing levels of fertility and mortality.

During the last 30 years or so there has been a dramatic increase in the number of elderly in the world. The whole group has increased by around 75 per cent while the number over the age of 80 has risen by 134 per cent. The difference in survival rates of the sexes accounts for the fact that females constitute 60 per cent of the elderly and 70 per cent of the very old.

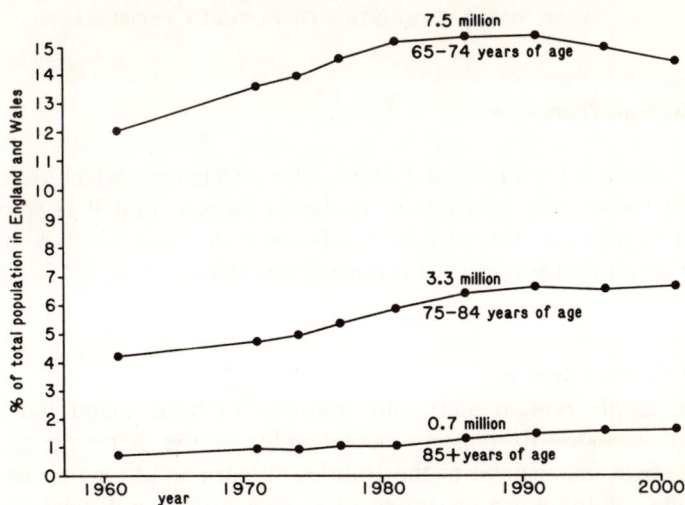

Figure 1.4　Distribution of elderly people in England and Wales

Between now and the turn of the century it is estimated that there will be a 60 per cent increase in the elderly population, 35 per cent in industrialised countries and 75 per cent in less well developed countries. It is expected that in the first quarter of the twenty-first century more than a fifth of the population in industrialised countries will be elderly. Those undergraduates reading this book will realise that most of their practising life will be influenced by this pattern. What proportion of this group will be edentulous remains to be seen. However, one can predict with reasonable confidence that a very high percentage of complete-denture provision will be required by them.

The vast majority of elderly people live in the community. A small percentage, estimated at between 12 per cent and 14 per cent, are house-bound because of physical or mental handicap. In Northern Europe, between 4 per cent and 7 per cent live in some form of institution. These figures are of particular relevance with respect to the delivery of care. The people living in some form of institution do have the advantage that their carers are in a position to recognise problems and to seek advice on their behalf. Of course, this presupposes that the carers have some knowledge of . prosthetic problems. Those elderly people who have some form of handicap and are living at home are perhaps the most vulnerable when it comes to dealing with prosthetic difficulties; frequently, the responsibility for initiating help and seeking treatment has not been accepted by any particular person.

SOME CHARACTERISTICS OF ELDERLY PEOPLE

Physiological Changes

Before describing some of the more relevant changes which occur generally in the elderly population, it should be said that it is sometimes difficult to separate truly physiological ones from those which result from disease. With that proviso the following points can be made.

Central Nervous System

Elderly people remain alert and continue to have sound judgement; however, a modest decrease in mental agility occurs. After the age of 70 there is slight impairment of the abilities to learn and to memorise. With increasing age there is a progressive loss of neurones and synapses in the cerebral cortex. As a result there is a slowing of the central processing facility with a consequential lengthening of reaction times and response to sensory stimuli.

Within the sensory system, age brings about a deterioration of the senses of smell and taste, the former being more affected. Hearing loss is reported in approximately 25 per cent of people over the age of 65.

With respect to the motor system, there tends to be impairment of balance and some postural tremor, both indicating deterioration of cerebellar function and of the extrapyramidal system. The elderly are less precise in controlling the contraction of muscles, such as the masseter muscles. It takes more time and effort before new dentures can be controlled automatically. Of course, an elderly patient has a great deal of experience to fall back on and if a new task is given which utilises previously acquired skills, difficulties will be minimised. However, problems are more likely to arise if the new task is more demanding than declining abilities are able to cope with. For example, previous denture experience can be of the greatest assistance when having to cope with new dentures, providing that major changes to the design of the dentures have not been introduced.

Denture-bearing Tissues

Age brings about some deterioration of the denture-bearing tissues. The epithelium becomes thinner, the connective tissue less resilient and the ability of the mucosa to heal is impaired. Osteoporosis is a common problem in old age, particularly affecting postmenopausal women, occurring in about one-third of women over 60. Not only is the skeleton affected but the lower jaw will show a decrease in bone density. The severity of osteoporosis is related not only to hormonal changes but also to long-term calcium deficiency and to loss of normal function. Regarding the latter point, it would be reasonable to suggest that the edentulous state adversely affects normal function of the mandible.

Saliva

There is no evidence to suggest that the rate of salivary secretion decreases with age. But as will be seen later, normal salivation can be adversely affected by drug therapy.

Systemic Disease

The following problems, which commonly occur in elderly people, can cause complications specifically related to the care and treatment of the edentulous patient.

Angina

Angina can cause pain which is experienced around the left body of the mandible or even the left side of the palate. This usually occurs in association with chest pain and the onset is usually related to physical exertion.

Congestive Heart Failure, Chronic Bronchitis and Emphysema

Elderly patients with these conditions are likely to become breathless if the dental chair is tipped back into the supine position.

Cerebro-vascular Accident

The occurrence of a 'stroke' may result in unilateral paralysis of the facial muscles, making it more difficult for the patient to control dentures, especially the lower denture. The patient may also have difficulty clearing food which has lodged in the buccal sulcus. Speech may be affected, making it difficult for the patient to communicate with the dentist.

Parkinson's Disease

This condition, as well as other tremors which are likely to occur in the elderly, can adversely affect the precise control of the mandible, making it more difficult to obtain an accurate recording of the jaw relationship. Parkinsonism can also cause difficulty in swallowing, leading to pronounced dribbling, which can be very distressing for the patient.

Diabetes

This condition occurs commonly in later life. It predisposes to infection in the mouth by *Candida albicans*, is a cause of a 'burning mouth' and can result in troublesome dryness.

Osteoporosis

Although this condition has already been mentioned with respect to the denture-bearing tissues, it is appropriate to mention that it can lead to a hunched posture, or kyphosis, which requires the dentist to ensure that work is undertaken with the patient in the sitting position with the head and neck adequately supported.

Arthritis

Elderly patients may suffer from osteoarthritis or rheumatoid arthritis. Either condition may have reached such an advanced state that the patient finds it extremely difficult, or even impossible, to attend the dental surgery. If either of these conditions affects the hands, it becomes increasingly difficult for the patient to clean dentures adequately. The patient can be helped by increasing the thickness of the brush handle so that it can be gripped without discomfort, by providing brushes which can be attached to a wash-basin and by recommending an effective cleansing solution which reduces the reliance on mechanical means of plaque removal.

Nutritional Deficiencies

Deficiencies of the vitamin B complex, folic acid and iron are not uncommon in the elderly. As will be described in later chapters, these deficiencies can lead to pathology of the mucosa and to widespread discomfort or burning.

Psychiatric Disorders

The prevalence of depression increases with age. It has been estimated that between 15 per cent and 30 per cent of elderly people suffer from this condition, which can result in poor appetite and weight loss, and can adversely affect motivation and self-care.

Dementia is found in 5–6 per cent of people over the age of 65 and in 20 per cent of the over-80s. This condition causes intellectual impairment, a poor memory (particularly for recent events) and poor concentration.

The implications that these conditions have for prosthetic treatment are self-evident. Additional problems may arise from the drug therapy given to these patients.

Drug Therapy

It has been reported that elderly patients are prescribed an average of 2.8 drugs per person. Poor compliance with medication is found in between 50 per cent and 60 per cent of patients; this is a particular problem among the elderly who are of course taking more drugs and may have some degree of intellectual impairment or poor recall.

The commonest drugs prescribed for elderly people, in descending order of frequency, are: diuretics, analgesics, hypnotics, sedatives, anxiolytics, antirheumatics and beta-blockers. Many of these drugs have side-effects which are relevant to the dentist about to undertake prosthetic treatment.

Xerostomia is produced by certain antidepressants, diuretics, antihypertensives and antipsychotics, some drugs having a more profound effect on secretion than others. Lack of saliva adversely affects the retention of dentures, increases the possibility of oral infection and, through the absence of lubrication, can result in generalised soreness or even a burning sensation.

Certain drugs, such as steroid inhalers used in the treatment of asthma, immunosuppressive drugs and broad spectrum antibiotics used over a long period, can alter the oral flora thus predisposing to candida infection.

Tardive dyskinesia is a condition characterised by spasmodic movements of the oral, lingual and facial muscles. These uncontrollable movements can make it extremely difficult, or even impossible, to provide stable dentures. The condition is brought on by extensive use of drugs such as antipsychotics and tricyclic antidepressants. It will occur in 20–40 per cent of patients who have been taking the drugs for longer than six months. In approximately 40 per cent of sufferers the condition is not reversible, even if the drug therapy is stopped.

Psychological Changes

Advancing age leads to certain inevitable changes which must be taken into account when treating the elderly patient. For example, the elderly patient finds it more difficult to perform tasks which depend upon rapid movements. Such tasks may well include the need to suddenly control a denture which has become destabilised during normal function. It should also be realised that elderly people take rather longer to learn to perform new tasks or to remember new information which is not put over clearly or which may not appear to be immediately relevant.

As mentioned earlier, depression is a common condition. One common cause is the changing role brought about by increasing age. For example, children are no longer dependent upon the parent, retirement brings about a new life with reduced income, life changes dramatically as a result of the death of the spouse, health deteriorates and the person is less able to care for him or herself. The greater the number of these life events, the more the person has to cope with. Of course, if the person is able to adapt to the changes, there is a reduced risk of depression developing.

Elderly people are less able to accept new situations, be they a change in denture shape, a new dentist or even the appointment time for treatment. There is a tendency for elderly people to become more self-centred. Discomfort, which at one time could be shrugged off, takes on a greater significance.

It will be appreciated that the clinician must take many aspects of the life of the patient into account when investigating a complaint. Of course, many problems will be straightforward, but some will be complicated by factors which are far removed from the oral cavity and the existing dentures. Unless their presence is suspected, there is a risk that prosthetic treatment alone will fail to deal with a problem.

Nutrition

A great deal has been written on the relationship between nutrition and the efficiency of the dentition, be it natural or artificial. It is not appropriate in this text to rehearse all the arguments. Instead, some of the more important conclusions will be listed.

Malnutrition among the elderly population living in a well-developed society is not common. One report quotes a prevalence of 2.5 per cent in the over-65s living at home. Nevertheless, it is important to be watchful for signs and symptoms which may suggest deficiencies of vitamins B and C and of iron. Those people more likely to have nutritional problems are the house-bound living at home, those with handicaps which make shopping and cooking difficult, alcoholics, people who suffer from mental illness or those who have been recently bereaved.

Although overt malnutrition is relatively rare, it should be pointed out that an inadequate diet can lead to reduced tolerance of the oral tissues to normal wear and tear and that this reduced resistance, in turn, can result in poor adaptation to dentures.

Absence of teeth or unsatisfactory dentures are likely to affect food consumption adversely by altering the choice of food; people with decreased masticatory function are likely to eat less dietary fibre, less meat, and fewer vegetables and fruit. Of particular importance is the fact that the natural enjoyment of eating is impaired.

It has been reported that inadequate masticatory ability is directly related to an increased prevalence of gastro-intestinal irritation and can adversely affect digestion if normal digestive capacity has already been impaired by another disease process. Finally, the point should be made that, in the absence of an effective dentition, there is a greater risk of a person choking on a large bolus of food which has not been adequately broken up.

THE CONDITION OF ELDERLY PEOPLE'S DENTURES

In recent years, there have been many surveys which have reported on the condition of the mouths and dentures of elderly people. Results indicate that most edentulous people over the age of 65 are wearing dentures which are more than 10 years old and that, as a result, mucosal changes are present in anything between 44 per cent and 63 per cent of cases. The need for treatment, based on clinical judgement, suggests that 40 per cent of five-year-old dentures and 80 per cent of 10-year-old dentures should be replaced. However, the picture is not that simple. Need can be measured in a variety of ways:

(a) 'Normative need' is the need defined by expert or professional opinion.
(b) 'Felt need' is the patient's subjective desire.
(c) 'Expressed need' is recorded when the 'felt need' is activated through the patient seeking treatment.

One estimate of 'normative need' has already been described. Others indicate that 70–85 per cent of elderly people's dentures require attention and that such need far exceeds the 'expressed need'. Elderly people are likely to consider that treatment is required as a result of experiencing pain, difficulty in chewing, a deteriorating appearance, or because the existing dentures are broken or have been lost. However, the 'felt need' may not be activated for a variety of reasons, including the following:

(a) The dental problem is low on the list of priorities compared with other problems.
(b) Inertia on the part of the patient.
(c) Ignorance of available services.
(d) Fear of treatment that may be required. It is important to remember that a large proportion of today's edentulous patients experienced dental treatment in less sophisticated times when pain was a frequent accompaniment.
(e) Inability to travel to a surgery because of ill health or problems of transportation.
(f) A feeling that nothing can be done anyway and that the dental problem is just one of the inconveniences of old age.
(g) Finance.

The effectiveness of some or all of these 'barriers to care' can be gauged from one survey which reported that of a group of 75-year-old people living independently, nearly half had an oral problem, one-third had pain and the majority had not visited a dentist for at least 10 years, and, what's more, did not plan to do so. Another interesting finding which highlights the transportation problem was that in a group of people over the age of 75, 40 per cent had difficulty in walking, 29 per cent experienced difficulty in climbing stairs, while 21 per cent had heart disease.

CARING FOR THE ELDERLY PATIENT: SOME PRACTICAL POINTS

Many of the subsequent chapters of the book refer to modifications to clinical technique which may be required to meet the particular needs of the elderly patient. This section mentions some aspects of management which naturally follow on from the previous discussion.

First, it should be stressed that to encourage elderly patients to attend for treatment, it is important to ensure that there is ready access to the surgery. A ground floor location is ideal, and both doors and corridors should be wide enough to provide access for wheelchairs. All members of the surgery team must have a sound understanding of the problems of the elderly and be sympathetic to their needs. For example, it should be recognised that the patient is likely to be anxious and unclear as to what might be involved at the first visit to the surgery. Sufficient time needs to be spent explaining the routine in order to put the patient at his or her ease. When settling the patient in the dental chair, it is important to warn the patient in advance of any movements of the chair that are about to be made and to remember that most elderly people will be more comfortable in the sitting rather than the supine position. In this respect, some designs of chair are more suitable than others.

It is imperative to develop appropriate communication skills so that the patient's problems can be assessed as accurately as possible, a realistic treatment plan evolved, and the patient made fully aware of what will be done and what may be the limitations of treatment. To this end, it is vital to carry out the discussion in a quiet, unhurried environment, to face the patient when talking and, if the patient is hard of hearing, to speak slowly and clearly but without undue exaggeration. It is also extremely important to allow plenty of time for listening to the patient's account of any problems so that he or she feels that sufficient opportunity has been given for matters of concern to be adequately explained to the dentist.

When information is being given to the patient, it should be relayed reasonably slowly, in a carefully structured manner, and without distraction or interruption. It is useful to back up verbal comment with written advice, recognising that the print should be large enough for those whose eyesight has deteriorated.

When obtaining a history, it is important to remember that elderly people have an increasing number of 'aches and pains', but regarding these problems as being a normal consequence of ageing can result in a risk of underdiagnosing. It must also be appreciated that chronic pain and depression commonly go together, so it is important to establish any predisposing factors. For example, widespread pain under a lower denture might be due to a clenching habit which has bruised the mucosa, and which has been initiated by worry at home; the pain is no less real, whatever the cause. In such circumstances, prosthetic treatment on its own is unlikely to offer long-term success; effective care is likely to require communication between the dentist and the patient's medical practitioner.

When deciding upon a course of treatment for an elderly patient, one must always have the original complaint at the forefront of one's mind and plan a programme of care which can be achieved in the circumstances. For example, the request to see the patient may come from a relative who has become increasingly embarrassed that dentures are not being worn on social occasions. The health of the patient may have deteriorated to such an extent that successful control of a new lower denture is clearly out of the question. It may be concluded that realistic treatment is the provision of an upper denture only, which will be worn for appearance's sake rather than for function. In such circumstances, it can be argued that the dentist is treating the relative as well as the patient, a course of action which surely is entirely justified. Although this particular illustration may be thought of as an extreme one, it is by no means uncommon and does serve to make the point that successful treatment is the 'art of the possible'.

In this section of the chapter dealing with the elderly patient, we have drawn attention to conditions which are likely to influence overall care. The reader should not progress to the remainder of the book with the impression that prosthetic treatment of the elderly patient is invariably going to be complicated by a long list of problems. It is important to put things in perspective by appreciating characteristics of normal ageing. Many of these characteristics are widely recognised but some have been less well accepted. Thus, in concluding this chapter we draw attention to studies which have investigated the level of knowledge that members of the health care team have about particular characteristics of elderly people.

Certain features which are well recognised include:

(a) The majority of elderly people are not senile, neither do they feel miserable for most of the time.
(b) Most old people can learn new things.
(c) Their reaction times tend to be slower.
(d) Physical strength tends to decline with old age; about 80 per cent are healthy enough to carry out normal activities.
(e) The majority like some kind of work to do.

Those features which are less well recognised include:

(a) All five senses tend to decline with age.
(b) Most elderly people are not set in their ways; they do, however, take longer to learn something new.

(c) The majority are seldom bored, and are neither socially isolated nor lonely.

(d) The majority of old people are seldom irritated or angry.

BIBLIOGRAPHY

Baillie, S. and Woodhouse, K. (1988) Medical aspects of ageing. *Dental Update*, **15**, 236–41.

Baker, K. A. and Ettinger, R. L. (1985) Intra-oral effects of drugs in elderly persons. *Gerodontics*, **1**, 111–16.

Bates, J. F., Adams, D. and Stafford, G. D. (1984) *Dental Treatment of the Elderly*. Wright, Bristol.

Bates, J. F. and Murphy, W. M. (1968) A survey of an edentulous population. *British Dental Journal*, **124**, 116–21.

Christensen, J. (1988) Domiciliary care for the elderly patient. *Dental Update*, **15**, 284–90.

Drummond, J. R., Newton, J. P. and Yemm, R. (1988) Dentistry for the elderly: a review and an assessment of the future. *Journal of Dentistry*, **16**, 47–54.

Fish, S. F., Bates, J. F. and Nairn, R. I. (1969) A study of prosthetic dentistry. *British Dental Journal*, **127**, 59–70.

Fiske, J., Gelbier, G. and Watson, R. M. (1990) The benefit of dental care to an elderly population assessed using a sociodental measure of oral handicap. *British Dental Journal*, **168**, 153–6.

Franks, A. S. T. and Hedegard, Bjørn (1973) *Geriatric Dentistry*. Blackwell Scientific Publications, Oxford, London, Edinburgh, Melbourne.

Grabowski, M. and Bertram, U. (1975) Oral health status and need of dental treatment in the elderly Danish population. *Community Dentistry and Oral Epidemiology*, **3**, 108–14.

Gray, P. G., Todd, J. E., Slack, G. L. and Bulman, J. S. (1968) Adult dental health in England and Wales in 1968. HMSO, London.

Hamilton, F. A., Sarll, D. W., Grant, A. A. and Worthington, H. V. (1990) Dental care for elderly people by general dental practitioners. *British Dental Journal*, **168**, 108–12.

Haraldson, T., Karlsson, U. and Carlsson, G. E. (1979) Bite force and oral function in complete denture wearers. *Journal of Oral Rehabilitation*, **6**, 41–8.

Heath, M. R. (1972) Dietary selection by elderly persons, related to dental state. *British Dental Journal*, **132**, 145–8.

Hoad-Reddick, G., Grant, A. A. and Griffiths, C. S. (1987) Knowledge of dental services provided: investigations in an elderly population. *Community Dentistry and Oral Epidemiology*, **15**, 137–40.

Holm-Pedersen, P. and Loe, H. (eds.) (1986) *Geriatric Dentistry*. Munksgaard, Copenhagen.

LeResche, L. and Dworkin, S. F. (1985) Evaluating orofacial pain in the elderly. *Gerodontics*, **1**, 81–7.

MacEntee, M. I. (1985) The prevalence of edentulism and diseases related to dentures – a literature review. *Journal of Oral Rehabilitation*, **12**, 195–207.

MacEntee, M. I., Dowell, T. B. and Scully, C. (1988) Oral health concerns of an elderly population in England. *Community Dentistry and Oral Epidemiology*, **16**, 72–4.

Murphy, W. M., Morris, R. A. and O'Sullivan, D. C. (1974) Effect of oral prostheses upon texture perception of food. *British Dental Journal*, **137**, 245–9.

Neill, D. J. and Phillips, H. I. B. (1972) The masticatory performance and dietary intake of elderly edentulous patients. *Dental Practitioner and Dental Record*, **22**, 384–9.

Office of Population Censuses and Surveys (1990) Adult dental health 1988. *British Dental Journal*, **168**, 279–81.

Osborne, J., Brill, N. and Hedegard, Bjørn (1966) The nature of prosthetic dentistry. *International Dental Journal*, **16**, 509–26.

Osborne, J., Maddick, I., Gould, A. and Ward, D. (1979) Dental demands of old people in Hampshire. *British Dental Journal*, **146**, 351–5.

Seymour, R. A. (1988) Dental pharmacology problems in the elderly. *Dental Update*, **15**, 375–81.

Shapiro, S., Bomberg, T. J. and Hamby, C. L. (1985) Postmenopausal osteoporosis: dental patients at risk. *Gerodontics*, **1**, 220–5.

Smith, J. M. and Sheiham, A. (1979) How dental conditions handicap the elderly. *Community Dentistry and Oral Epidemiology*, **7**, 305–10.

Storer, R. (1966) Geriatric dentistry. *British Dental Journal*, **121**, 547–52.

Strayer, M. S., DiAngelis, A. J. and Loupe, M. J. (1986) Dentists' knowledge of aging in relation to perceived elderly patient behavior. *Gerodontics*, **2**, 223–7.

Todd, J. E. and Walker, A. M. (1980) *Adult Dental Health*, Vol. 1: England and Wales, 1968–78. HMSO, London.

Walls, A. W. G. and Barnes, I. E. (1988) Gerodontology: the problem? *Dental Update*, **15**, 186–91.

WHO (1982) Introductory document: demographic considerations. World Assembly on Aging, Vienna.

(1990) Elderly people: Their medicines and their doctors. *Drug and Therapeutics Bulletin*, **20**, 77–9.

2 The Patient's Contribution to Prosthetic Treatment

The successful outcome of prosthetic treatment depends upon a three-person effort – that of the dentist in making a diagnosis, preparing a treatment plan and undertaking the clinical work; that of the dental technician in constructing the various items which lead up to the finished dentures; and that of the patient in adapting to the dentures and accepting their limitations. In this chapter, we consider the patient's contribution.

ADAPTING TO DENTURES

The ability of the patient to adapt is vital to success for two main reasons. First, the change in the oral environment is so great when two large foreign bodies are inserted into the mouth that a positive effort has to be made to come to terms with it. Second, the wearing of these foreign bodies is in the complete control of the patient. At any time the dentures can be removed from the mouth, considered, discussed, compared and even set aside.

To come to terms with the drastic change within the oral cavity, the patient must:

(a) become accustomed to the sensation of the dentures, a process known as habituation;
(b) learn to control the dentures;
(c) come to terms with the new appearance.

Habituation

Habituation has been defined as a gradual diminution of responses to continued or repeated stimuli. When new dentures are placed in the mouth, they stimulate mechanoreceptors in the oral mucosa. Impulses arising from these receptors, which record touch and pressure, are transmitted to the sensory cortex with the result that the patient can 'feel' the dentures. However, continuous stimulation of these receptors does not result in a corresponding continuous stream of impulses. The receptors adapt to the new environment and so, likewise, the patient begins to lose conscious awareness of the new shapes in the mouth. Of course, if replacement dentures are constructed whose shape is dissimilar to existing ones, a new set of stimuli will be evoked and the process of habituation starts all over again. This concept is one of the main reasons for copying dentures, using a method such as that described in Chapter 7.

In addition to the mechanoreceptors in the oral mucosa being stimulated by the new dentures while the patient is at rest, further stimulation arises as a result of contact of the occlusal surfaces during function. The forces generated by contraction of the muscles of mastication are transmitted through the dentures to the underlying tissues. The pattern of the stimulation of the mechanoreceptors enables the patient to recognise the presence or absence of occlusal harmony. This is dealt with in greater detail in Chapter 13.

Control of the Dentures

A discussion of the behaviour of sensory receptors is equally relevant when considering the patient's ability to control dentures; the successful manipulation of dentures depends upon purposeful and effective muscular activity, which in turn is related to adequate sensory feedback. It has been shown that when sensory nerve endings in the oral cavity are anaesthetised, the retention of complete lower dentures is reduced. In other words, loss of sensory input results in a lower level of purposeful muscle activity.

The patient's ability to control dentures involves a learning process which, initially, is a conscious endeavour. The first few faltering steps of the inexperienced denture wearer are often discouraging to the clinician. However, it is comforting to realise that the vast majority of these patients return to the surgery after a few days showing few signs of their initial difficulty. The learning process has come to the rescue; as a result of repetition, new reflex arcs have been set up in the central nervous system and the conscious effort has been replaced by a subconscious behaviour pattern. Constant repetition of impulses lowers the synaptic resistance and facilitates the formation of conditioned reflexes. At the same time, however, it must be realised that the synaptic resistance will be increased in the absence of these repeated stimuli. In other words, practice makes perfect while idleness leads to decay.

Appearance

'Beauty is in the eye of the beholder', and in the prosthetic context one is concerned with the patient looking at the new dentures in a mirror. Because pleasing appearance is a subjective evaluation, there is obviously room for disagreement between dentist and patient. Open disagreement does not lead to successful treatment and so it is vitally important that the dentist should take careful notice of a patient's views on appearance. This does not mean, however, that the dentist should meekly follow the patient's requests if they are likely to lead to a poor aesthetic result. Indeed, advice and demonstration may well succeed in convincing the patient that a more pleasing appearance may be obtained by introducing irregularities into the positioning of the front teeth and by choosing a darker and more natural shade. However, if such modifications meet with a lukewarm response then it is obvious that the patient's mind is made up and that success will be obtained only if an appearance is produced which conforms with the original request.

Some patients, when asked about the characteristics of their natural teeth, volunteer the information that 'My teeth were white, even and small'. Observations of natural dentitions of all ages suggest that this viewpoint is a wish rather than a statement of fact. Why then is such an artificial appearance requested? One possible reason is that such an appearance is considered to be more 'healthy' than their previously neglected mouths for which extraction of all teeth was the only possible treatment. A second possibility is that the artificial appearance is in fact a fashion and that many people are happier if they keep up with the edentulous 'Joneses' in the neighbourhood. If this is indeed the case, one hopes that with more effective persuasion and education the majority of edentulous patients will be persuaded to accept more natural-looking dentures.

Although the point has been made that, after appropriate advice and demonstration by the dentist, the patient has the final word on the appearance of the dentures, there are some clinical situations where the dentist's opinion should take precedence. This would be the case, for example, when the patient requests a particular arch form which is likely to prejudice the stability of the dentures. Because of age changes in the soft tissues surrounding the mouth, patients occasionally request that new dentures should be designed so as to 'iron out' a few wrinkles on the face. Occasionally, it is possible to improve the appearance by a judicious expansion of the upper dental arch or by thickening the denture border. However, complications may arise from excessive post-extraction resorption of the alveolar ridge with a resulting decrease in prospects for retention. If the dental arch is expanded, the increased lip pressure on the labial face of the upper denture may be enough to lead to instability. On these occasions, it is advisable to explain and even demonstrate the difficulties to the patient and to indicate tactfully that it may be necessary to balance the advantages of a stable denture against the presence of a few skin creases. The clinical demonstration can be carried out on the old dentures at the patient's first visit; wax additions can be made to simulate the requested change and to see whether alteration is likely to have any beneficial effect on facial shape (Figure 2.1). This gives the dentist the opportunity of discussing the difficulties and perhaps pointing out the limitations of dentures in dealing with the general problem of ageing. A

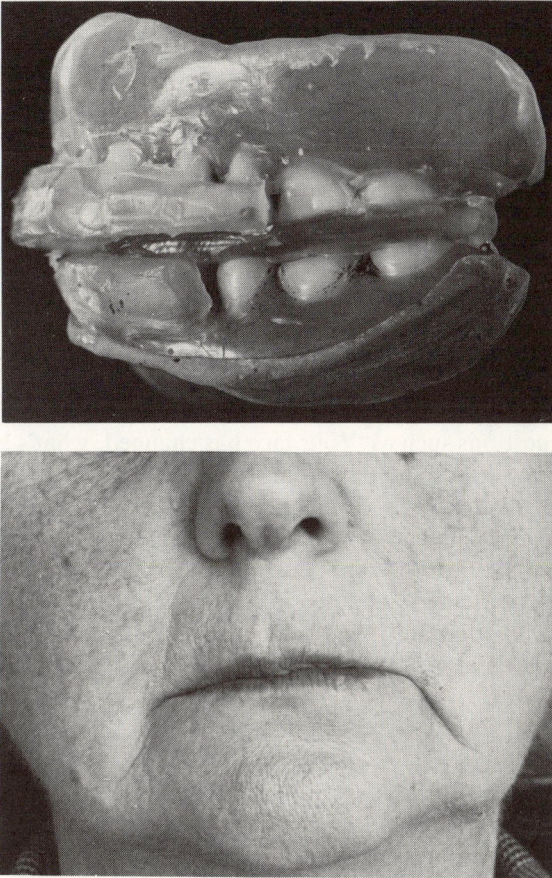

Figure 2.1   *Top*: The patient requested that replacement dentures be made to eliminate marked creasing at the angles of the mouth. Possible alterations in design were demonstrated by the addition of wax to the existing dentures; the dental arches were expanded and the occlusal vertical dimension increased. *Bottom*: With the modified dentures in the mouth it was possible to show the patient that her request could not be met and that the creases were, in fact, an age change

second case in point is where it is necessary to construct replacement dentures with a lower occlusal plane so that the tongue, by resting on the occlusal surface, can be more effective in stabilising a lower denture whose prognosis for retention is poor. Although such a modification will improve stability, the altered appearance may lead to objections from the patient.

On all these occasions where it is necessary to seek a compromise between function and appearance, the ability of the patient to adapt to the modified appearance will depend just as much on the effectiveness of the dentist's words as on his or her deeds. Having said this, one must always be aware of the occasional patient who will not accept advice. In this case, the dentist has the choice of refusing to undertake a form of treatment which is considered to be against the patient's best interests, or of making the dentures after warning the patient of the possible outcome and ensuring that he or she accepts responsibility for the design. Occasionally, it is possible to satisfy the awkward patient by constructing two sets of dentures, one set with which to eat and one set in which to be seen!

One further aspect of appearance is worthy of consideration. It is not uncommon for patients to seek replacement dentures in circumstances where the existing set has deteriorated to such an extent that a great deal of lip support and occlusal vertical dimension has been lost. Replacement dentures will undoubtedly make a dramatic change to appearance – a change hopefully appreciated by the patient. However, there is the risk that the appreciation will be lessened if the patient meets friends or acquaintances who perhaps stare rather pointedly, or even somewhat tactlessly ask questions such as 'Your face has changed, what's happened?' or even 'Have you had some new dentures?' Such unwelcome comments can undermine the patient's confidence because they indicate that the friend perhaps recognises that the patient is a denture wearer. When obvious but necessary changes are being made, it is therefore a wise policy to warn the patient in advance of possible reactions from friends so that he or she is mentally prepared for them and therefore less likely to be discouraged by them.

CLINICAL ASSESSMENT OF ADAPTIVE CAPABILITY

The discussion so far has ranged around the problems posed by new dentures. Inevitably, the success with which patients cope with these problems varies enormously. Fortunately, the majority of patients have very little difficulty in adapting to an artificial dentition. If one accepts the view that a coarse measure of success is whether or not the dentures are worn throughout the day, evidence from surveys of adult dental health and of patients treated in dental schools suggests a success rate of 85 per cent. It has also been shown that although very high levels of satisfaction are frequently recorded immediately after new dentures have been fitted, a significant deterioration occurs after one year. Most of the dissatisfaction is blamed on the fit and comfort of the lower denture. This comment emphasises the importance of recalling patients and maintaining the dentures (Chapter 14). Some patients present very considerable difficulties which can in fact be treated successfully by using special techniques. However, there remain a few patients who never really learn to become successful denture wearers. It is therefore very important that the dentist should be able to recognise the 'chronic' denture patient before treatment is commenced as the treatment plan should reflect the problems that lie ahead.

How can one assess the adaptive capability of prosthetic patients? Various attempts have been made to tease out the factors which might be taken into account when trying to make this difficult judgement. The present state of knowledge does not enable us to select certain pointers and to say with absolute confidence that if any one or a combination of pointers occurs in a patient then one can safely predict that, on the one hand, treatment will be an almost impossible task or, on the other, that success is a foregone conclusion. The best one can do in attempting to estimate the probable outcome of treatment is to build up a general picture made up of clues from such factors as the patient's psychological make-up, general health, the existence of social problems or upsets, previous prosthetic experience and the technical quality of previous dentures. The relationship between dentist and patient can also be a potent factor; empathy is likely to encourage success whereas indifference, impatience or frank hostility is more likely to spell disaster. The various aspects can be conveniently grouped together under the following headings:

(a) age of the patient,
(b) patient's motivation,
(c) previous denture experience,
(d) health of the patient.

Age of the Patient

In general, as patients grow older, it becomes more difficult for them to adapt successfully to new dentures for the reasons already discussed in Chapter 1. As the rate of ageing varies greatly between individuals, the actual age of a patient may be an unreliable guide to adaptive potential. A better basis for this assessment is the biological age which may be estimated by judging how old the patient looks. It is not uncommon for the biological and actual ages to differ markedly. For example, when comparing the two people in Figure 2.2, one would not expect the woman to have greater difficulty in adapting to the dentures in spite of the fact that she is 29 years older than the man.

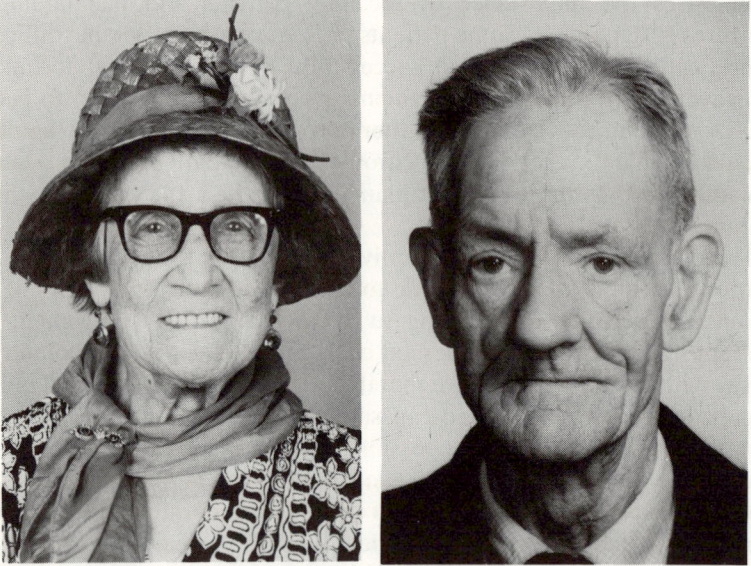

Figure 2.2   Variation of biological age with actual age. The woman, aged 95, is 29 years older than the man

The influence of advancing age is seen in the denture-bearing tissues as well as the central nervous system. Atrophy of the oral mucosa, resorption and osteoporosis of the alveolar bone, and a reduced ability to repair damaged tissues create a situation where the denture-bearing tissues may be less able to withstand the masticatory stresses. All these factors lead to a situation in which the treatment of the elderly edentulous patient presents its own set of problems. With advances in preventive dentistry and an increased expectancy of life, one can foresee the possibility of people being faced with their first set of complete dentures much later in life. The problems of adaptation with which prosthetic dentistry will be faced are therefore likely to increase in the future.

Having said all this, increasing age should not be linked automatically with worsening adaptation; rather, it should be looked at as offering advantages as well as disadvantages. Whereas on the one hand there is a greater chance of such features as debilitating chronic disease, a reduced efficiency in the functioning of the central nervous system and a dry mouth resulting from drug therapy, on the other hand the patient is likely to be able to draw upon previous denture experience which, if favourable, can play an extremely valuable part in achieving ultimate success. A further point is that the older patient may have more realistic expectations as to the prognosis of replacement dentures.

Patient's Motivation

Most patients requesting their first complete dentures do so because they are concerned about their appearance and their inability to chew efficiently; such motivating factors are powerful and are likely to enhance the adaptive capability.

Patients requesting replacement dentures generally do so for reasons of function and appearance; function includes fit and comfort of the dentures as well as the ability to eat effectively. Studies have shown that a satisfactory outcome to treatment is strongly related to the level of function achieved and to the technical quality of the dentures. It is of interest to note that concern over appearance seems to be under-reported, both before and after treatment. If functional requirements have been satisfied by the new dentures, patients may be inclined to look more closely at appearance. If they are unhappy with what they see, there is occasionally a reluctance to complain directly. Instead, patients may resort to making complaints about function to draw the dentist's attention to their real concern in a somewhat roundabout way. Functional complaints which seem to have no logical cause should always be considered in this particular light.

Poor motivation will be expected from those patients who are badgered into seeking treatment by their relatives when it is apparent that they themselves are perfectly content with both comfort and function of their existing dentures. Deterioration in appearance is the usual cause of pressure from relatives. On occasions, one meets an elderly person who is quite content with the edentulous state but has been instructed to obtain complete dentures before a major family event such as the grandchild's wedding. Inevitably, motivation is very weak in this instance and, in all probability, the new dentures will be placed in the bottom drawer once the family celebration is over.

Previous Denture Experience

The picture obtained of the patient's reactions to previous dentures is frequently of value. The significance of the past dental history can be appreciated by considering two common, yet contrasting situations. There are those patients who seek new dentures to replace existing ones which have been worn for very many years. So often it is apparent that the old dentures are ill-fitting and the occlusion no longer balanced, and yet the patient has tolerated an increasing inadequacy for some time. Although this state of affairs indicates a well-marked ability to adapt to dentures and to overcome difficulties, such a level of perseverance can be dangerous as it can result in accelerated resorption of the underlying bone and may induce pathological changes in the mucosa. This example of stoicism is in marked contrast to the second group made up of patients who have been provided with several sets of dentures in a short period of time. Such a story of repeated failure should always be a warning to the dentist as it may indicate a patient who is unable or unwilling to accept complete dentures. Some reasons for this difficulty will be discussed in the next section dealing with general health. There are, however, other reasons for constant failure of prosthetic treatment. For example, it may become apparent during examination of the various old dentures that there are obvious errors in design and construction. If patients receive inadequate treatment on one or more occasions and are told that the problems experienced are due to them, confidence in prosthetic treatment is lost rapidly and a mental barrier is built up against dentures. Problems of tolerance can also originate through lack of communication between dentist and patient. In cases where examination of the denture-bearing tissues indicates that the prognosis for satisfactory stability is poor, it is essential for the dentist to warn the patient in advance of the difficulties and to describe the steps which will be taken to minimise them. If a patient is not advised of the limited prognosis in the particular circumstances, any shortcomings in performance may be blamed on the dentures and the patient becomes discouraged prematurely.

Many patients use their friends' prosthetic experiences as the yardstick for their own expectations. On recognising this state of affairs through the patient's remarks, the dentist must ensure that this impression is altered and the patient encouraged to appreciate that no two mouths present the same degree of difficulty. If steps are taken to keep a patient fully informed as to the problems and the methods that are to be used to deal with them, there is a much greater chance of limitations being accepted and cooperation being given.

Health of the Patient

Clinically, it is recognised that significant impairment of general bodily or mental health is likely to affect the learning process adversely, with the result that the patient experiences considerable difficulty in mastering new dentures; in this respect it should be remembered that the chances of impairment of health increase as people grow older. When assessing a patient it is therefore very important to note details of the medical history, such as a chronic debilitating illness, which may reduce the patient's stamina to such an extent that there is little left to cope with the demands of new dentures. For example, patients suffering from any form of arthritis may be persistently troubled with pain to the extent that it becomes a depressing and overwhelming part of life. Chronic bronchitis and the iron-deficiency anaemias result in a general feeling of tiredness and lassitude. These three conditions occur more frequently in the middle-aged or elderly, the same groups for whom one most commonly constructs complete dentures. The ability to manipulate dentures may be reduced severely by various neurological disorders, such as the muscle tremor and reduced muscular power of Parkinson's disease and the muscle weakness of myasthenia gravis or bulbar palsy.

Gastric and duodenal ulceration are characterised by frequent bouts of pain. Patients suffering from these conditions are often referred to the dentist by their doctor with the request that dentures should be constructed in order to improve mastication. It is not known whether the provision of new dentures materially assists digestion of the special diet prescribed in these instances. However, it can be argued with conviction that an increase in masticatory efficiency may reduce the burden placed on the mucosa of the alimentary tract. The problem for dentists, in such instances, is that they are being asked to produce dentures for a person whose adaptive capability may have been reduced by the disease for which the dentures are being prescribed.

Gastric and duodenal ulceration are known to have a strong connection with emotional stress, a factor which itself adversely affects adaptation. Any set of circumstances which impairs mental health may create a situation whereby anxiety, depression or other neurotic states may result in the patient being unable or unwilling to tolerate new dentures. Clues that such adverse psychological factors exist may be supplied by the medical history; for example, the patient may be taking tranquillisers or sedatives. Further information can be difficult to obtain because patients may suspect a dentist of being unnecessarily inquisitive if personal questions are asked. This stems from the fact that many patients are not aware of the influence their general condition may have on the outcome of prosthetic treatment. To assist dentists in recognising behavioural problems, various question-naires have been designed to measure characteristics of personality and the levels of anxiety or depression. The results from these self-administered tests can help to build up a picture of the individual patient and assist the dentist in making a judgement as to the prognosis of the proposed treatment.

BIBLIOGRAPHY

Basker, R. M. (1966) Adaptation to dentures. *British Dental Journal*, **120**, 573–6.

Berg, E. (1984) The influence of some anamnestic, demographic, and clinical variables on patient acceptance of new complete dentures. *Acta Odontologica Scandinavica*, **42**, 119–27.

Berg, E. (1988) A 2-year follow-up study of patient satisfaction with new complete dentures. *Journal of Dentistry*, **16**, 160–5.

Berg, E., Backer Johnsen, T. and Ingebretsen, R. (1984) Patient motives and fulfillment of motives in renewal of complete dentures. *Acta Odontologica Scandinavica*, **42**, 235–40.

Berg, E., Backer Johnsen, T. and Ingebretsen, R. (1985) Social variables and patient acceptance of complete dentures. *Acta Odontologica Scandinavica*, **43**, 199–203.

Berry, D. C. and Mahood, M. (1966) Oral stereognosis and oral ability in relation to prosthetic treatment. *British Dental Journal*, **120**, 179–85.

Brill, N., Tryde, G. and Schübeler, S. (1959) The role of exteroceptors in denture retention. *Journal of Prosthetic Dentistry*, **9**, 761–8.

Brill, N., Tryde, G. and Schübeler, S. (1960) The role of learning in denture retention. *Journal of Prosthetic Dentistry*, **10**, 468–75.

Crum, R. J. and Loiselle, R. J. (1972) Oral perception and proprioception: A review of the literature and its significance to prosthodontics. *Journal of Prosthetic Dentistry*, **28**, 215–30.

Fish, S. F. (1969) Adaptation and habituation to full dentures. *British Dental Journal*, **127**, 19–26.

Langer, A. (1979) Prosthodontic failures in patients with systemic disorders. *Journal of Oral Rehabilitation*, **6**, 13–19.

Newton, A. V. (1975) The difficult denture patient, a review of psychological aspects. *British Dental Journal*, **138**, 93–7.

Reeve, P. E., Watson, C. J. and Stafford, G. D. (1984) The role of personality in the management of complete denture patients. *British Dental Journal*, **156**, 356–62.

Storer, R. (1965) The effect of the climacteric and of ageing on prosthetic diagnosis and treatment planning. *British Dental Journal*, **119**, 349–54.

Weinstein, W., Schuchman, J., Lieberman, J. and Rosen, P. (1988) Age and denture experience as determinants in patient denture satisfaction. *Journal of Prosthetic Dentistry*, **59**, 327–9.

Zigmond, A. S. and Snaith, R. P. (1983) The hospital anxiety and depression scale. *Acta Psychiatrica Scandinavica*, **67**, 361–70.

3 Transition from Natural to Artificial Dentition

For most people, the prospect of losing all their remaining natural teeth, particularly the anterior teeth, and having nothing with which to replace them immediately after extraction is unacceptable. Fortunately, this situation can usually be avoided by fitting a denture immediately following tooth removal. This transition to the completely artificial dentition is a major and irreversible procedure for the patient in which both timing of extractions and the provision and maintenance of dentures must be planned with great care.

The transition is a critical stage in the patient's treatment which can have far-reaching effects and may influence the success of subsequent complete dentures. The level of anxiety with which people face the prospect of losing their teeth and being provided with complete dentures was reported in the UK Adult Dental Health survey of 1978 (Table 3.1). As one would expect, nearly 60 per cent of those who expected to keep their teeth found the thought of losing them and having complete dentures very upsetting. Yet, as many as 30 per cent of those who expected to have to make the transition at some time had the same feeling. The aim of this chapter is to outline the principles of treatment contributing to a successful transition. Details of clinical techniques are, in the main, omitted.

Table 3.1

Attitude to having complete dentures	Proportion (%) who expect to:	
	Keep natural teeth all their lives	Have complete dentures
Very upsetting	58	30
A little upsetting	24	27
Not at all upsetting	18	43

From Todd *et al.*, 1982

METHODS OF TRANSITION

The various methods of making the transition from natural to artificial dentition may be considered under the following headings.

Transitional Partial Dentures

Such partial dentures restore existing edentulous areas; they may be worn for a short period of time before the remaining natural teeth are extracted and the dentures converted accordingly.

Overdentures

These are dentures which are fitted over retained roots and which derive some of their support from that coverage. As will be described later, special attachments may be fixed to the root faces to provide mechanical retention for the denture. If, in due course, the roots have to be extracted, the overdenture can be converted into a complete denture.

Immediate Dentures

These dentures are constructed prior to the extraction of the natural teeth and are inserted immediately after removal of those teeth.

Clearance of Remaining Natural Teeth prior to Making Dentures

This approach differs from all those mentioned previously in that, after the extractions, time is allowed for initial healing and alveolar bone resorption to occur before providing complete dentures.

FACTORS INFLUENCING THE DECISION OF WHETHER OR NOT TO EXTRACT THE REMAINING TEETH

When the patient's dentition has reached the stage where it appears that complete dentures will be necessary in the foreseeable future, the dentist must consider carefully the timing of extraction of the remaining teeth. The following considerations will influence the decision.

The Condition of the Teeth and Supporting Tissues

The prognosis of each remaining tooth should be assessed carefully. Useful teeth can be retained as long as it is feasible to undertake appropriate treatment to eliminate disease and if there is confidence in the patient's ability to maintain good oral health.

In contrast, the presence of gross caries or advanced periodontal disease, coupled with the proven reluctance of the patient to respond to oral hygiene instruction, makes the decision of whether or not to extract the teeth a simple one; early extraction in such circumstances is clearly inevitable. Such a decision is perhaps especially important in the case of advanced periodontal disease where any undue delay will result in further destruction of what will become the bony denture foundation.

Natural Teeth Opposing an Edentulous Ridge

The situation where one arch only is rendered edentulous can eventually lead to major prosthetic complications. The combination most commonly found is a complete upper denture opposed by a number of lower natural teeth. A most unfavourable situation develops in which the natural teeth generate high occlusal loads and excessive horizontal displacement of the denture, which cause rapid destruction of the denture-bearing bone and the production of a flabby ridge (see Chapter 15). Additional problems include complaints of a loose denture, a deteriorating appearance as the denture sinks into the tissues, and fracture of the denture base. The problems are accentuated in the lower jaw where the denture-bearing area is smaller.

Serious consideration should be given to reducing such problems by either utilising selected teeth as overdenture abutments or, in extreme cases, extracting the remaining teeth. The least that should be done is to warn the patient of the possible consequences and arrange for regular inspection and maintenance so as to 'nip in the bud' any possibility of rapid, damaging resorption.

When faced with a patient who has a few remaining teeth in one jaw opposing many natural teeth in the other, the dentist should seek ways of retaining some or all of the few teeth and employing them to support and stabilise an overdenture, thus avoiding the damaging situation previously described.

Age and Health of the Patient

As mentioned in Chapter 2, advancing years, coupled frequently by worsening health, reduce the patient's ability to adapt successfully to complete dentures. This consideration should be borne in mind when planning the extraction of teeth of uncertain prognosis. The teeth may, for example, be expected to have a few more years of useful life, but delaying extractions until absolutely necessary may postpone the patient's first experience of complete dentures to a time when adaptive capability is seriously reduced; as a consequence the patient may have difficulty in coping with complete dentures or, indeed, may fail totally.

It may therefore be argued that the correct approach under such circumstances is to extract the teeth at an earlier age when the patient stands a better chance of adapting successfully to complete dentures.

However, the decision to carry out such extraction of reasonably sound teeth as a preventive measure can be an extremely difficult one to make. As the rate of biological ageing and reduction in adaptive capability vary greatly from one patient to another, it is not possible to identify accurately a cut-off point in years at which such extractions should be carried out. It is true that early extractions may reduce problems of adaptation to dentures, but this advantage must be balanced against the immediate probability of reduced oral function and comfort in a patient who is happy with a few remaining natural teeth and, maybe, a partial denture. The correct way out of the dilemma of whether or not to take the irrevocable step of a dental clearance may be clarified by delaying the decision and placing the patient on a programme of annual review appointments. At each appointment, an assessment can be made of the rate of deterioration of the patient's dentition and the standard of oral hygiene, and thus a clearer picture will emerge of the probable life of the teeth and their value to the patient. A somewhat crude judgement is to assess the health of the patient and the teeth and to try to answer the question 'Is the patient likely to outlive the remaining useful natural teeth, or is the reverse more likely to occur?' In the first case, serious thought should be given to whether the transition to artificial dentition should be made earlier rather than later.

TRANSITIONAL PARTIAL DENTURES

Transitional partial dentures are of particular value in those cases where problems of adaptation to, or tolerance of, complete dentures are anticipated. The transitional partial denture provides a training period which allows the patient to acquire the skills of denture control and to adapt to the presence of a prosthesis in the mouth before having to face the much more demanding task presented by complete dentures, once the stabilising effect of the remaining teeth has been lost.

The chance of success of a transitional partial denture is influenced to a large extent by the particular teeth which remain in the mouth. For example, stability of a lower denture will be increased if an anterior saddle is present because the existence of the labial flange and contacts with the mesial surfaces of the abutment teeth will resist posterior displacement. Also, as the denture carries anterior teeth, the patient will be better motivated to persevere with the denture in the face of any initial difficulties. Thus, the retention of $\overline{43/34}$ rather than $\overline{321/123}$ is likely to be more successful.

Although transitional partial dentures are a potentially valuable means of smoothing the passage from the partially dentate to the edentulous state, they can compound the difficulties of complete dentures unless correctly designed and adequately maintained. A partial denture which is underextended, poorly fitting or which has an incorrect occlusion is likely to be unstable and uncomfortable, thus undermining the patient's confidence in denture wearing. Also, if the patient perseveres with the partial denture in spite of the difficulties, destruction of the denture-bearing tissues is likely to occur, creating a more unfavourable foundation for subsequent complete dentures. It should be remembered that the tissue-borne transitional partial denture is virtually always provided for a patient whose dental awareness is highly suspect. The effects of increased plaque formation and lack of adequate support can cause severe tissue destruction in a relatively short time (Figure 3.1). In this particular case, a high-risk denture has been provided for a high-risk patient.

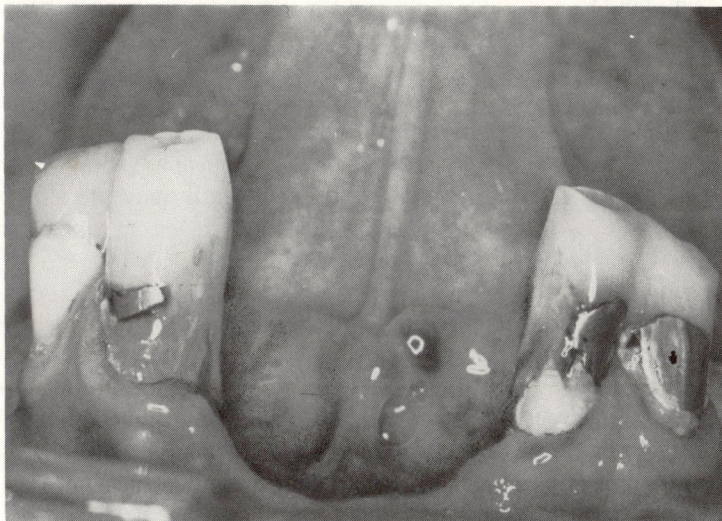

Figure 3.1   Severe tissue destruction caused by a tissue-borne partial denture

OVERDENTURES

In the transitional dentition the overdenture, like the partial denture, can be used to provide a training period, allowing the patient to prepare for the more demanding task imposed by future complete dentures. If the life of teeth is limited, treatment should normally be kept as simple as possible. However, as even the simplest overdenture treatment usually entails root filling and decoronating two or three abutment teeth, this type of denture tends to be reserved for cases where the teeth have a somewhat better prognosis than is acceptable for transitional partial dentures. In fact, because the loading of the teeth is more advantageous, the simple overdenture may well extend the life of the teeth.

Advantages of Overdentures

Preservation of the Ridge Form
Efficient support of the overdenture by the root faces of the abutment teeth reduces the loading of the edentulous areas and therefore the rate of bone resorption is likely to be less. This factor is the most important advantage of the overdenture, particularly for the lower jaw where it has been shown that preserving the canine roots as abutments can reduce the rate of resorption approximately eight times. This preservation of alveolar bone has obvious benefits in providing support and promoting stability of dentures. If the retained roots are in the anterior region, the preservation of bone will help to maintain support of the lips and thus will contribute to facial appearance.

Minimising Horizontal Forces on the Abutment Teeth
The reduction in crown length of the abutment teeth and the production of a domed shape to the root face reduces the mechanical advantage of these damaging forces. The life of the abutment teeth may therefore be prolonged.

Proprioception
While the roots and their periodontal ligaments remain, periodontal mechanoreceptors are said to allow a finer discrimination of food texture, tooth contacts and levels of functional loading. A better appreciation of food and a more precise control of mandibular movements is therefore possible than is provided for by receptors in the denture-bearing mucosa of edentulous patients.

Correction of Occlusion and Aesthetics
Overdentures have a particular advantage over partial dentures in those cases where the crowns of the remaining few teeth pose problems either in

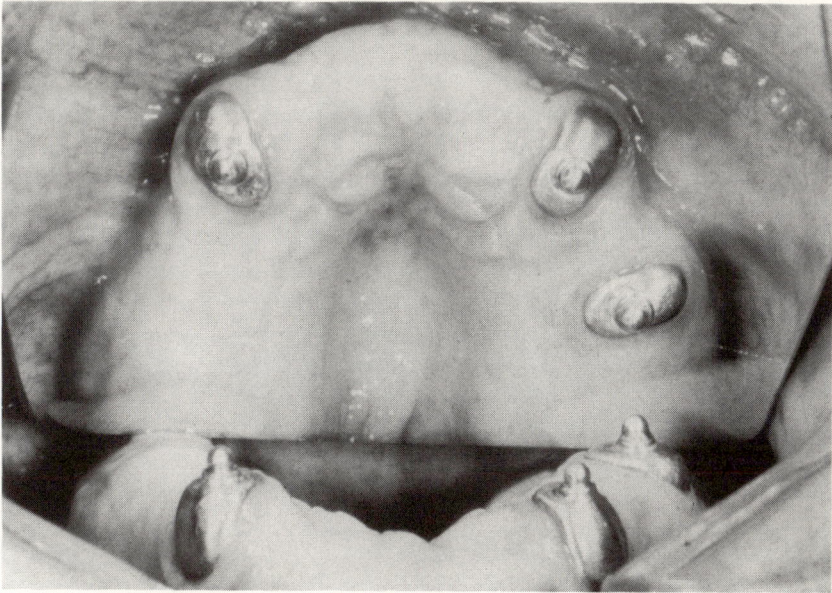

Figure 3.2   Stud attachments on the abutment teeth are engaged by spring clips
within the overdenture to provide positive retention

terms of occlusion or appearance. Removal of the offending crowns and covering the roots with an overdenture provide the freedom in tooth arrangement necessary to correct the undesirable features of the natural dentition.

Denture Retention

As mentioned earlier, more positive retention of the denture to the root faces may be obtained by means of precision attachments (Figure 3.2). However, in many instances such additional retention is not needed. It can be argued, in fact, that precision attachments are contraindicated for overdentures which are provided as a transitional stage of limited duration en route to complete dentures. First, as attachments add additional expense, they are not cost effective if used on abutments of poor prognosis. Second, the retention achieved can be too good, thus inhibiting the development of the patient's neuromuscular skills which will be required to control the future complete dentures.

An alternative method of augmenting retention is to use rare earth magnets as illustrated in Figure 3.3. These devices are less expensive than many of the precision attachments. As the magnet applies less force to the abutment tooth, it can be used in situations where much of the periodontal attachment has been destroyed.

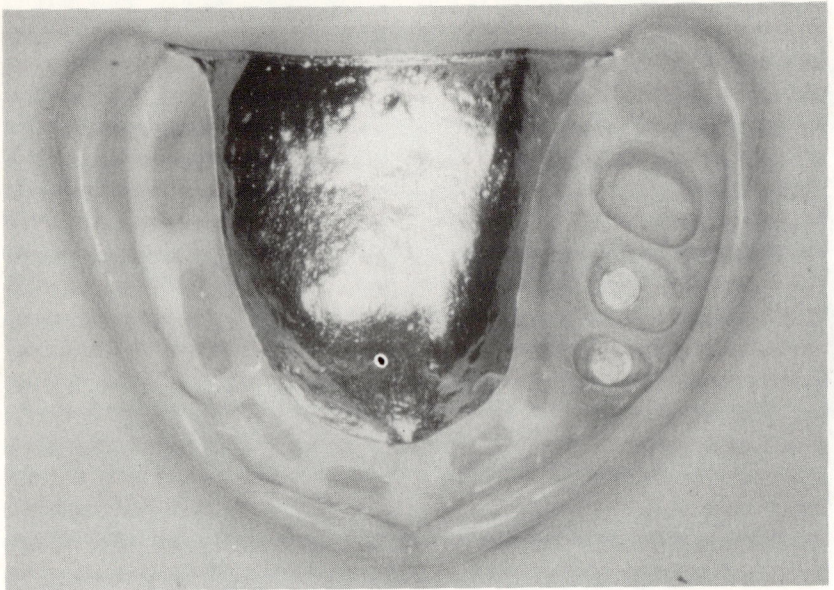

Figure 3.3   A complete upper overdenture with rare earth magnets placed in |56. The copings covering the abutment teeth are constructed in a special alloy appropriate to the system

Psychological Benefits

The complete, irrevocable loss of all teeth can be a serious blow to a patient's morale signalling, perhaps, that a major milestone in life has been reached and that all that is left is senile decay. The retention of remnants of the natural dentition in the form of overdenture abutments can soften the blow and allow a period of mental adjustment before the edentulous state is reached. The patient's attitude to treatment and to the ultimate complete dentures may thus be more favourable. This particular benefit is not, in the authors' opinion, a common one. However, when it does arise it can be of considerable value to both patient and dentist.

Disadvantages of Overdentures

Root Canal Therapy

The preservation of roots as overdenture abutments usually necessitates endodontic treatment, thus extending the course of treatment and increasing its cost. The technical difficulty of achieving a satisfactory root filling may be increased because of partial obliteration of the root canal by secondary dentine due to ageing or in response to excessive loss of tooth substance.

Caries
Covering root faces with an overdenture can increase the rate of carious attack of these surfaces to an unacceptable degree. The conclusions from a number of surveys reveal a caries prevalence ranging from 15 per cent to 36 per cent. Protection of the root faces is therefore required in addition to oral hygiene instruction and dietary advice. Such protection is more simply provided by regular applications of topical fluoride using a fluoride varnish in the surgery and a fluoride toothpaste at home. Effective plaque control of abutment teeth and denture is of fundamental importance. If caries develops, the alternative and more costly approach is to cover the root face with a gold coping.

Periodontal Disease
Covering the gum margins of abutment teeth with an overdenture has the potential for initiating periodontal disease or aggravating any existing disease process. There have been reports of gingival bleeding around all abutment teeth after four years and of obvious inflammation around 12 per cent of abutment teeth after three years. To reduce the risk, meticulous plaque control is required. Fortunately, the simple shape of a root face places fewer demands on a patient's oral hygiene technique than does the more complex tooth crown.

Overdenture Technique

The summary which follows outlines a simple technique appropriate for the construction of a complete overdenture.

Selection of Abutments
As the mandibular residual ridge provides a less favourable foundation for a complete denture than the maxillary ridge and hard palate, the indications for retaining roots as overdenture abutments are stronger in the lower jaw.

Although any tooth amenable to root canal therapy may be retained as an overdenture abutment, single-rooted teeth are preferable on the grounds of simplicity. Teeth such as the canines, lower first premolars and upper central incisors are thus particularly suitable. Lower incisors and upper lateral incisors are not ideal abutments because of their small periodontal ligament area. Extraction of these teeth may, in fact, facilitate the task of cleaning adjacent abutments. Such extractions will usually be carried out at the appointment for fitting the overdenture.

Clinical and Laboratory Stages

After endodontic treatment of the abutment teeth has been carried out, the production of an overdenture follows the stages of conventional partial denture technique until the try-in stage has been completed. The working cast is then modified by cutting off the crowns of the chosen abutment teeth and undertrimming the root faces to produce a domed preparation slightly more supragingival than is intended for the actual root faces. It is useful to measure the height from the top of the dome to a fixed point at the gingival margin with dividers and to note this measurement in order to guide the preparation of the natural tooth at the next clinical visit. The crowns of any teeth to be extracted at the time of fitting the denture are also cut off the cast. The denture is then processed in the normal way.

At the appointment for fitting the denture, the crowns of the abutment teeth are removed and the root faces are domed, using the measurement made on the working cast. The openings of the root canals are then sealed with either glass–ionomer cement or amalgam. The other teeth are extracted and the immediate overdenture fitted.

When the denture is checked at the next appointment, the restorations and the root faces are polished and fluoride varnish applied to the dentine. An accurate fit of the denture to the root faces is achieved by placing cold-curing acrylic resin within the recesses in the impression surface corresponding to the roots. Correct seating of the denture under occlusal pressure is facilitated by drilling a vent hole from each of the recesses to the polished surface to allow escape of any excess acrylic resin (Figure 3.4).

Maintenance of the Overdenture

It is important to arrange a programme of review appointments to allow proper maintenance of the overdenture. This will involve maintaining oral and denture hygiene and reinforcing when necessary. Regular applications of topical fluoride should be made to the abutments. Temporary or permanent relining procedures will be required to compensate for alveolar resorption in regions where extractions were carried out at the time of fitting the denture. If caries of the root faces poses a problem in spite of topical fluoride applications, gold copings can be considered as a secondary procedure. If the patient is unable to control the denture as well as had been anticipated, magnets or stud attachments may be placed on the abutments to enhance retention.

IMMEDIATE DENTURES

Providing the patient with immediate dentures is one of the most commonly practised methods of effecting the transition from the natural to the

excess
acrylic
resin

vent

glass–ionomer
restoration

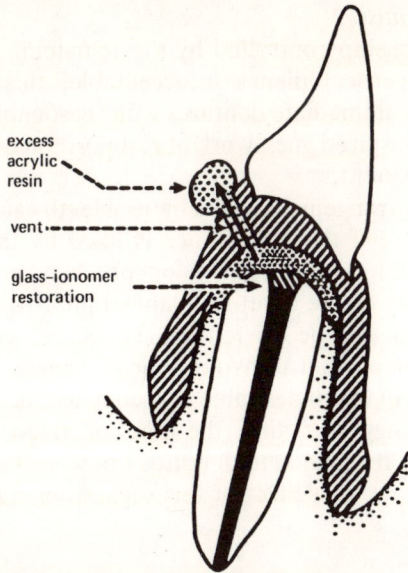

Figure 3.4   Cross-section of overdenture and abutment tooth showing correction
of fit by addition of cold-curing acrylic resin

artificial dentition. It was once said that this method was the appropriate
treatment for those in the professions who could not do without teeth for
any length of time. The typical list would usually include vicars, doctors
and business people – dentists were never mentioned! Times and outlooks
have changed and today the preservation of appearance is an almost
universal wish. It is true that in certain circumstances immediate dentures
are not indicated, but it is also true that people in the UK are being
gradually educated to expect and accept this form of treatment.

Advantages of Immediate Dentures

Related to the Patient
Maintenance of dental appearance and facial contour.
Minimising disturbances of mastication and speech.
Facilitating adaptation to dentures.
    Difficulties with adaptation occur more commonly if the patient
    experiences an edentulous period of several months before dentures are
    fitted.
Maintenance of the patient's physical and mental well-being.

Related to the Dentist

If the jaw relationship controlled by the remaining natural teeth in both horizontal and vertical planes is acceptable, this relationship can be transferred to the immediate dentures with reasonable accuracy, obviating the need for the inspired guesswork of rest position estimation required for the edentulous patient.

The form and arrangement of the natural teeth can be reproduced in the immediate denture if the appearance is liked by the patient. When the appearance of the natural teeth is poor, or when their positions are likely to cause instability of the denture, planned improvements of the anterior tooth arrangement can be carried out. However, when such changes are anticipated it is important to avoid radical changes in incisal relationship which may result in the undesirable consequences described in Chapter 11.

It has been suggested that the rate of ridge resorption following extractions is less if immediate dentures are worn than if no dentures are fitted. However, the evidence for this suggestion is inconclusive.

Disadvantages of Immediate Dentures

The main disadvantage of immediate dentures is that a number of visits are required after extraction of the teeth to allow for maintenance of the dentures. Such maintenance may include temporary and permanent relines, occlusal adjustment and also the addition of a labial flange in the case of an open-face denture (page 43). If the dentures are not properly maintained, extensive destruction of the denture-bearing tissues usually results. Thus, before embarking upon treatment it is essential to make the patient aware of the need for maintenance. Only patients who are prepared to attend for such additional treatment should be accepted for immediate dentures.

The patient who is a candidate for immediate dentures should also accept that replacement dentures may be required sooner than would be the case for a complete denture fitted some months after extractions had been carried out.

Because of the overwhelming advantages of immediate dentures, this form of treatment should be offered to the vast majority of patients for whom the transition from natural to artificial dentition must be made. There are relatively few circumstances in which the immediate denture is contraindicated.

Types of Immediate Denture

There are basically two types of immediate denture – the flanged and the open-face. The flanged denture may be subdivided into two types: the complete flange and partial flange. The former has a labial flange fully extended to the depth of the sulcus, whereas the latter has a flange usually finished with the border extended about 1 mm beyond the maximum bulbosity of the ridge. In the open-face denture there is no labial flange and the anterior teeth extend a few millimetres into the labial aspect of the sockets of their natural predecessors (Figure 3.5).

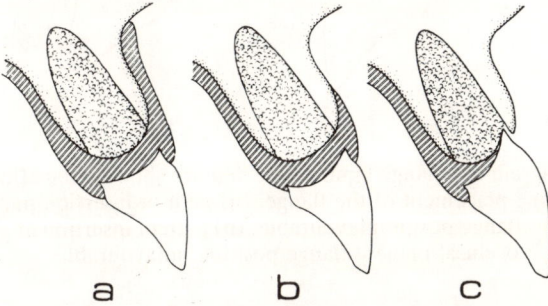

Figure 3.5   Types of immediate denture: (a) complete flange; (b) partial flange; (c) open-face

Comparison of Flanged and Open-face Dentures

Appearance
The appearance of a flanged denture does not alter after fitting whereas the appearance of an open-face denture, although good initially, can deteriorate rapidly as resorption causes a gap to appear between the necks of the teeth and the ridge. Also, the flange design, unlike the open-face denture, allows considerable freedom in positioning the anterior teeth for optimum effect. For these reasons the flange design is preferable; however, it is essential that the flange is kept thin and positioned correctly against the labial surface of the ridge, otherwise distortion of the lip will result in poor facial appearance. In this context, selection of the correct path of insertion of the denture is essential (Figure 3.6). Where the ridge morphology produces a deeply undercut area, it may not be possible to fit a full labial flange unless there is surgical reduction of that undercut. Under such circumstances, a partial flange may be acceptable unless the patient has a smile line high enough to reveal the edge of that flange.

Stability
The flanged denture promotes a more effective border seal than an open-face denture. The labial flange also resists posterior displacement of the denture resulting in greater stability, a point of particular importance for the lower denture.

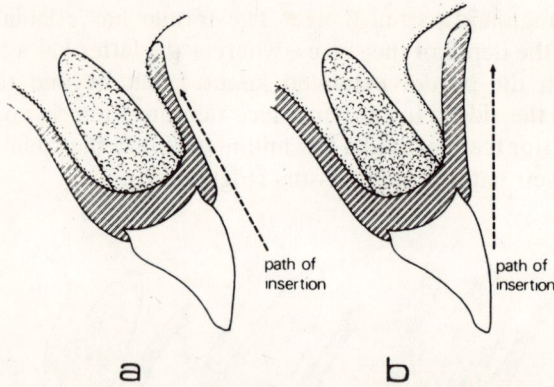

Figure 3.6   Diagram of a flanged immediate denture showing the effect of the path of insertion on the placement of the flange: (a) path of insertion parallel to labial surface of ridge – flange position favourable; (b) path of insertion at right angles to occlusal plane – flange position unfavourable

Strength
The presence of a labial flange produces a denture which is less likely to fracture as a result of accidental impacts or high occlusal loads. The denture will also resist flexing so that the danger of a mid-line fatigue fracture is minimised.

Maintenance
As the bone resorbs following extraction of the teeth, the immediate denture becomes loose and a reline is required. The presence of a labial flange makes it particularly easy to add either a short-term resilient lining material or a cold-curing poly(butylmethacrylate) relining material as a chairside procedure. Such convenience is appreciated by both the dentist and the patient.

Haemostasis
The flanged denture covers the clots completely and protects them more effectively than does an open-face denture. The flanged denture also exerts pressure on both lingual and labial gingivae reducing the likelihood of post-extraction haemorrhage.

Remodelling of the Ridge
There is always the danger that the patient will fail to attend for a maintenance appointment. The consequent wearing of an ill-fitting denture will, if it is open-faced, produce a scalloped ridge in the region of the socketed teeth (Figure 3.7). This danger is avoided in the case of a flanged denture which, in addition, has the advantage of distributing the functional

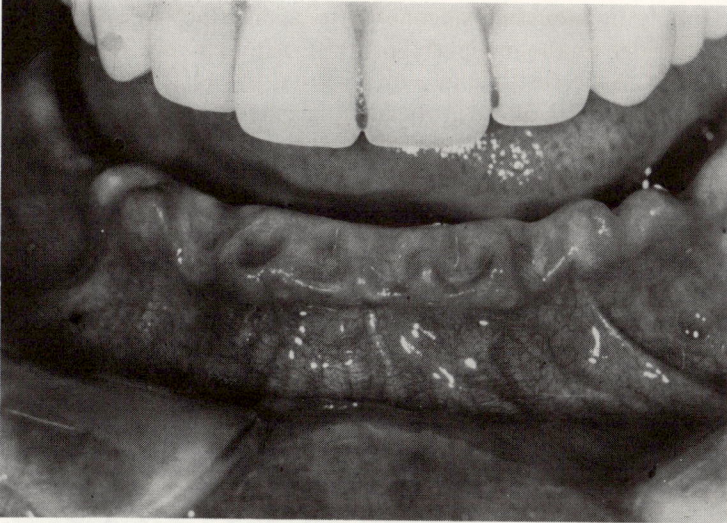

Figure 3.7 Tissue damage produced by an open-face lower immediate denture

loads more favourably to the underlying ridge, thus minimising bone resorption.

A frequent clinical problem is the difficulty that patients experience in accepting a labial flange on a replacement denture when the immediate denture had an open face. Although the flange replaces bone which has resorbed, its presence in the richly innervated oral cavity frequently promotes a complaint of 'fullness' of the upper lip. If a flanged denture had been worn from the very beginning, there is no problem with adaptation.

An Outline of Relevant Clinical and Technical Procedures

The essential steps in the construction of immediate dentures follow the same sequence as those for conventional partial dentures until after the try-in stage. The subsequent conversion of the try-in to the complete denture requires modification of the cast in the laboratory. The nature of the modification depends upon whether the denture is to be flanged or open-face.

Flanged Dentures

Extraction without Alveolar Surgery
If the arrangement of the natural anterior teeth is to be reproduced in the denture, a record of their position must be obtained by producing a labial index before the teeth are cut off the cast. The index can be produced

quite simply by moulding silicone putty against the labial surface of the teeth and ridge on the model (Figure 3.8). Alternatively, the teeth may be removed from the cast one at a time so that the adjacent teeth serve as a guide to the position of the artificial replacement. Information on anterior tooth position can also be recorded by guide-lines scribed on the cast (Figure 3.9). Once the artificial teeth have been positioned, the flange is added in wax prior to the denture being processed.

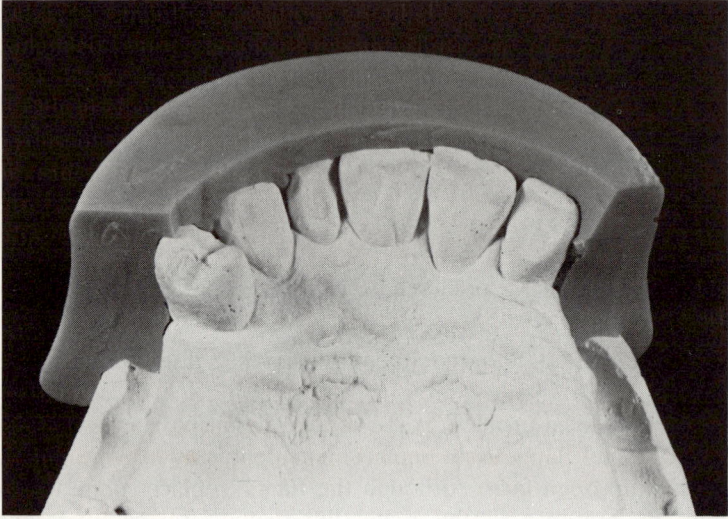

Figure 3.8   Position of the anterior teeth recorded by a silicone putty index

Alveolotomy Following Interseptal Alveolectomy
This procedure is intended to eliminate moderate undercuts in the alveolus, usually in the upper anterior region, so that a flanged denture can be used without that flange distorting the upper lip unduly. In simple terms, surgery involves the extraction of the teeth and removal of the associated interseptal bone. The labial cortical plate of bone, together with the mucoperiostium, is then collapsed back into the gutter so formed and the wound is closed.

The denture will be constructed on a working cast which is now trimmed to the anticipated contour of the alveolus after surgery. Once the gingival margins have been marked and the teeth have been removed, guide-lines are drawn on the cast (Figure 3.10). One line, drawn on the crest of the ridge, passes across the centre of the sockets of the incisors and through the junction of the labial third and palatal two-thirds of the canine sockets. A second line is drawn horizontally along the labial aspect of the ridge; it is placed approximately two-thirds down the length of the shortest

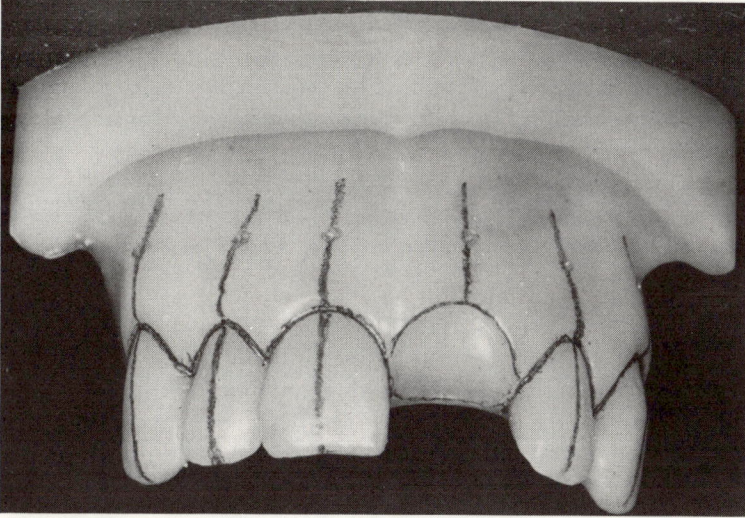

Figure 3.9   Long axes of the teeth marked on the cast to assist in placing the artificial teeth in similar positions. The location of incisal edges can be determined by direct measurement with dividers

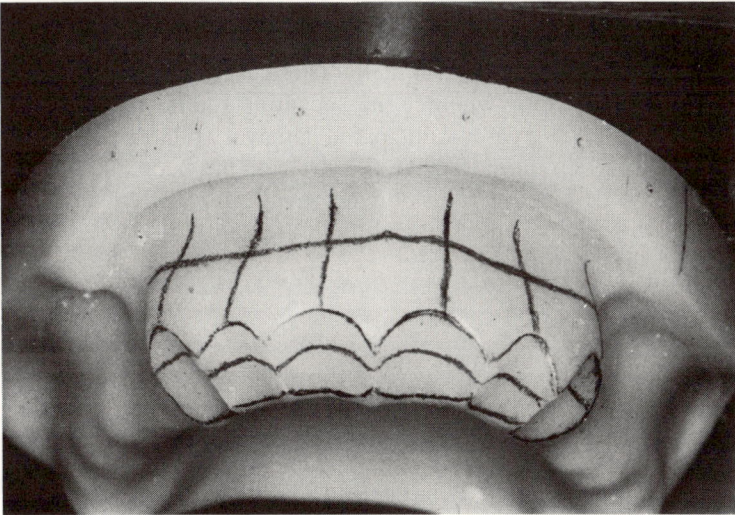

Figure 3.10   Alveolotomy following interseptal alveolectomy: lines drawn on the cast to guide model trimming (see text for details)

root, usually the lateral incisor, and is continuous around all the teeth at that level. All that part of the cast contained within these two lines is trimmed away and the edges rounded over. A clear acrylic template is processed on a duplicate of this cast and is used as a guide when the bone is removed at the time of operation. Blanching of the mucosa occurs beneath the clear acrylic template in any areas where there is excessive pressure due to inadequate bone removal. Further bone removal is then undertaken in these areas until insertion of the template ceases to cause blanching. Once the sockets have been sutured, the immediate denture is inserted.

Alveolectomy

The most common indication for an alveolectomy in association with the fitting of immediate dentures is the reduction of a prominent premaxilla to allow a more favourable placing of anterior teeth on the dentures.

A clear acrylic template is processed on a duplicate of the working cast trimmed to produce the desired ridge form. The template is used as a guide to bone removal during surgery in the same way as that for an alveolotomy following interseptal alveolectomy, as previously described.

Open-face Dentures

The purpose of socketing anterior teeth on an open-face denture is to maintain an acceptable appearance for a few weeks by allowing for the gingival collapse that occurs after extractions. Without socketing, an unsightly gap would soon appear between tooth and mucosa. The amount of gingival collapse will depend on the degree of pocketing and bone loss that is present around the natural teeth. These aspects should therefore be assessed before deciding whether the socketing should be to a depth of 2 mm or whether a greater anticipated gingival collapse indicates that deeper socketing is required. When this decision has been taken, the teeth are cut off the cast and a recess of the required depth cut in the labial aspects of the sockets. The artificial teeth are carefully positioned in the sockets and the denture processed.

Contraindications to Immediate Dentures

Patients at Risk from a Bacteraemia

Some clinicians believe that movement of an immediate denture can disturb the clots and surrounding tissues sufficiently to precipitate a bacteraemia. There is a strong body of opinion opposed to the provision of immediate dentures for patients such as those who have a history of rheumatic fever with cardiac damage, or those with heart valve or hip prostheses.

Patients with a Genuine History of Post-extraction Haemorrhage

As multiple extractions of anterior teeth are generally required when immediate dentures are fitted, such treatment is inappropriate when there is a proven history of post-extraction haemorrhage which has been difficult to control. A more cautious approach is indicated, involving the extraction of a few teeth at a time followed by suturing the sockets. Dentures are then fitted at a later date when the initial healing is complete.

The Presence of Gross Oral Sepsis

Although it is possible to provide immediate dentures for a neglected mouth it is generally unwise to do so. The anterior teeth are often unsightly because of surface deposits, caries, gingival inflammation or recession; their retention for aesthetic reasons is therefore unjustified. Furthermore, a patient who has neglected the mouth in this way is often unconcerned about appearance anyway. The benefits of an immediate denture are therefore reduced significantly.

CLEARANCE OF TEETH WITHOUT IMMEDIATE PROVISION OF DENTURES

When a decision is taken to extract the remaining teeth prior to denture construction, it is common practice for a period of several months to be allowed for healing and initial alveolar modelling. This delay before taking impressions will produce more stable supporting areas for the dentures, although it must be accepted that resorption will continue indefinitely but at a slower rate. The main advantage of this method, that the initial dentures retain their fit for a longer period, is outweighed by the following disadvantages:

(a) Loss of masticatory function and appearance during the waiting period.
(b) The undesirable mental and physical effects on a patient that the absence of teeth creates.
(c) Tongue and cheeks may invade the future denture space making adaptation to subsequent dentures more difficult.
(d) Difficulty in assessing vertical and horizontal jaw relationships when constructing new dentures.
(e) The difficulty in restoring appearance if all information on the natural dentition has been lost.

The last two disadvantages can be overcome by using a method whereby pre-extraction records can be kept and transferred to the subsequent dentures using the following procedure:

Clinic: Take stock tray impressions and record shade of teeth.
Laboratory: Construct record rims to fill edentulous spaces.
Clinic: Record occlusion. Extract remaining teeth.

Laboratory: Leave record blocks on the casts and add wax 'flanges' on the buccal side of the standing teeth. Obtain an impression of the whole assembly in a duplicating flask. Remove the assembly, cut the teeth off the cast and adapt a shellac baseplate to what is now an edentulous cast. Replace cast and attached baseplate in the duplicating flask, and cut channels in the surrounding impression material to allow molten wax to flow into the space previously occupied by the record rim and natural teeth to produce what will be the record block to be used once the patient's ridges have healed sufficiently.

Clinic: Record the jaw relationship with the pre-prepared rims which will act as useful guides to the positions of the natural teeth before they were extracted. Take wash impressions in the record blocks.

Subsequent treatment: Progress to the conventional trial and fit stages. If necessary, further wash impressions can be taken in the trial dentures if further rapid resorption has taken place.

This technique eliminates a good deal of the guesswork in assessing jaw relationships and tooth positions in the situation where immediate dentures are contraindicated.

It is surprising, in view of these disadvantages, that the more efficient alternative method of making the transition from the natural to the artificial dentition via immediate dentures is not used routinely unless definite contraindications exist.

BIBLIOGRAPHY

Anderson, J. N. and Storer, R. (1981) *Immediate Replacement Dentures*, 3rd edn. Blackwell Scientific Publications, Oxford.

Basker, R. M., Harrison, A. and Ralph, J. P. (1988) *Overdentures in General Dental Practice*, 2nd edn. British Dental Association.

Bates, J. F. and Stafford, G. D. (1971) *Immediate Complete Dentures*. The British Dental Association, London.

Brewer, A. A. and Morrow, R. M. (1980) *Overdentures*, 2nd edn. The C. V. Mosby Company, Saint Louis.

Demer, W. J. (1972) Minimising problems in placement of immediate dentures. *Journal of Prosthetic Dentistry*, **27**, 275–84.

Johnson, K. (1977) A study of the dimensional changes occurring in the maxilla following open-face immediate denture treatment. *Australian Dental Journal*, **22**, 451–4.

Johnson, K. (1978) Immediate denture treatment for patients with Class II malocclusions. *Australian Dental Journal*, **23**, 383–8.

Murphy, W. M., Huggett, R., Handley, R. W. and Brooks, S. G. (1986) Rigid cold curing systems for direct use in the oral cavity. *British Dental Journal*, **160**, 391–4.

Mushimoto, E. (1981) The role in masseter muscle activities of functionally elicited periodontal afferents from abutment teeth under overdentures. *Journal of Oral Rehabilitation*, **8**, 441–55.

Nairn, R. I. and Cutress, T. W. (1967) Changes in mandibular position following removal of the remaining teeth and insertion of immediate complete dentures. *British Dental Journal*, **122**, 303–6.

Preiskel, H. W. (1979) *Precision Attachments in Dentistry*, 3rd edn. Kimpton, London.

Preiskel, H. W. (1985) *Precision Attachments in Prosthodontics: Overdentures and Telescopic Prostheses*, Vol. 2. Quintessence, Chicago.

Quinn, D. M., Yemm, R., Ianetta, R. V., Lyon, F. F. and McTear, J. (1986) A practical form of pre-extraction records for construction of complete dentures. *British Dental Journal*, **160**, 166–8.

Ralph, J. P. and Basker, R. M. (1989) The role of overdentures in gerodontics. *Dental Update*, **16**, 353–60.

Tallgren, A. *et al.* (1980) Roentgen cephalometric analysis of ridge resorption and changes in jaw and occlusal relationships in immediate complete denture wearers. *Journal of Oral Rehabilitation*, **7**, 77–94.

Todd, J. E., Walker, A. M. and Dodd, P. (1982) *Adult Dental Health*, Vol. 2: United Kingdom, 1978. HMSO, London.

4   Stability of Dentures

A stable denture is one which moves little in relation to the underlying bone during function. It is perhaps surprising that dentures stay in place at all, since they simply rest on mucous membrane and lie within a very active muscular environment. They stay in place if the retentive forces acting on the dentures exceed the displacing forces and the dentures have adequate support. This support is determined by the form and consistency of the denture-bearing tissues and the accuracy of fit of the denture. The relationship of these factors is as follows:

$$\begin{array}{ccccc}
\text{Retentive} & > & \text{Displacing} & + & \text{Adequate} & \to & \text{Stability} \\
\text{forces} & & \text{forces} & & \text{support} & &
\end{array}$$

RETENTIVE FORCES

Retentive forces offer resistance to dislodgement of a denture from the underlying mucosa and act through the three surfaces of a denture:

(a) *Occlusal surface*: That portion of the surface of a denture which makes contact or near contact with the corresponding surface of the opposing denture or dentition.

(b) *Polished surface*: That portion of the surface of a denture which extends in an occlusal direction from the border of the denture and includes the palatal surface. It is that part of the denture base which is usually polished, includes the buccal and lingual surfaces of the teeth, and is in contact with the lips, cheeks and tongue.

(c) *Impression surface*: That portion of the surface of a denture which had its contour determined by the impression. It includes the borders of the denture and extends to the polished surface.

The retentive forces which act upon each of these surfaces (Figure 4.1) are of two main types, muscular forces and physical forces. Muscular forces are exerted by the muscles of the lips, cheeks and tongue upon the polished surface of the denture and by the muscles of mastication indirectly through the occlusal surface. Physical forces are associated with the properties of

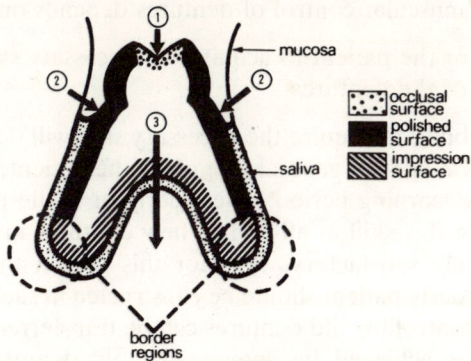

Figure 4.1   Retaining forces acting on a denture: (1) force of the muscles of mastication acting through the occlusal surface; (2) muscular forces of lips, cheeks and tongue acting through the polished surface; (3) physical forces acting through the impression surface

the film of saliva present between the denture and mucosa. They act primarily between the impression surface of the denture and the underlying mucosa, and are to a large extent dependent on the maintenance of a seal between the mucosa and the border regions of the denture.

Muscular Forces

Patients who wear their dentures successfully do so because they have learnt to control them with their lips, cheeks and tongue. This skill may be developed to such a high degree that a denture which appears loose to the dentist may be perfectly satisfactory from the patient's point of view. There are instances of patients who can eat without difficulty in spite of the fact that the denture has broken into two pieces. These observations indicate that the muscular control of dentures can be sufficient to allow satisfactory denture function without the assistance of physical retentive forces.

The physical retention of dentures depends on the maintenance of an intact seal around the border of the denture. Cineradiographic studies show that a large proportion of complete dentures moves several millimetres in relation to the underlying tissues during mastication. Loss of physical retention therefore occurs frequently during mastication as movement of this extent breaks the border seal. Muscular control is therefore extremely important, particularly in the case of the lower denture where the reduced area of the impression surface and the difficulty of obtaining a border seal reduce the amount of physical retention that can be obtained.

The successful muscular control of dentures depends on two factors:

(a) the ability of the patient to acquire the necessary skill,
(b) the design of the dentures.

The patient's ability to acquire the necessary skill will depend to a large extent on biological age. In general, the older the patient, the longer and more difficult the learning period. The elderly or senile patient may not be able to acquire this skill at all and so new dentures may fail although they are technically satisfactory. It is for this reason that replacement dentures for an elderly patient should be constructed in such a way that the patient's skill in controlling old dentures can be transferred directly to the new ones. This is achieved by copying the old denture as closely as possible, ideally using a technique such as that described in Chapter 7.

A specific example of the muscular control of dentures is seen when a patient incises (Figure 4.2). The forces tend to tip the upper denture, causing the posterior border to drop. This movement can be resisted by the dorsum of the tongue which presses against the denture and reseats it. Patients who complain of difficulty when incising with dentures which otherwise appear to be satisfactory should be examined very carefully to establish whether or not tongue control is present. If it is not, it is essential for the dentist to draw the patient's attention to the problem and to institute appropriate training. Unless purposeful muscular activity is learnt, replacement dentures will fail to overcome the patient's complaint.

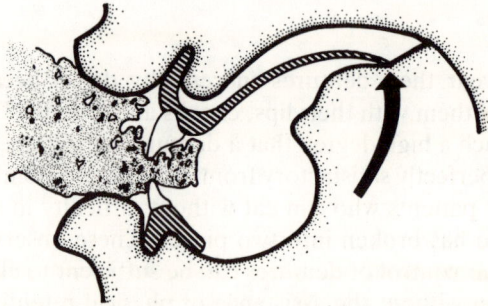

Figure 4.2   As the patient incises, the upper denture is controlled by the tongue pressing against the posterior border

The second factor which contributes to effective muscular control is the design of the dentures. During mastication the cheeks, lips and tongue control the bolus of food, move it around the oral cavity and place it between the occlusal surfaces of the teeth. In so doing, they exert pressure against the polished surfaces of the dentures. If these surfaces are correctly shaped with the buccal and lingual surfaces converging in an occlusal direction, this pressure will contribute to the retention of the dentures

(Figure 4.3). In addition to this active muscular fixation of the dentures during function, there will be a certain amount of passive fixation when the muscles are at rest, the relaxed soft tissues 'sitting' on the dentures thereby maintaining them in position.

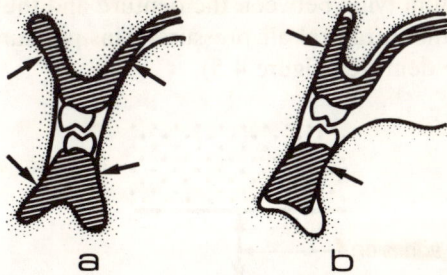

Figure 4.3   Influence of soft tissue forces on dentures: (a) seating the dentures when the polished surfaces are correctly shaped; (b) displacing the dentures when the polished surfaces are incorrectly shaped

When dentures are first fitted, muscular control takes some time to develop and is therefore likely to be inefficient. If, in addition, the physical retention is poor the resulting looseness of the dentures may lead to their rejection by the patient. Thus, it is during this initial learning period that the physical forces of retention are particularly important. The stronger these forces are, the smaller will be the demand on the patient's skill in controlling the dentures.

As alveolar resorption progresses, the fit of the dentures deteriorates with a consequent reduction in physical retention. This will not necessarily result in a reduction in the overall retention, however, as there will have been a compensating increase in the level of muscular control. However, the fit may eventually become so poor that complete compensation is no longer possible and movement of the dentures begins to increase. The degree of denture mobility which elicits a complaint of looseness will vary considerably between individuals; some patients are quite happy with dentures which perform 'acrobatics' in the mouth while others complain bitterly about dentures which hardly move at all.

Physical Forces

These are *adhesion* – the force of attraction between dissimilar molecules such as saliva and acrylic resin or saliva and mucosa – and *cohesion* – the force of attraction between like molecules.

The adhesive forces influence the wetting of the denture and the mucosal surfaces while the cohesive forces maintain the integrity of the saliva film.

Thus, these intermolecular forces form a chain between the denture and the mucosa which tends to retain the denture in position (Figure 4.4).

The forces of adhesion and cohesion give rise to two properties of saliva, *surface tension* and *viscosity*, which are thought to contribute to the retention of complete dentures. As a result of these properties the pressure within the saliva film lying between the denture and the mucosa becomes less than that of the intra-oral air pressure. This pressure differential will help to retain the denture (Figure 4.5).

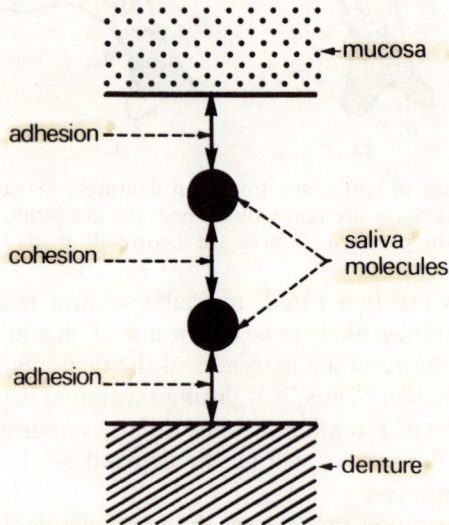

Figure 4.4   The chain of intermolecular forces between the denture and the mucosa contributing to retention

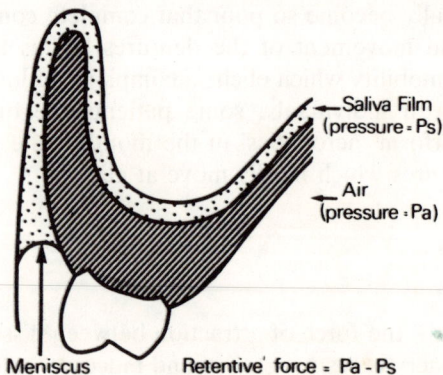

Figure 4.5   Retention due to the pressure differential between the saliva film and the air

As soon as a denture is seated in the mouth, a pressure differential between the saliva film beneath the denture and the intra-oral air pressure is established. It has been suggested that this persistent pressure differential is the product of the surface tension of saliva. Surface tension is the result of cohesive forces acting at the surface of a fluid. In the case of saliva, these cohesive forces are less than the forces of adhesion between the molecules of the saliva film and its two containing surfaces, the denture and the mucosa. Under these circumstances, a concave meniscus should theoretically form at the surface of the saliva in the border region. When a fluid film is bounded by a concave meniscus the pressure within the fluid is less than that of the surrounding medium; thus, in the intra-oral situation a pressure differential will exist between the saliva film and the air. However, the opposing view, that surface tension does not contribute to denture retention, has been put forward. It has been argued that all the denture surfaces are covered by a film of saliva and that therefore a true meniscus does not form in the mouth.

Whereas the retentive force attributed to surface tension acts continuously, retention due to saliva viscosity only operates during displacement of the denture. As a denture is pulled away from the tissues, saliva is drawn into the space created beneath the denture. A retentive force is generated by a resistance to this flow of saliva, resulting from the viscous properties of the saliva and the dimensions of the channel through which it is flowing (Figure 4.6). It follows that the narrower the channel and the greater the viscosity of the saliva, the more effective should be the retention. This certainly holds true clinically for the dimensions of the channel, but it appears that very viscous saliva is associated with relatively poor retention. It may be that the resistance to flow is low in this instance because the excessive viscosity of the saliva results in a thick and possibly discontinuous film between the denture and the mucosa.

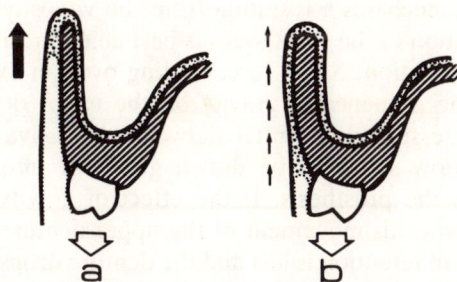

Figure 4.6   Relationship between the width of the buccal channel and resistance to flow of saliva: (a) wide channel, rapid flow, poor retention; (b) narrow channel, slow flow, good retention

It is important to appreciate that the walls of the buccal channel through which the saliva flows differ from each other. The denture flange is rigid while the soft tissues of the cheeks or lips are movable. If the denture is displaced, the pressure within the saliva film drops and the mucosa is drawn tightly against the denture surface so that the channel between the two becomes very narrow indeed. This causes a greatly increased resistance to the flow of saliva and a corresponding increase in retention (Figure 4.7). If, however, the denture is constructed with flanges which are too thin, resulting in a wide buccal channel (Figure 4.6(a)), impaction of the buccal mucosa will not occur, and saliva and air will be rapidly drawn towards the impression surface as the denture is displaced. Retention in this instance will be poor.

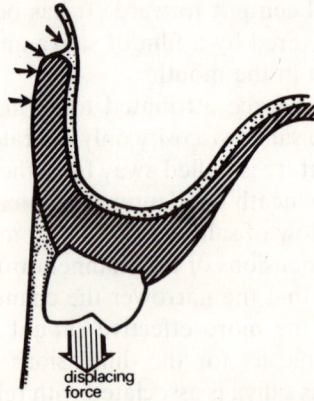

displacing
force

Figure 4.7   Drop in pressure of the saliva film beneath the denture causing impaction of the buccal mucosa and greatly increased retention

The retentive mechanism resulting from the viscosity of the saliva and the valve-like action of the soft tissues is best able to resist large displacing forces of short duration. Small forces acting over an extended period of time, such as the influence of gravity on the upper denture, result in a much smaller pressure differential between the saliva film and the air because they allow saliva to be drawn gradually into the space being created beneath the prosthesis. If the effect of gravity is unopposed, a progressive downwards movement of the upper denture is likely to occur until eventually all retention is lost and the denture drops. In this situation, however, occlusal forces are important in restoring the denture to its former position. Whenever the patient occludes (for example, during swallowing), excess saliva which has accumulated beneath the denture is squeezed out again and the denture reseated.

OBTAINING OPTIMUM PHYSICAL RETENTION

There is a lack of general agreement in the dental literature as to the relative importance of the physical factors responsible for retention. This, however, is not of great importance clinically as those features of complete dentures which result in good physical retention influence both surface tension and viscosity effects. These features include:

(a) border seal,
(b) area of impression surface,
(c) accuracy of fit.

Border Seal

For optimum retention, the denture border should be shaped so that the channel between it and the sulcus tissues is as small as possible.

It is not possible to maintain a close approximation between the border of a denture and the mucosal reflection in the sulcus at all times because the depth of the sulcus varies during function. The denture has to be constructed so that the border conforms to the shallowest point the sulcus reflection reaches during normal function. This means that for some of the time when the patient is at rest the denture will be slightly underextended. If the denture were extended further in an attempt to produce a more consistent seal in this area, displacement might occur when the sulcus tissues moved during function. The problem of achieving a constant border seal is overcome by extending the flanges of the denture laterally so that they contact and slightly displace the buccal and labial mucosa to produce a facial seal (Figure 4.8).

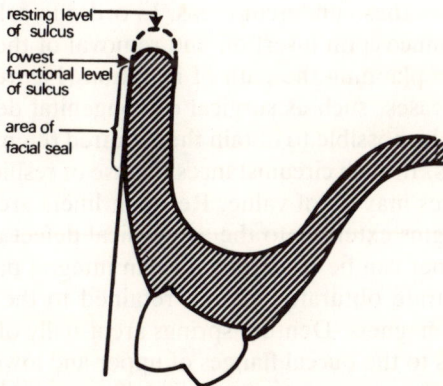

resting level
of sulcus

lowest
functional level
of sulcus

area of
facial seal

Figure 4.8   Lateral extension of the buccal flange to produce a facial seal

It is not possible to produce a facial seal along the posterior border of the upper denture as it crosses the palate. In this area, a border seal is obtained by cutting a groove known as a post-dam in the working cast (Chapter 10). The posterior border of the finished denture then has a raised lip which becomes embedded a little way into the palatal mucosa. As the palatal mucosa does not surround the posterior border, a valve mechanism cannot operate in this region and consequently even a small downwards movement of the posterior border of the denture will result in breaking of the seal and a loss of retention.

Area of Impression Surface

It has been shown that the degree of physical retention is proportional to the area of the impression surface. It is important therefore to ensure maximum extension of the dentures so that the optimum retention for a particular patient may be obtained.

Accuracy of Fit

The thinner the saliva film between the denture and underlying mucosa, the greater the forces of retention. It is therefore important that the fit of the dentures is as accurate as possible. A poor fit will increase the thickness of the saliva film and increase the likelihood of air bubbles occurring within the film. These bubbles will further reduce the retention of the denture. In addition, as the pressure of the saliva film drops due to displacing forces acting on the denture, the air bubbles will expand and may extend to the border area, resulting in a breaking of the border seal.

If bony undercuts exist, retention may be enhanced by designing a denture that utilises these undercut areas. In order to achieve this without traumatising the mucosa on insertion and removal of the denture, special care is required in planning the path of insertion (Figure 4.9).

In exceptional cases, such as surgical or congenital defects of the hard palate, it may not be possible to obtain the required retention using routine clinical techniques. In such circumstances the use of resilient liners, springs or denture fixatives may be of value. Resilient liners are designed so that free, flexible margins extend into the anatomical defect and engage tissue undercuts. The liner can be constructed as an integral part of the denture base or as a separate obturator section retained to the denture base by cobalt–samarium magnets. Denture springs are usually of coil type and are attached by pivots to the buccal flanges of upper and lower dentures in the premolar region. The springs are often partially covered by acrylic flanges, or 'hooded', to stabilise the springs and reduce irritation of the buccal mucosa. The springs exert a force which acts to separate the dentures and

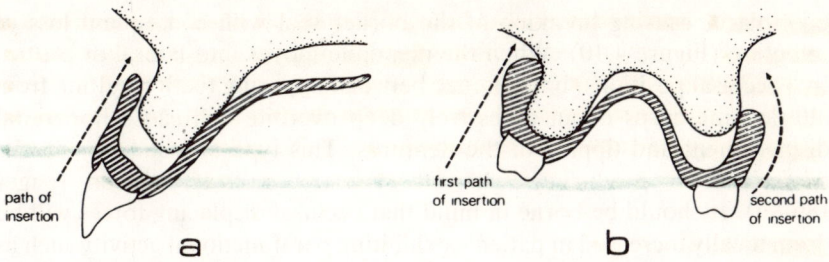

Figure 4.9 Selection of path of insertion to improve retention by utilising undercuts: (a) single path of insertion to engage labial undercut; (b) dual path of insertion to engage unilateral buccal undercut

thus helps to maintain the dentures in contact with the supporting tissues. A denture fixative can be an invaluable aid to retention under difficult anatomical circumstances. Fixatives come in powder, paste or sheet form, the latter having the advantage of staying longest beneath the denture.

Other approaches to providing increased retention include microvalves which may be inserted into an upper denture base. The working principle of these valves is that the patient actively evacuates air and saliva from beneath the denture by employing a sucking action. Movement of air and saliva beneath the denture towards the microvalves is facilitated by the provision of channels created in the impression surface of the denture. For the valves to be of any benefit, an efficient facial seal and post-dam is essential. However, clinical experience suggests that the beneficial effect is short-lived, probably because the mucosa proliferates into the suction channels created in the denture.

In the past, rubber suction discs have been used to increase the retention of upper dentures. However, these discs are extremely destructive to the underlying soft and hard tissues; indeed, there have been reports of perforation of the hard palate and malignant change in the denture-bearing mucosa as a consequence of the continuous local irritation from such discs. Therefore, suction discs are only mentioned here in order to condemn them outright.

DISPLACING FORCES

Acting through the Occlusal Surface

Imbalance
If, when the dentures occlude, tooth contact on one side of the dental arch is not balanced by contact on the other side, tipping of the dentures will

take place, causing breaking of the border seal with consequent loss of retention (Figure 4.10). When the mandible moves into lateral or protrusive occlusal positions, interference between opposing teeth resulting from interlocking cusps or an excessively deep overbite will cause horizontal displacement and tipping of the dentures. This type of instability can be minimised by producing balanced occlusion and articulation (pages 186–93). It should be borne in mind that occlusal displacing forces will be dramatically increased in patients exhibiting parafunctional activity such as bruxism.

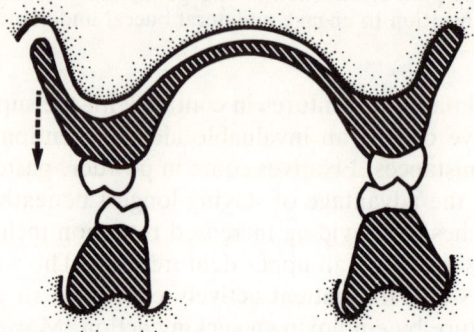

Figure 4.10   Tipping of the denture due to an unbalanced occlusal contact

Food

During mastication, pressure exerted by the food on the teeth tends to displace the denture. This problem may influence the positioning of artificial teeth. For example, stability of the lower denture can be improved by careful consideration of the posterior extension of the occlusal table. If that table extends to the steeply sloping part of the ridge posteriorly, pressure from the bolus will cause the denture to slide forwards (Figure 4.11). The occlusal table should therefore terminate in the relatively horizontal part of the ridge where effective support is available and displacement prevented. Occasionally, the problem might create a conflict of interests between the requirements of optimum appearance and denture stability. This is illustrated by the example of the experienced denture wearer who expresses a strong preference for having upper anterior teeth placed close to the crest of the ridge where strong incising forces can be applied with minimal leverage effects, in spite of the fact that lip support and appearance would be compromised. In the face of such a clearly stated preference it is usually wise for the dentist to comply with the patient's request.

During the opening phase of the masticatory cycle, when the teeth begin to separate after penetrating a bolus of food, the adhesive properties of the

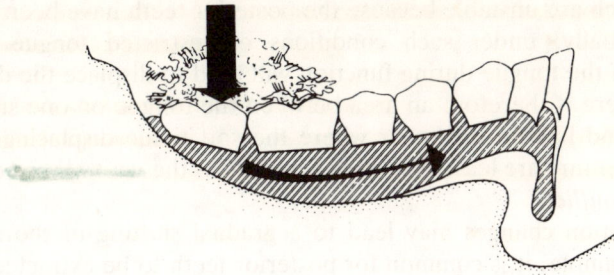

Figure 4.11 Pressure from the bolus on the posterior part of the lower occlusal table, which overlies a sloping part of the ridge, causes the lower denture to slide forwards

food generate a displacing force in an occlusal direction. Sticky foods therefore tend to move the dentures away from the mucosa.

Acting through the Polished Surface

The muscles of the lips, cheeks and tongue, in addition to being of fundamental importance in the retention of dentures, are also capable of causing denture instability. Displacement will occur, as mentioned earlier, if the polished surfaces have an unfavourable slope (Figure 4.3(b)) and also if the denture interferes with the habitual posture and functional activity of the surrounding musculature. For example, distal movement of a lower denture may be produced by the lower lip if the anterior teeth are placed too far labially (Figure 4.12). The teeth should therefore be placed just far enough lingually to prevent this displacement but not so far as to allow excessive tongue pressure to develop. It is not uncommon to see lower

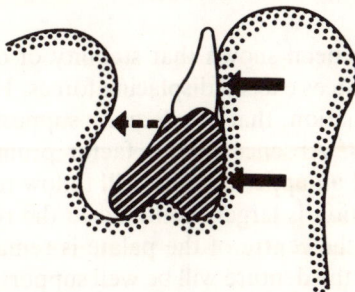

Figure 4.12 Distal displacement of the lower denture caused by placing teeth too far labially

dentures which are unstable because the posterior teeth have been placed too far lingually; under such conditions of restricted tongue space, movement of the tongue during function will tend to displace the denture upwards. There is therefore an area between the tongue on one side and the cheeks and lips on the other where the soft tissue displacing forces acting on a denture are least. This area is known as the *neutral zone* or *zone of minimal conflict*.

Post-extraction changes may lead to a gradual shifting of the neutral zone. For example, it is common for posterior teeth to be extracted some considerable time before the anterior teeth. If a partial denture is not fitted, the tongue spreads laterally into the edentulous space; this, in effect, moves the neutral zone laterally as well as reducing its buccolingual dimension. In other words, there is a reduced space in which to place a denture. Comparable changes in the neutral zone between the lower lip and the tongue occur as a result of post-extraction changes affecting the mentalis muscle; resorption of the alveolar bone leads to the superior fibres of the origin of the mentalis muscle lying on top of the residual ridge and a lingual migration of the neutral zone. Certainly, in these circumstances, it is no longer possible to position the artificial teeth where once the natural ones were situated.

Gravity

The effect of gravity on an upper denture has been described on page 58. In order to minimise this effect it is important that the upper denture is of light construction. Heavy denture base materials, such as cobalt–chromium alloy, should be avoided unless other requirements, such as strength, are of overwhelming importance.

SUPPORT

In this chapter, it has been shown that stability of dentures can only be obtained if retentive forces exceed displacing forces. However, there is one more factor in the equation, that of adequate support for the dentures by the underlying tissues. Absence of this factor promotes instability. For example, instability of an upper denture will follow resorption of supporting bone. This resorption is largely confined to the region of the alveolar ridges as the bone in the centre of the palate is remarkably stable. Thus, after a period of time, the denture will be well supported by the hard palate but there will be no contact between the impression surface of the denture and the alveolar ridges. In these circumstances, occlusal contact readily produces tipping, with the denture pivoting about the mid-line of the palate. Similarly, support will be inadequate if the ridges are small because resistance to lateral displacing forces will be poor. As a final example, support will be reduced if the ridges are flabby (page 261); the denture will move considerably during function even though the retention may be good and contact with the mucosal surface maintained.

BIBLIOGRAPHY

Barbenel, J. C. (1971) Physical retention of complete dentures. *Journal of Prosthetic Dentistry*, **26**, 592–600.

Brill, N. (1967) Factors in the mechanism of full denture retention – a discussion of selected papers. *Dental Practitioner and Dental Record*, **18**, 9–19.

Culver, P. A. J. and Watt, I. (1973) Denture movements and control – a preliminary study. *British Dental Journal*, **135**, 111–16.

Davenport, J. C. (1984) Clinical and laboratory procedures for the production of a retentive silicone rubber obturator for the maxillectomy patient. *British Journal of Oral and Maxillofacial Surgery*, **22**, 378–86.

Lindstrom, R. E., Pawelchak, J., Heyd, A. and Tarbet, W. J. (1979) Physical–chemical aspects of denture retention and stability. A review of the literature. *Journal of Prosthetic Dentistry*, **42**, 371–5.

Sheppard, I. M. (1963) Denture base dislodgement during function. *Journal of Prosthetic Dentistry*, **13**, 462–8.

Tyson, K. W. (1967) Physical factors in retention of complete upper dentures. *Journal of Prosthetic Dentistry*, **18**, 90–7.

5 Jaw Relations – Theoretical Considerations

The clinical procedure of recording the jaw relationship enables the dentist to provide the dental technician with the following information:

(a) The correct vertical and horizontal relationship of the mandible to the maxilla.
(b) The desired shape of the dentures.

This information is given to the technician in the form of wax record rims which enable the models to be mounted on an articulator. The technician then possesses a blueprint to guide him or her in the preparation of the trial dentures.

This chapter is devoted to a discussion of the theoretical background to occlusion and the points arising from the discussion are used to justify the clinical techniques described in Chapter 10.

BASIC MANDIBULAR POSITIONS

When a patient is relaxed the mandible takes up a relatively constant position known as the *rest position* in which the teeth are out of contact. The rest position can be defined as the position the mandible assumes when the mandibular musculature is relaxed and the patient is upright.

The space between the occlusal surfaces of the teeth when the mandible is in the rest position is known as the *freeway space* or inter-occlusal rest space. The space is wedge-shaped, being larger anteriorly where the separation between the teeth is normally within the range 2–4 mm.

If the mandible is raised from the rest position by balanced muscular activity, the point at which initial tooth contact is made is called the *muscular position*. In the denture wearer, the muscular position should coincide with the *intercuspal position* which is the jaw relationship in which maximum occlusal contact occurs.

With light tooth contact maintained, movement of the mandible in a posterior direction from the intercuspal position is usually possible. This posterior position is known as the *retruded contact position* and is separated from the intercuspal position by approximately 1 mm. Further retrusion of the mandible is prevented by the lateral ligaments of the temporomandibular joints.

With the condyles maintained in the retruded position, the movement of the mandible, as it opens, is a hinge movement until jaw separation in the incisal region is approximately 20 mm. The path taken by the mandible up to this point is known as the *retruded arc of closure*. Further opening of the mandible results in a forwards and downwards translation of the condyles. The interrelationship of the mandibular positions is shown in Figure 5.1.

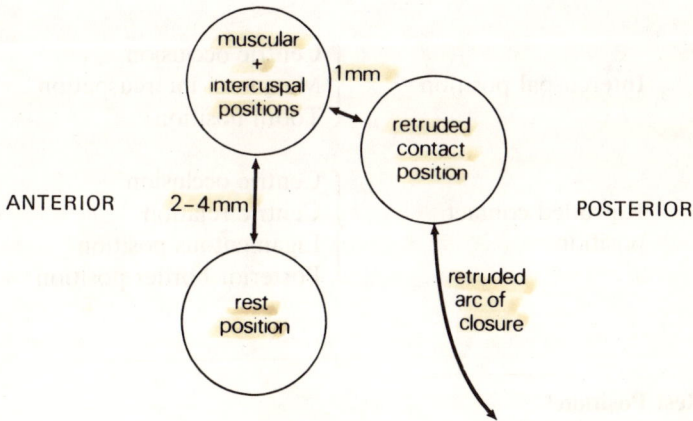

Figure 5.1   Diagrammatic representation of the basic positions of the mandible in the sagittal plane

The distance between two selected points, one on the maxilla and one on the mandible, when the teeth are in contact is known as the *occlusal vertical dimension*. When the mandible is in its resting position, this distance is the *rest vertical dimension* (Figure 5.2). The difference between the measurements is the freeway space.

In the past, there has been much confusion with regard to nomenclature with the result that the same term has been used to describe entirely different positions of the mandible. The terms used in this book, together with the alternatives commonly used elsewhere in the dental literature, are shown below.

Rest position   Physiologic rest position

Muscular position   Habitual position

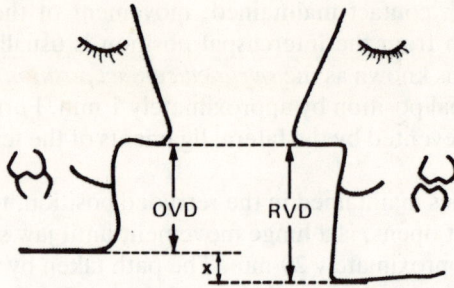

Figure 5.2   The difference between the rest vertical dimension (RVD) and the occlusal vertical dimension (OVD) is the freeway space (X)

Intercuspal position
{
Centric occlusion
Maximum intercuspation
Tooth position

Retruded contact position
{
Centric occlusion
Centric relation
Ligamentous position
Posterior border position

The Rest Position

Clinical Significance

In order to establish an acceptable occlusal vertical dimension in the edentulous patient, it is necessary to refer to the rest position because, once the rest vertical dimension has been measured, an occlusal vertical dimension can be derived and an adequate freeway space provided.

The presence of a freeway space allows relaxation of the masticatory apparatus; when the mandible is in the rest position and the teeth are out of contact, the tissues which support the dentures are not loaded, there is no strain on the temporomandibular joint capsules and only minimal, if any, activity in the elevator and depressor muscles of the mandible. If new dentures have no freeway space, the denture-bearing tissues are subjected to excessive loading, the elevator muscles are unable to return to their normal resting length, and the continuous muscular activity results in an accumulation of metabolites and subsequent pain in the affected muscles. If an excessive freeway space is provided, the load on the tissues is of course reduced. At the same time, however, there is a reduction in masticatory efficiency and the appearance of the patient may be adversely affected.

Control of the Rest Position

The rest position of the mandible at any one time is the result of a balance of forces as shown in Figure 5.3. Both passive and active forces are described. The relative importance of active and passive forces in determining the rest position is a controversial issue. One school of thought maintains that active forces are the major factor, another that passive forces alone are responsible for the true rest position, while yet a third school suggests that the rest position is the product of both active and passive forces in combination.

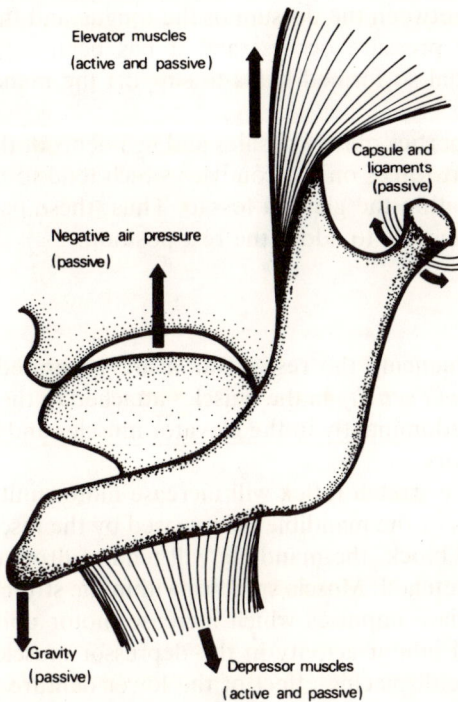

Elevator muscles
(active and passive)

Capsule and
ligaments
(passive)

Negative air pressure
(passive)

Gravity
(passive)

Depressor muscles
(active and passive)

Figure 5.3   Forces which determine the rest position of the mandible

Passive Forces

Passive forces arising from the *muscles* result from the elastic nature of the muscle fibres and of the connective tissue elements. Although it has been suggested that, in the truly relaxed state, the passive forces inherent in the muscles are able to maintain the rest position, this state is rarely evident and many variables, such as change in posture or emotional state, affect the equilibrium of passive forces, resulting in the introduction of active forces to stabilise the rest position.

The force of *gravity* is a constant factor. However, its influence on the balance of forces acting on the mandible varies with the position of the head in the gravitational field and with the mass of the mandible. Thus, the gravitational effect will be reduced when the patient is supine, when lower teeth are extracted or when a lower denture is removed from the mouth.

A contribution to the balance of forces may come from *negative air pressure* within the oral cavity which, in the majority of people, is a closed box when the mandible is in the rest position and the patient is breathing through the nose. Anteriorly, a seal is produced by the lips while posteriorly the soft palate is in contact with the dorsum of the tongue. There is a space between the dorsum of the tongue and the hard palate in which a negative pressure occurs, and it has been suggested that the pressure differential so formed helps to support the mandible in the rest position.

The elastic properties of the capsules and ligaments of the temporomandibular joints exert forces on the condyles which tend to return them to a central position within the glenoid fossae. Thus, these passive forces will encourage the mandible to adopt the rest position.

Active Forces

Active forces influencing the rest position are generated by continuous low-grade *motor unit activity* in the muscles attached to the mandible. This activity is seen predominantly in the elevator muscles and is influenced by the following factors.

Activation of the stretch reflex will increase motor unit activity. If, for example, the mass of the mandible is increased by the insertion of a lower denture or record block, the mandible will tend to drop and the elevator muscles will be stretched. Muscle spindles within the stretched muscles are activated and initiate impulses which increase motor unit activity in the same muscles and inhibit activity in the depressor muscles. This activity acts to oppose the displacing effect of the lower denture and returns the mandible towards its original rest position.

Other mechanoreceptors which may play a part in maintaining the status quo following changes in position of the mandible, or of the head as a whole, are to be found in the temporomandibular joint, the middle ear and the cervical spine.

External factors are able to influence motor unit activity via the reticular system; the effect may be either facilitatory or inhibitory. For example, the amount of jaw separation at rest is reduced by pain, drugs such as adrenalin and caffeine, and emotional stress. Emotional stress itself may be caused by factors in the patient's own domestic environment, or by disturbing visual, auditory or olfactory stimuli in the dental surgery. Jaw separation is increased during sleep or by drugs such as diazepam and the barbiturates.

The rest position of the mandible has been considered from an entirely different viewpoint, its association with the function of respiration. When a patient is at rest, respiration is the primary function affecting the oral region. It has been suggested that the rest position of the mandible is determined by the demands of the tongue in performing its respiratory function of completing the anterior wall of the pharyngeal part of the respiratory tract (Figure 5.4(a)). Following extraction of teeth and resorption of the alveolar bone, the tongue spreads laterally into the edentulous space. When the resorption of bone is extensive, the tongue spreads to such a degree that the posterior oral seal cannot be maintained (Figure 5.4(b)). The reaction of the mandible in this situation is to rise, thus allowing the posterior oral seal to be re-established (Figure 5.4(c)). A

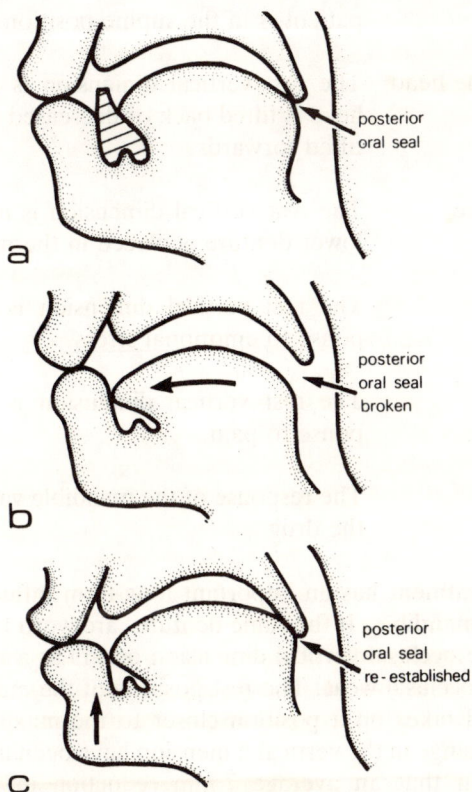

Figure 5.4 The association of the tongue with respiration and its influence on the rest position of the mandible: (a) posterior oral seal established between the soft palate and the tongue – lower denture *in situ*; (b) the tongue spreads into the area vacated by the denture; the posterior oral seal cannot be maintained; (c) the mandible is raised so that the posterior oral seal can be re-established (the rest vertical dimension when the denture is in the mouth is therefore larger than when it is removed)

lower denture replaces the natural teeth and alveolar bone and, when inserted into the mouth, controls the lateral tongue spread and allows the mandible to return to a lower resting position while still maintaining the posterior seal.

Summary

At one time, the rest position of the mandible was thought to be constant throughout life. From the foregoing description, it is apparent that this is not so. The rest position of the edentulous patient can be affected by short- and long-term variables.

The short-term variables include:

Position of the body	The rest vertical dimension is reduced if the patient is in the supine position.
Position of the head	The rest vertical dimension is increased as the head is tilted back or decreased when the head is tilted forwards.
Lower denture	The rest vertical dimension is increased when a lower denture is placed in the mouth.
Stress	The rest vertical dimension is reduced in response to emotional stress.
Pain	The rest vertical dimension is reduced in response to pain.
Drugs	The response of the mandible varies according to the drug.

Prosthetic treatment has an important long-term influence on the rest position of the mandible. If the same dentures are worn for many years, a reduction in the occlusal vertical dimension occurs as a result of alveolar resorption and occlusal wear. The rest position of the mandible adapts to this change and takes up a position closer to the maxilla. Longitudinal studies of the change in the vertical dimension have been undertaken and it has been shown that an average 7 mm reduction in occlusal vertical dimension occurs in as many years (Figure 5.5). The rest vertical dimension responds in a similar manner, although to a lesser degree. As a result, the freeway space becomes larger. Where these changes have taken place in young patients, it is often possible to recover much of the lost ground when new dentures are constructed. However, with the elderly patient, any attempt to restore the occlusal vertical dimension to its original level

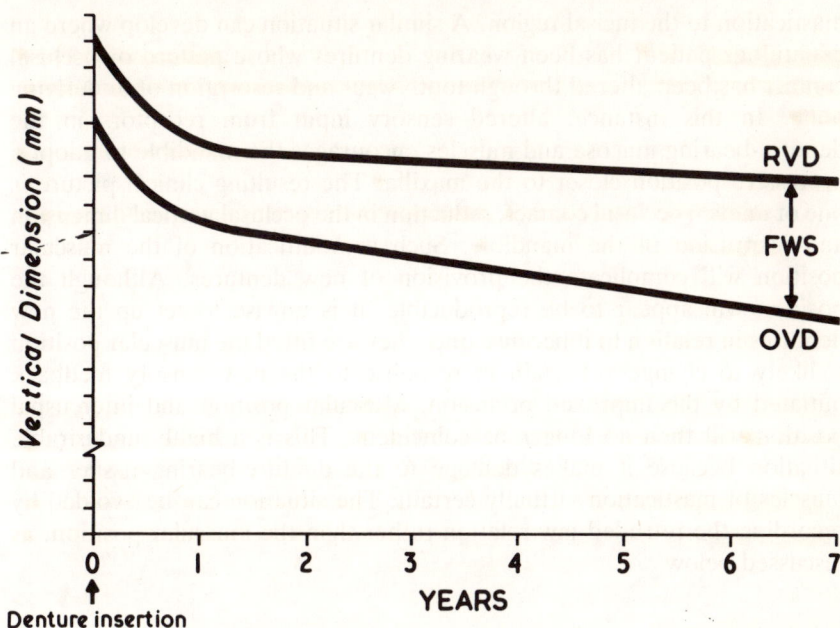

Figure 5.5   Average change in vertical dimension after fitting complete dentures (modified after Tallgren, 1966)

may be met with problems, which are discussed more fully in Chapter 7. Extensive loss of occlusal vertical dimension is the result of lack of maintenance of the dentures, and the lesson to be learnt is all too obvious.

The existence of the variables discussed in no way reduces the value of the rest position as a reference point in establishing the occlusal vertical dimension. Any long-term variable is unlikely to affect the reproducibility of the rest vertical dimension during the relatively short time of a course of treatment, while the influence of short-term variables can be minimised by careful clinical procedures, which will be discussed in Chapter 10.

The Muscular and Intercuspal Positions

The precise nature of the muscular and intercuspal positions in a dentate subject depends upon the arrangement of the natural teeth and the proprioceptive impulses arising from receptors in the periodontal ligaments and muscles of mastication. The muscular position is not constant and may be modified by sensory feedback resulting from changes in intercuspal position. For example, a protrusive relationship may be adopted following loss of posterior teeth and consequent restriction of mastication to the incisal region. A similar situation can develop where an edentulous patient has been wearing dentures whose pattern of occlusal contact has been altered through tooth wear and resorption of underlying bone. In this instance, altered sensory input from receptors in the denture-bearing mucosa and muscles encourages the mandible to adopt a protrusive position closer to the maxilla. The resulting clinical picture is one of uneven occlusal contact, reduction in the occlusal vertical dimension and protrusion of the mandible. Such a modification of the muscular position will complicate the provision of new dentures. Although the position will appear to be reproducible, it is unwise to set up the new dentures in relation to it because once they are fitted the muscular position is likely to change yet again in response to the new sensory feedback initiated by the improved occlusion. Muscular position and intercuspal position will then no longer be coincident. This is a highly undesirable situation because it makes damage to the denture-bearing tissues and muscles of mastication virtually certain. The situation can be avoided by recording the retruded jaw relation rather than the muscular position, as discussed below.

The Retruded Jaw Relation

This relation is determined by the lateral ligaments of the temporomandibular joints and does not depend upon the presence of teeth. It does not therefore alter when the natural teeth are extracted or when a new occlusal surface replaces an unsatisfactory one. It has been suggested that the retruded position has practical significance during normal functional movements, as tooth contact in this position is the termination of the heavy masticatory strokes needed to break up pieces of hard food.

REFERENCE POSITIONS OF THE MANDIBLE TO BE USED WHEN RECORDING
THE JAW RELATIONSHIP

When providing complete dentures the relationship of the mandible to the maxilla in both horizontal and vertical planes must be determined. In the vertical plane, it is of prime importance that the occlusal vertical dimension of the dentures allows for an adequate freeway space. In the absence of clues from existing dentures, the occlusal vertical dimension must be created artificially, and it is obvious that the reference position of the mandible in the vertical plane can only be the rest position.

The issue is perhaps less clear-cut with respect to the jaw relationship in the horizontal plane. Some authorities prefer to record the anteroposterior relationship of the mandible to the maxilla in the muscular position, while others describe techniques for obtaining the retruded position.

Evidence indicates that it is possible to record the retruded position with greater consistency than the muscular position. Furthermore, it has also been shown that variation of the muscular position in the anteroposterior plane is especially affected by the posture of the patient whereas the reproducibility of the retruded position remains high. In addition, it is quite possible that the muscular position may have been influenced by an abnormal occlusion and may alter once the new occlusal surface has been provided. Because of the uncertainty of the muscular position, the authors recommend using the retruded position as the point of reference in the horizontal plane. However, when positioning the artificial teeth, allowance must be made for the patient to adopt the muscular position. This concept is considered further in Chapter 10.

BIBLIOGRAPHY

Brill, N. and Tryde, G. (1974) Physiology of mandibular positions. *Frontiers of Oral Physiology*, **1**, 199–237.

Brill, N., Lammie, G. A., Osborne, J. and Perry, H. (1959) Mandibular positions and mandibular movements. A review. *British Dental Journal*, **106**, 391–400.

Crum, R. J. and Loiselle, R. J. (1972) Oral perception and proprioception: A review of the literature and its significance to prosthodontics. *Journal of Prosthetic Dentistry*, **28**, 215–30.

Faigenblum, M. J. (1966) Negative oral pressures. A research report. *Dental Practitioner and Dental Record*, **16**, 214–16.

Fish, S. F. (1961) The functional anatomy of the rest position of the mandible. *Dental Practitioner and Dental Record*, **11**, 178–88.

Fish, S. F. (1964) The respiratory associations of the rest position of the mandible. *British Dental Journal*, **116**, 149–59.

Helkimo, M., Ingervall, B. and Carlsson, G. E. (1971) Variation of retruded and muscular position of mandible under different recording conditions. *Acta Odontologica Scandinavica*, **29**, 423–37.

Nairn, R. I. and Cutress, T. W. (1967) Changes in mandibular position following removal of the remaining teeth and insertion of immediate complete dentures. *British Dental Journal*, **122**, 303–6.

Posselt, U. (1952) Studies in the mobility of the human mandible. *Acta Odontologica Scandinavica*, **10,** supplement 10.

Preiskel, H. W. (1965) Some observations on the postural position of the mandible. *Journal of Prosthetic Dentistry*, **15**, 625–33.

Tallgren, A. (1957) Changes in adult face height due to ageing, wear and loss of teeth and prosthetic treatment. *Acta Odontologica Scandinavica*, **15**, supplement 24.

Tallgren, A. (1966) The reduction in face height of edentulous and partially edentulous subjects during long-term denture wear. *Acta Odontologica Scandinavica*, **24**, 195–239.

Yemm, R. (1969) Variations in the electrical activity of the human masseter muscle occurring in association with emotional stress. *Archives of Oral Biology*, **14**, 873–8.

Yemm, R. (1972) Stress-induced muscle activity: A possible etiologic factor in denture soreness. *Journal of Prosthetic Dentistry*, **28**, 133–40.

Yemm, R. and Berry, D. C. (1969) Passive control in mandibular rest position. *Journal of Prosthetic Dentistry*, **22**, 30–6.

6 Assessment of the Patient

INTRODUCTORY REMARKS TO THE CLINICAL CHAPTERS

It is much more common for a dentist to have to provide complete dentures as replacements for old dentures than to provide them for a patient who has not worn such dentures before.

What is the reason for this pattern of treatment? Clearly, one of the main factors is that the average life expectancy of patients receiving complete dentures for the first time is considerably greater than the average life expectancy of the dentures themselves. This is, of course, particularly the case if the patient's first complete dentures were immediate restorations whose useful life is relatively short. Thus, dentures are likely to be replaced several times during the life of the patient.

The remaining chapters of this book are largely concerned with clinical procedures and, because of the pattern of demand mentioned above, the major emphasis is placed on the treatment of patients requiring replacement dentures.

After this chapter dealing with the first stage of treatment, namely history, examination and treatment planning, there follows a discussion of the use of old dentures, as their existence affects treatment from the outset. The next logical step is to consider the measures that may be required to prepare the oral tissues before continuing with the stages of denture construction.

Of course, there are patients who are provided with their first complete dentures, in which case the initial state of assessment is usually a far less complicated procedure. After mouth preparation, the conventional clinical stages of treatment are followed, as described in the appropriate chapters.

A thorough and systematic history and examination will ensure that all relevant details are recorded, thus enabling a diagnosis and treatment plan to be formulated and a prognosis made. The purpose of this chapter is to describe a systematic approach to this all-important stage preceding treatment. The significance of the information obtained is discussed more fully in other chapters of the book.

Obtaining a history and carrying out an examination involve contact with the patient. Therefore, before undertaking such procedures, it is essential that the dentist has a thorough knowledge and understanding of the significance and control of cross-infection.

THE CONTROL OF CROSS-INFECTION

The appearance of HIV infection and AIDS has focused attention on the control of cross-infection within the dental environment.

There are a number of excellent publications which provide clear guide-lines for the control of cross-infection and the reader is referred to these for background information. However, the practice of dental pros-thetics presents particular problems of its own and it is therefore appropriate that these are addressed before proceeding with the clinical stages of complete-denture provision.

Rubber Gloves

Rubber gloves should be worn for all clinical procedures. However, these can represent a hazard for the dentist. Many prosthetic techniques require the warming of materials such as wax and compound. If a naked flame is used for this purpose, great care needs to be taken to ensure that the gloves do not catch fire and cause serious burns. The risk can be reduced by placing a bowl of water within easy reach so that the gloved hand can be plunged into it if the worst happens. Alternatively, the risk can be avoided by using a hot-air heater instead of a naked flame. The former will soften the materials without reaching a temperature sufficient to ignite the gloves.

Rubber gloves can also be an inconvenience in that many techniques require the manipulation of materials with the fingers. Unfortunately, many of these materials adhere tenaciously to rubber gloves, creating impossible working conditions. The problem can usually be overcome by individual experimentation to discover the least troublesome permutation of gloves, materials and techniques. For example, smearing the gloves with petroleum jelly will help to prevent them sticking to softened greenstick compound when the material is being applied to an impression tray.

Silicone putty impression materials are generally best mixed by kneading with the fingers. However, the setting of the addition-cured type is inhibited by certain types of rubber glove. Therefore, appropriate glove selection is required when using these materials; alternatively, they can be mixed by a dental surgery assistant who has removed the gloves.

Handling Materials

When handling prosthetic materials, it is important to develop a regime that avoids contamination of stocks and unacceptable levels of wastage.

Careful advance planning for each prosthetic appointment so that, as far as possible, all the required materials and instruments are placed ready is the key to minimising the chance of contaminating stock. However, even then it is difficult to avoid the situation where it is necessary to collect additional items part-way through a procedure. This can only be done by decontaminating or changing the gloves, or by placing a barrier between the contaminated gloves of the dentist and the stock. This barrier may take the form of a 'clean' dental surgery assistant to hand the item to the dentist, cheap vinyl over-gloves which are subsequently discarded, or sterile forceps. Rummaging through stocks with contaminated gloves clearly creates a breach in any cross-infection policy.

Care needs to be taken not to breach cross-infection procedures when using impression compound. This material is usually softened in a thermostatically controlled water-bath. However, these baths must be regarded as contaminated once the impression has been completed, and must therefore be emptied, cleaned and disinfected before being used for another patient – a cumbersome procedure. The situation can be simplified by softening the compound in bowls which can be autoclaved after use.

It is important for economic reasons to minimise wastage. Dispensing prosthetic materials, such as the various waxes in portions appropriate for single use, keeps the residue of unused materials to a level at which they can be discarded without incurring an unacceptable financial penalty. The less satisfactory alternative is to design a procedure for disinfecting the surplus before returning it to stock.

The Dental Laboratory

The dental technician is an integral member of the dental team, and the dental laboratory, wherever it is situated, is an integral part of the dental environment. It is therefore essential that cross-infection policies are fully discussed, understood and agreed by both technician and clinician. Without this close cooperation, the chain upon which cross-infection control depends will be broken and the mutual protection lost.

The key to preventing transmission of infection between the two areas is a disinfectant 'barrier' through which all items must pass before being dispatched in either direction. The precise nature of this barrier will vary according to the item involved, but it commonly consists of thorough rinsing in water, immersion in dilute hypochlorite solution and then sealing in a plastic bag. It is recommended that the disinfection is generally carried out by the sender rather than the recipient.

Solutions which have been recommended for disinfecting impressions are chlorinated disinfectants containing 10 000 ppm available chlorine and 2 per cent glutaraldehyde. Some alginate impression materials are damaged by the chlorinated disinfectants at the recommended concentration while others are not, even when the immersion period is as long as 10 minutes. Therefore, the choice of brand of alginate is important in this context. Soaking alginates in these aqueous solutions for longer than 10 minutes is inadvisable because of the danger of dimensional change in the impression caused by imbibition.

Zinc oxide–eugenol pastes, and silicone and polysulphide elastomers are all compatible with these disinfectants at the recommended concentrations and immersion times. The polyethers, on the other hand, absorb water and will distort if soaked in aqueous solutions for long periods. Where uncertainty exists regarding compatibility of impression material and disinfectant, the impression can be simply washed before being sent to the laboratory, provided the technician is informed of the situation. The technician then pours up the impression while wearing rubber gloves and subsequently disinfects the model in hypochlorite.

Cross-infection within the dental laboratory can be a problem. One study attributed a high prevalence of eye infections among technicians to contaminated pumice. It was found that the pumice was heavily infected but that the bacterial count could be significantly reduced by mixing up the slurry with a solution of a commercially available disinfectant. It was concluded that untreated pumice slurries presented an unacceptable risk of cross-infection.

HISTORY

Reason for Attendance

After noting personal particulars such as name, address, age and occupation, the dentist should record the complaint in the patient's own words. For example, if the patient says that the denture is loose, it may be positively misleading if the dentist records the comment as 'the denture lacks retention'. The denture may, in fact, exhibit excellent physical retention but is being displaced by an uneven occlusal contact.

History of the Present Complaint

It is important to ascertain full details of any complaint. If, for example, the complaint is of pain in relation to a denture, the location, character and timing of the pain should be determined; relieving and aggravating factors should also be recorded.

If a denture is loose, it is important to enquire when the looseness was first noticed. If one discovers that the denture has been worn satisfactorily for several years, it will be essential, at the examination stage, to note the good features of the denture as well as discovering the defect which has led to the complaint. On the other hand, if the looseness was present from the time the denture was fitted, the cause may be attributed to a basic design fault in the denture, to unfavourable anatomical factors or perhaps to the inability of the patient to adapt to dentures. Until an examination is made, it is not possible to distinguish between these causes.

Dental History

When recording a patient's dental history, it is necessary to ascertain when the natural teeth were extracted, why they were extracted and whether there were any surgical complications. The dentist should then determine how many dentures have been provided subsequently, whether any previous dentures have been worn successfully or whether major problems have been experienced with all previous sets. This information is useful on three counts:

(a) The history of tooth loss may provide a basis on which to make an assessment of the current rate of bone resorption. If extractions were carried out in the previous few months, resorption will still be continuing at a rapid rate; if dentures are to be provided at this time, they will soon become loose and the patient should be warned of this likelihood. If, however, the teeth were extracted several years ago, the alveolar bone will have reached a relatively stable state and the life of a replacement denture will therefore be considerably extended.

(b) If there is a history of difficult extractions, it will be advisable to obtain radiographs in order to check for the presence and location of retained roots.

(c) Clues are obtained to the adaptive capability of the patient. For example, if three sets of dentures have been worn successfully over a period of, say, 15 years, it may be assumed that adaptation has been satisfactory, whereas if the same number have been provided over the last two or three years and each has been troublesome, adaptation must be suspect. However, it is vitally important not to jump to conclusions and to put the blame on the patient until one is satisfied that the complaint cannot be related to defects in the design of previous dentures. It is thus wise practice to ask the patient to bring all available sets of dentures when attending for the initial assessment, as inspection of them can yield valuable clues and increase the accuracy of the diagnosis.

Medical History

Notes should be made of a patient's past and present medical history relevant to future dental treatment. Information should include particulars of drug therapy and, where considered necessary, the name of the doctor. A patient for whom sedatives and tranquillisers are being prescribed may have a reduced capacity in adapting to dentures, as may a person suffering from a protracted chronic disability. It should also be noted that a number of antidepressants and tranquillisers produce xerostomia. This condition may reduce the physical retention of a denture and may cause a generalised soreness of the denture-bearing mucosa. It has also been reported that certain antidepressants and tranquillisers may affect adversely the tonicity of the facial muscles and may produce facial grimacing and trismus or bizarre tongue movements. It can be helpful when taking a medical history to work with a questionnaire.

EXAMINATION

Extra-oral Examination

Simply by talking to the patient and making careful observations at the same time, the dentist may obtain important clues which will help in treatment planning.

Any discrepancy between the actual age and biological age should be noted; this factor is important in assessing adaptive capability and is discussed more fully in Chapter 2. The skeletal relationship of the patient should be assessed because this will provide information as to the appropriate incisal relationship (Chapter 11). The appearance of the face may provide valuable evidence as to the occlusal vertical dimension of existing dentures (Figure 6.1). If loss of occlusal vertical dimension is noted, correction may be required before new dentures are started (see page 94). If the patient already has dentures, the appearance of these can

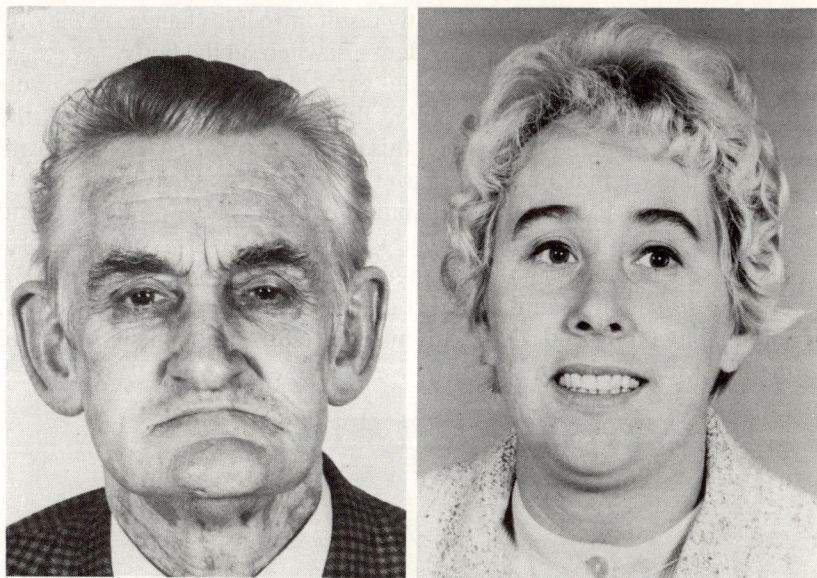

Figure 6.1   Both patients are wearing complete dentures which are in occlusion. The man shows obvious signs of a gross loss of occlusal vertical dimension; the freeway space is approximately 10 mm. On the other hand, the woman's facial appearance leads one to suspect that the occlusal vertical dimension of her dentures is excessive

be evaluated at this stage in the examination. Features such as inadequate lip support or poor appearance of the anterior teeth should be noted. Inflammation and fissuring at the corners of the mouth (angular stomatitis) may be present; the significance and treatment of this condition are described on page 127. While the patient is talking it may be possible to detect any obvious looseness of dentures or whether the patient is having difficulty in controlling the prostheses.

Intra-oral Examination

In broad terms, this part of the examination determines:

(a) whether there is any pathology in the mouth,
(b) what the prospects are for the new dentures providing a satisfactory level of comfort and function.

The mouth has been aptly described as a mirror which reflects the state of health of the individual. When systemic disease develops, the powerful combination of micro-organisms, normal wear and tear, and moisture and warmth present in the mouth frequently result in visible changes in the oral tissues before signs of disease are evident elsewhere in the body. Investigation of these changes may allow an early diagnosis of the systemic condition to be made. For example, there may be a change in the population of papillae on the tongue; this change occurs first on the tip and sides, the areas of maximum trauma. The filiform papillae are progressively lost so that the fungiform papillae become more noticeable and produce the appearance of a 'pebbly' tongue; eventually, the fungiform papillae also disappear and the tongue becomes smooth (Figure 6.2). These changes should lead the dentist to suspect deficiencies such as iron, vitamin B12 and folic acid. Diagnosis may be confirmed by the appropriate haematological investigations.

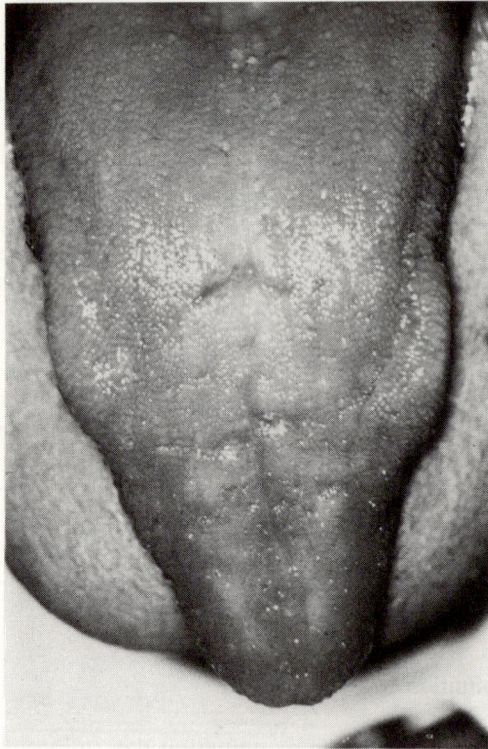

Figure 6.2   Alteration in population of filiform and fungiform papillae as a result of a folic acid deficiency

Dentists, because of their training, experience and equipment, are uniquely qualified to examine the oral cavity thoroughly and to recognise any features which are outside the range of normal variation. Large numbers of people are examined dentally each year; the dentist therefore plays the central role in screening the population for oral manifestations of systemic disease. Of particular relevance in the elderly complete-denture patient is the presence of oral malignancy. It has been reported recently that the oral cavity and pharynx combined constitute the sixth commonest site for cancer and that oral cancer is increasing in a number of countries in both the developed and developing world. Although the overall prevalence of oral cancer is low, 95 per cent of cases, excluding salivary gland tumours, occur in patients who are over 45 years of age. Early detection by the dentist increases the chance that treatment may effect a cure. Any ulceration, change in character of the mucosa, or swelling, whose presence cannot be readily explained, should be regarded with suspicion (Figure 6.3); in all instances, appropriate steps such as radiographic examination, biopsy or immediate referral should be undertaken.

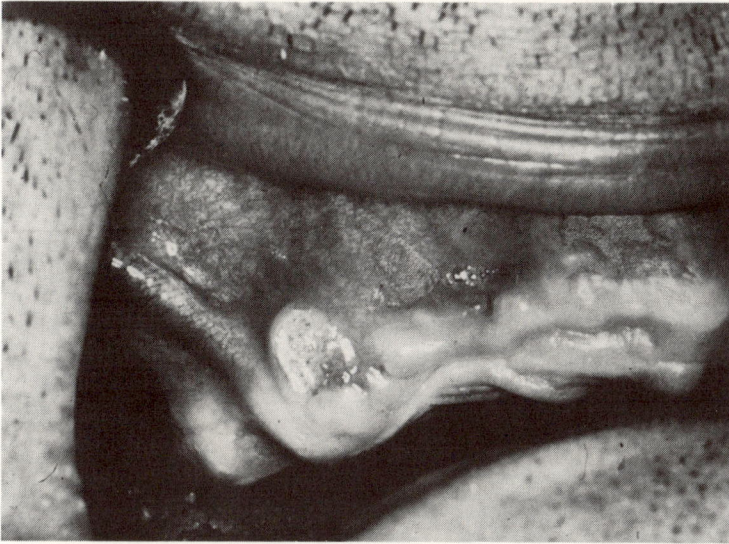

Figure 6.3   The ulcer in the upper right canine region has a raised, rolled margin; there was no history of trauma. Biopsy confirmed a malignant change

If there are no signs of systemic disease, the findings of the intra-oral examination assume a primarily local significance by helping to diagnose the patient's dental complaint, to formulate a treatment plan and to determine a prognosis. Features of interest are: the shape and size of ridges, palate and tuberosities; the degree of compressibility of the denture-bearing mucosa determined by palpation; the depth and width of the sulci, including the presence of prominent frena; the size of the tongue; the quality and quantity of saliva. The relevance of such observations to the stability of complete dentures is discussed more fully in Chapters 4 and

9. The oral mucosa should be examined for inflammatory or hyperplastic change and for the presence of sinuses or swellings which lead one to suspect pathology within the underlying bone; if pathological conditions of the underlying bone are suspected, radiographs must be taken. These conditions, described in Chapter 8, should normally be treated before starting prosthetic treatment so that a stable and healthy denture foundation is produced.

Examination of Dentures

A detailed and systematic extra-oral examination of the impression, and the polished and occlusal surfaces of existing dentures should be made. With regard to the impression surface, the presence or absence of a post-dam (see page 172) and palatial relief (see page 179) should be noted. The amount and distribution of plaque on denture surfaces, an important cause of denture stomatitis (Chapter 8), may be shown by a disclosing solution. The inclination and shape of the polished surfaces should be noted. The occlusal surface should be examined for the degree of wear, whether there are shiny wear facets produced by parafunction and whether porcelain or acrylic teeth have been used.

Each denture is then placed in the mouth separately and examined for stability, retention and border extension. The correct border extension of dentures is described in Chapter 9.

A rough assessment of stability and retention can be made by carrying out the following simple tests.

(a) The upper denture is seated in the mouth and an attempt made to rotate it in the horizontal plane. Any resulting lateral movement of the mid-line is noted. Some movement is inevitable because of the compressibility of the mucosa, but a movement of 3 mm or more either side of the mid-line is an indication of loss of fit or the presence of a flabby ridge.

(b) A further test is to seat the upper denture and attempt to dislodge it by pulling vertically downwards on the incisor teeth. Lack of resistance indicates poor retention. This latter test has little significance for lower dentures where physical retention is usually minimal.

(c) Each denture is seated in turn on the denture-bearing tissues and the patient is asked to open the mouth until the incisal separation is 2–3 cm. If this causes displacement of a denture in an occlusal direction, an error in either the impression or the polished surface should be suspected.

An assessment should be made of the height of the occlusal plane of the lower denture and whether it is in such a position that the tongue is able to rest on the occlusal surface and thus play a part in stabilising the denture.

Both dentures are next examined together in the mouth and a check made on occlusal balance and the presence of an adequate freeway space. Every effort should be made to obtain an accurate estimation of the freeway space at this stage because the result will be of fundamental importance both in the diagnosis and in the formulation of a treatment plan; the clinical techniques for obtaining this information are described in Chapter 10. However, it should be remembered that an assessment of the freeway space at this stage may, in some instances, only be a rough estimate because it may be impossible to induce a relaxed state at the patient's first visit. Further estimations will be made when the occlusion is recorded and will serve to check on the accuracy of the original assessment.

Mention was made earlier of the value of having the dentures available for examination. Diagnosis of the present complaint may well be made easier by referring to them. A comparative examination of these old dentures should be carried out in the manner just described. Even when a patient has old unsatisfactory dentures, they should be examined so that the faults may be noted and thus avoided in future treatment.

Special Tests

It may be necessary to take radiographs, organise blood tests, arrange for microbiological examination of swabs or smears, or to carry out diagnostic modifications of existing dentures. The reasons for undertaking any of these procedures are discussed in the relevant sections of the book.

DIAGNOSIS

By correlating the findings of the examination and special tests with the patient's history, the cause of the complaint should be identified and recorded. It is important to realise that, unless a diagnosis is made, there is little prospect of solving a patient's problems by providing new dentures and, in some cases, it is unwise to embark on such treatment.

TREATMENT PLAN

Following the diagnosis, a treatment plan is formulated. If this involves making replacement dentures, it may be necessary to carry out preparatory treatment such as border and occlusal adjustment or modification of the impression surface of the present dentures with a short-term resilient lining material (Chapter 7).

If replacement dentures are to be made, it is of great value to make a note of the features in the existing dentures which must be modified in order to overcome the patient's complaint. It is just as important to make a note of those aspects of the existing design which have proved to be successful. Such written comments serve as an invaluable checklist during subsequent clinical stages.

Alternative treatment may be simple modification of the existing dentures to correct minor faults, relining or rebasing (Chapter 14), or the use of a copying technique (Chapter 7). Thus, it will be appreciated that the provision of new dentures is but one of the treatment options.

There are several approaches to designing complete dentures: the dentist should make a positive decision at the treatment plan stage as to which is appropriate for the patient.

The shape, or design, of the dentures may be determined by the dentist carving the record rims as described in Chapter 10, so that the upper rim provides adequate lip support and the lower rim lies in the neutral zone.

Another approach to design involves the use of biometric guides – measurements from certain anatomical landmarks which allow the denture teeth and base to be placed in positions similar to those formerly occupied by the natural teeth and alveolar bone. The desirability of so doing has been a source of controversy for many years but has received a considerable measure of support. Anatomical guide-lines have now been researched which allow the dentist to achieve this aim with a reasonable degree of certainty (Chapter 9).

Where dentures have provided satisfactory service for the patient in the past, it may be advisable to base the design of replacement dentures on the well-accepted features of the old ones. Although such an approach is particularly appropriate for the treatment of elderly patients who have a markedly reduced ability to adapt, it can also be of value in a number of other clinical situations.

A potentially accurate method of maintaining the well-accepted features of existing dentures is to use a copy technique (Chapter 7). However, carving record blocks by eye to a shape similar to the old dentures is an acceptable alternative technique in cases where minor differences between old and new dentures are not of critical importance.

When there are particular problems in achieving stability of a lower denture, for example, if there is abnormal muscular activity or intra-oral anatomy, the dentist can record the neutral zone by getting the patient to mould a soft record rim into a position of stability between the tongue and cheeks and lips by means of swallowing and speaking. Details of this technique are described in Chapter 11.

All these approaches to complete-denture design are based on sound clinical principles and require an adequate prescription to be sent by the dentist to the laboratory. In the absence of such a prescription, the technician may have to produce a denture design which is essentially mechanistic with the teeth placed on the crest of the ridge. The greater the amount of resorption that has occurred, the greater the problem this approach can create. This is because the pattern of bone resorption of the residual ridges is not uniform. Although in the mandible the bone loss is fairly even and the crest of the ridge moves little in the horizontal plane as resorption progresses, the picture is very different in the maxilla. Here the bone loss is predominantly from the buccal and labial aspects of the ridge, causing its crest to progressively migrate palatally. Setting the upper teeth on the crest of the ridge as shown in Figure 6.4 has the following undesirable consequences:

(a) Poor facial appearance due to inadequate lip and cheek support.
(b) Reduced physical retention associated with an inefficient or absent facial seal.
(c) Encroachment on tongue space, resulting in denture instability, tongue soreness and interference with tongue function during speech and food transport.

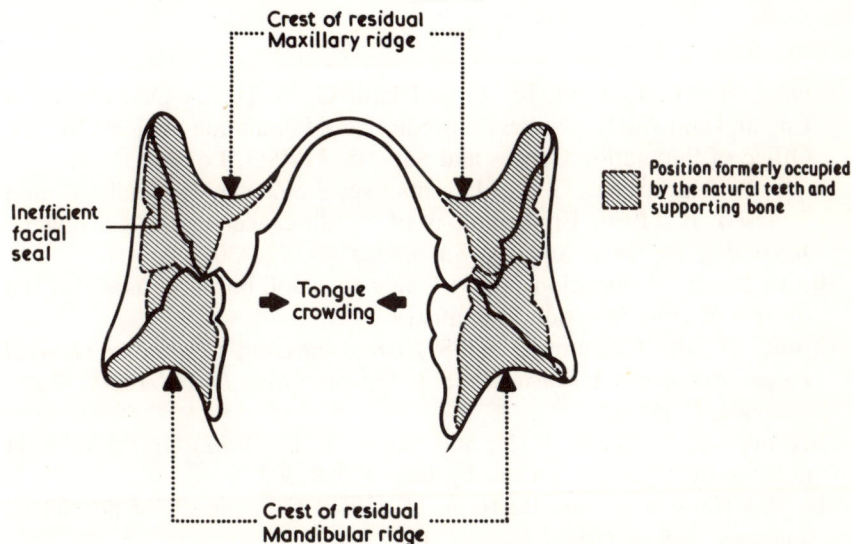

Figure 6.4   Pattern of resorption in the maxilla and mandible following loss of the natural teeth. A mechanistic upper denture has been produced with teeth on the crest of the residual ridge. Occlusion with the lower denture has been achieved by producing a cross-bite on the patient's right and excessive lingual placement of the lower teeth on the left

(d) Problems in achieving a satisfactory occlusal relationship with the lower denture. For example, in Figure 6.4 the alternatives are to accept a posterior cross-bite or place the lower teeth so far lingually that instability of the lower denture is bound to result.

In view of these undesirable consequences, it can be argued that a mechanistic approach, which results from the dentist omitting to supply a design prescription to the laboratory, is an avoidance of professional responsibilities by the dentist, who alone has the clinical information necessary to make an informed decision on the design.

PROGNOSIS

The findings of the history and examination will enable the dentist to assess the degree of success the proposed line of treatment is likely to achieve. If problems are anticipated, they should be explained to the patient before treatment proceeds. The patient is then more likely to cope with the unavoidable limitations of the new dentures.

BIBLIOGRAPHY

Binnie, W. H., Cawson, R. A. and Hill, G. B. (1972) Oral cancer in England and Wales. Studies on Medical and Population Subjects No. 23. Office of Population Census and Surveys, HMSO, London.

Boyle, P., Macfarlane, G. J., Maisonneuve, P., Zheng, T., Scully, C. and Tedesco, B. (1990) Epidemiology of mouth cancer in 1989: a review. *Journal of the Royal Society of Medicine*, **83**, 724–30.

British Dental Association (1988) Guide to blood-borne viruses and the control of cross-infection in dentistry.

Croser, D. and Chipping, J. (1989) *Cross-infection Control in General Dental Practice – A Practical Guide for the Whole Dental Team*. Quintessence, London.

Duxbury, A. J., Leach, F. N. and Smart, T. E. (1982) Oral dyskinesia induced by Tryptizol. *Dental Update*, **9**, 299–302.

Hjørting-Hansen, E. and Bertram, U. (1968) Oral aspects of pernicious anaemia. *British Dental Journal*, **125**, 266–71.

Jones, J. H. (1973) The oral mucous membrane markers of internal disease. *British Dental Journal*, **134**, 81–7.

Likeman, P. R. and Watt, D. M. (1974) Morphological changes in the maxillary denture bearing area. *British Dental Journal*, **136**, 500–3.

Scully, C., Cawson, R. A. and Griffiths, M. (1990) Occupational hazards to dental staff. *British Dental Journal.*

Tyldesley, W. R. (1973 and 1974) Oral medicine for the dental practitioner. *British Dental Journal*, **135**, 405–11; 449–55; 494–8; 537–41. **136**, 23–7; 68–72; 111–16; 151–4.

Watt, D. M. (1977) Tooth positions on complete dentures. *Journal of Dentistry*, **6**, 147–60.

Watt, D. M. and Likeman, P. R. (1974) Morphological changes in the denture bearing area following the extraction of maxillary teeth. *British Dental Journal*, **136**, 225–35.

Wilson, S. J. and Wilson, H. J. (1987) The effect of chlorinated disinfecting solutions on alginate impressions. *Restorative Dentistry*, **3**, 86–9.

Witt, S. and Hart, P. (1990) Cross-infection hazards associated with the use of pumice in dental laboratories. *Journal of Dentistry*, **18**, 281–3.

7 The Relevance of Existing Dentures

Patients requiring replacement dentures can be placed in one of three broad groups. In the first are those patients who were provided with immediate dentures. The second group consists of people who have worn complete dentures with satisfaction but seek replacement dentures to overcome symptoms of relatively recent origin. In sharp contrast are those in the third group who have had persistent trouble with a number of sets and for whom consideration will be given to construct new dentures in an attempt to solve their problems.

Existing dentures, whether successful or unsuccessful, provide invaluable evidence when planning their replacement. Furthermore, use can be made of the old dentures during the various stages of constructing the new ones.

ASSESSMENT OF THE DENTURES

Patients requesting replacement of their immediate dentures do so usually because the post-extraction resorption of bone has led to a loss of retention and stability. Apart from a desire for better fitting dentures, most of these patients are anxious that the appearance of the original dentures should be maintained, and the dentist must satisfy these demands if success is to be achieved. Improving the fit is seldom a problem, but considerable care is needed to maintain the other well-accepted characteristics, such as position and arrangement of the artificial teeth. These difficulties are best overcome by using a copying technique which is described later in the chapter.

It is important when providing prosthetic treatment for those patients whose dentures have been satisfactory for a number of years that all successful features of the old dentures are retained and that alterations are made only to those aspects which have produced symptoms. Clearly, these judgements can be made only if an accurate diagnosis has been established as a consequence of a detailed history and examination. Lack of attention to this principle, which is particularly relevant to the treatment of elderly patients who do not readily adapt to change, leads to the construction of poorly tolerated dentures and accounts for a proportion of patients in the third group who have experienced persistent denture problems.

For those patients with chronic denture problems, it is again vitally important to establish an accurate diagnosis. This is best achieved by asking the patient to bring in all sets of dentures in their possession so that the previous attempts can be analysed. In the end, the fundamental question which must be answered is 'Are there errors in the design of the previous dentures which have led to the problems experienced by the patient and is it likely that the complaints can be treated by correcting these errors?' Within each of the groups described, clinical situations occur in which the dentist observes a shortcoming in the denture design which has not troubled the patient. Should alteration be made, or not? It is impossible to be dogmatic in answering this question, particularly when treating elderly patients. If it is decided to make an alteration then it is essential to explain the reasons to the patient. In all instances, the dentist must assess whether it is possible to retain the error and at the same time be in a position to make new dentures which successfully overcome the patient's symptoms.

The positioning of the posterior border of the upper denture is just one example of this problem. Frequently, it is necessary to make replacement dentures for a patient complaining of a loose upper denture in which the posterior border is not extended to the vibrating line (Chapter 9). If the denture has been worn for several years and the symptom is of recent origin, then it is unlikely that the position of the posterior border of the denture has contributed to the trouble. If this state of affairs is confirmed by clinical examination, it is wise practice to maintain the posterior border in the well-tolerated position as any change, especially in the older patient, is likely to induce a new complaint, that of nausea. On the other hand, if the patient has experienced poor retention of the upper denture since it was fitted, then it is likely that the incorrectly placed posterior border has contributed to this problem. The approach, in this instance, is to make good the deficiency after explaining to the patient the reason why the modification is necessary.

Having assessed the patient's problems, the treatment plan is likely to fall into one of the following categories:

(a) Make permanent modifications to the existing dentures (for example, rebase or modify the occlusion).
(b) Make temporary modifications to the existing dentures to confirm a diagnosis.
(c) Construct replacement dentures using conventional techniques.
(d) Construct replacement dentures using a copy technique.
(e) No treatment, or referral for specialist advice. Such a decision may be made when the dentist assesses that new dentures will not

overcome the patient's complaint or where a diagnosis cannot be established with confidence, and thus there is a real risk of new dentures being no more successful than any of the existing ones.

PREPARATION OF THE MOUTH

The existing dentures may be of value when treating inflammation of the denture-bearing mucosa or when modifying an unsatisfactory jaw relationship.

Treatment of Inflammation of the Denture-bearing Mucosa

The commonest causes of this condition are trauma from an existing denture and the proliferation of micro-organisms on the impression surface of the denture. Denture trauma may be the result of an ill-fitting denture, an unbalanced occlusion which causes movement of the denture, or lack of freeway space.

It is important that the inflammation of the mucosa is resolved before the final impressions are taken for construction of new dentures. If not, the well-fitting denture seated on the inflamed tissue surface is likely to affect some recovery of the condition. The change in shape of the denture-bearing surface will result in lack of fit of the new dentures, re-establishing one of the causative factors. Although the simplest method of treatment is to instruct the patient not to wear the dentures, this advice is unacceptable to the majority of patients; therefore, the dentures can be corrected as part of the treatment.

The fit of a denture can be improved quickly and effectively by temporarily relining it with a short-term resilient lining material (page 115). Occlusal imbalance can be corrected either by selective grinding or by applying a layer of cold-curing acrylic resin to the occlusal surface of the posterior teeth of one of the dentures, provided that the addition leaves an adequate freeway space. Methods of eliminating infection by micro-organisms are described on page 125.

Modification of an Unsatisfactory Jaw Relationship

Some patients still believe that once complete dentures have been provided there is no need for further treatment. As a result, examples are seen where, through lack of maintenance, there have been considerable changes in occlusal vertical dimension and in the intercuspal position. Severe wear of the acrylic occlusal surface and resorption of alveolar bone leads to a situation where the freeway space may be 10 mm or more. Patients seeking new dentures at this advanced stage of occlusal derangement may make such statements as 'I can't chew my food so well', or 'My teeth don't show as much as they used to'. Little imagination is required on the part of the dentist to appreciate the basis of their complaints (Figure 7.1). However, patients are not fully aware of the problems produced in allowing the tooth contact position to deteriorate to such a degree.

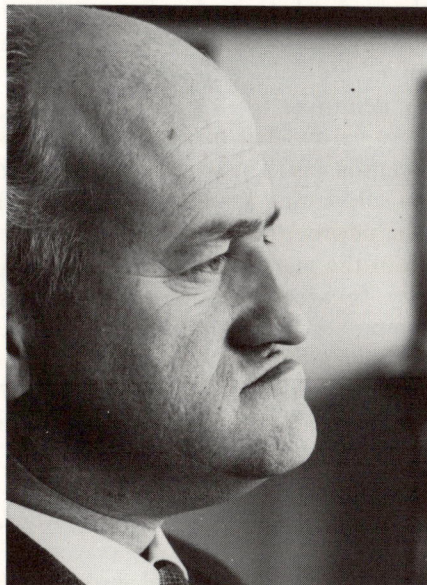

Figure 7.1   The patient is occluding on his complete dentures. Lack of maintenance has led to gross loss in occlusal vertical dimension and protrusion of the mandible

The difficulties in restoring the situation are two-fold. First, a decision has to be made on the amount of reduction in the freeway space that will be tolerated when the occlusal vertical dimension is altered. If one attempts to reduce the freeway space to 3 mm, then, in many cases, the occlusal vertical dimension has to be increased by 7 mm or more. This magnitude of change results in increased masticatory stress being transmitted to the denture-bearing tissues, but in many elderly patients changes in the mucosa have reduced the ability to accept such stresses. Furthermore, it has been pointed out that a patient possessing a large freeway space has been able to eat large mouthfuls of food without having to open the mandible much beyond the rest position. If the same dietary habits continue once the new dentures are fitted, the increased jaw opening may well produce pain in the muscles of mastication.

The second problem arises from the pattern of mandibular movement acquired by these patients. As a result of loss in occlusal vertical dimension and disturbance of occlusal contacts, there is protrusion of the mandible, which is partly anatomical and partly habitual, which may make it difficult, or even impossible, to record the retruded position. Retrusion of the mandible to some degree is instantaneous on restoration of the occlusal vertical dimension because of the anatomy of the temporomandibular joint. Correcting the habitual element is a more gradual process. If the new occlusal surface is, in fact, provided by replacement dentures, the gradual retrusion of the mandible will result in a long programme of occlusal adjustment to these dentures.

This situation may be avoided by modifying the old dentures before recording the jaw relationship. The occlusal vertical dimension is increased by adding a layer of cold-curing acrylic resin to the occlusal surface of one of the dentures. The new occlusal pattern initiates the breakdown of the habitual protrusion of the mandible as well as allowing an assessment of the patient's ability to accept a known increase in occlusal vertical dimension. The temporary occlusal surface can be modified to accommodate the gradual change in the jaw relationship. New dentures can be constructed when one is satisfied that the planned increase in vertical dimension is acceptable and the protrusion of the mandible has been abolished.

Clinical Procedure for the Addition of Cold-curing Acrylic Resin to the Occlusal Surface

It is usual to apply the resin to the occlusal surface of the lower denture as the addition is less likely to be visible. The occlusal surface of acrylic resin teeth on which the resin will be placed is dried. If the dentures have porcelain teeth, it is necessary to provide a mechanical attachment for the acrylic resin onlays. This can be done by grinding retentive holes interstitially in the premolar and molar regions. A separating medium, petroleum jelly, is smeared over the opposing occlusal surface. Cold-curing resin is placed on the occlusal surface of the lower denture in the premolar and molar regions. The denture is placed in the mouth when the dough stage is reached so that the flow of the resin can be easily controlled. The patient is instructed to close into the resin and is stopped at the required increase in occlusal vertical dimension, as judged by the amount of occlusal separation in the incisal region. The occlusion is adjusted to produce even contact and to allow freedom of movement in an anteroposterior direction, to accommodate the change in tooth position that will occur as the protrusion is corrected (Figure 7.2).

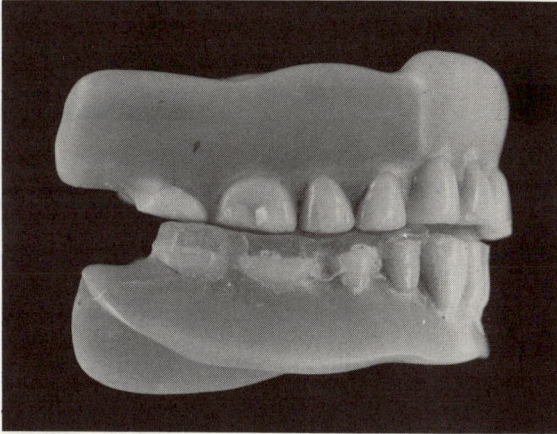

Figure 7.2   Occlusal vertical dimension corrected by the addition of a layer of cold-curing acrylic resin applied to the occlusal surface of the lower denture

IMPRESSION PROCEDURES

Clinical experience indicates that, in general, it is far more difficult to provide a satisfactory replacement for a previously successful lower denture than an upper. As the upper denture covers the palate, there are usually few problems in obtaining adequate retention and distribution of the masticatory forces. However, the narrower confines of the denture-bearing tissues in the lower jaw result in these requirements being far more critical. A lower denture, which has previously been satisfactory but is now loose, can be used as an impression tray which is likely to be better than a tray obtained by resorting to conventional impression techniques.

The old lower denture can be used in one of the following ways:

(a) as a basis for a functional impression,
(b) as an impression tray using a 'wash' impression technique,
(c) for copying the existing impression surface.

Use of the Lower Denture for a Functional Impression

When using the conventional impression techniques described in Chapter 9, the shape of the denture-bearing tissues is influenced by the force exerted by the operator seating the impression tray and by the amount of extracellular fluid present in the tissues at that time. The magnitude and direction of the operator's force is unlikely to be similar to that experienced during mastication, while the distribution of extracellular fluid varies throughout the day. Both these factors lead to a situation where a 'snapshot' of the tissues is obtained at one moment in time, under conditions of artificial loading. By using a functional impression material, it is possible to record the shape of the denture-bearing tissues over a period of time and under conditions of functional normality. Moreover, this technique allows one to gauge the patient's reaction to the new fitting surface over a period of time. If, for example, a new lower denture is being provided for a patient who has experienced comfort and stability from the existing denture, but with a history of recent instability which the operator attributes to shortcomings in the impression surface, a layer of functional impression material can be added to the denture. If the patient comments favourably on the result at a subsequent appointment, the operator has gained valuable first-hand information that the new impression surface is compatible with comfortable, normal function and that a new denture made to this new surface is likely to be equally well tolerated. Using this technique, one can follow the dictates of the saying 'the proof of the pudding lies in the eating'.

Functional impression materials are discussed more fully on page 118.

Use of the Lower Denture as an Impression Tray using a 'Wash' Impression Technique

In some instances, the operator may wish to use the old lower denture as an impression tray, realising however that corrections may have to be made to the existing borders. For example, it may be decided that further extension over the all-important retromolar pads will improve the stability of the new dentures. If it is necessary to increase the extension of the border by more than 2 mm, it is advisable to use one of the rigid border-trimming materials which are discussed on page 157.

Where necessary, the borders should be corrected for overextension. Any undercuts in the impression surface must be removed so that when the cast is poured, the dentures can be removed without damage to either cast or denture (Figure 7.3). The impression surface of the denture should be dried thoroughly to ensure that the impression material adheres firmly to the denture. Either a low viscosity silicone impression material or a zinc oxide–eugenol impression paste may be used to record the detail of the denture-bearing mucosa. Both materials are accurate when used in thin section but the former has the advantages of being tasteless, elastic and relatively clean to use. The denture is returned to the patient after the cast has been poured and the impression material has been removed. If it is found that the amount of acrylic cut away has reduced the retention of the

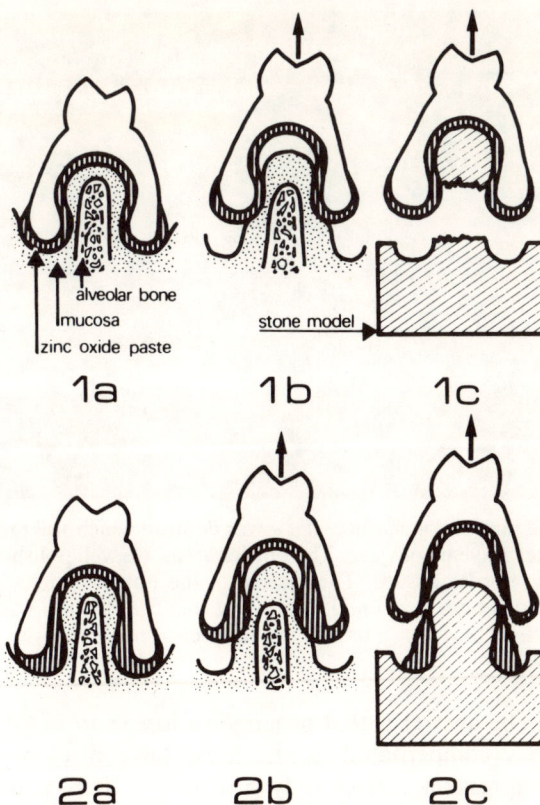

alveolar bone
mucosa
zinc oxide paste

1a

stone model

1b

1c

2a   2b   2c

Figure 7.3 1(a)–(c): Undercuts not removed from the impression surface. Mucosal compressibility allows removal of the denture from the mouth. Subsequent removal from the cast is impossible without damage. 2(a)–(c): Undercuts removed prior to taking the impression. Denture can be removed successfully both from the mouth and from the cast

denture, a short-term resilient lining material can be applied in order to overcome the problem until the new denture is fitted.

Copying the Existing Impression Surface of the Lower Denture

Attention has been drawn to the occasions when a replacement lower denture is constructed and the patient returns to the surgery with the comment that 'The old plate was much more comfortable'. This set of circumstances is seen more often in the patient who has given a history of comfort and stability which conflicts with the clinical assessment. Why do the reactions of the patient differ from the evidence of the clinical

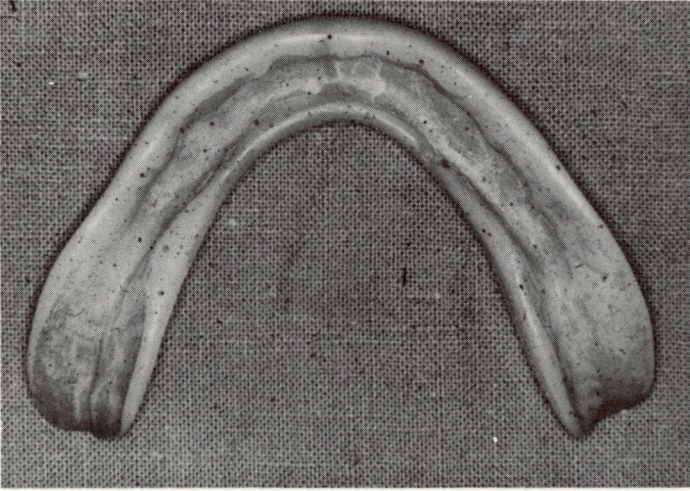

Figure 7.4   The impression surface of a lower denture which still provides comfort and stability after 10 years of wear. The border areas are well polished by continual contact with the border tissues. The middle of the impression surface is covered with calculus and is heavily stained, indicating that the denture no longer fits the tissues in that area

examination? The answer is that progressive loss of fit of the denture has been adequately compensated by the muscular control of the denture. Perhaps the impression surface only contacts the border tissues (Figure 7.4); however, the reactions of the patient and the appearance of the mucosa show that this state of affairs is perfectly acceptable. If a new denture is constructed with an accurate impression surface, the masticatory forces will be transmitted to tissues which, for a long time, have not been stressed; the mucosa overlying the ridge may have become thinner and may no longer be able to accept the forces. If, therefore, one is faced with an old denture whose impression surface is well tolerated by the patient and which has not caused mucosal damage, dental stone can be poured directly into it and the new denture constructed on the cast. It may be advisable, for psychological reasons, to take a lower impression but to discard it when the patient has departed.

RECORDING JAW RELATIONS

If replacement dentures are being made using conventional techniques, it is when recording jaw relations that reference to previous dentures is particularly rewarding. During this clinical stage, one is producing a blueprint for the technician so that he or she can construct dentures which faithfully follow the design concepts decided at the chairside. In the case of a patient requiring replacement dentures, the dentist possesses the advantage of a previous blueprint, the old dentures, which will yield valuable information.

Assessing Occlusal Vertical Dimension

The various clinical methods of assessing occlusal vertical dimension are based on intelligent guesswork. Any opportunity of minimising one's reliance on this quality is therefore desirable and existing dentures are of great help in this respect. If, from the patient's comments and one's own observations, the intercuspal position of the existing dentures appears to allow adequate freeway space, a recording can be made of the occlusal vertical dimension and the new recording rims carved to produce the same dimension. On the other hand, if the patient complains of symptoms which signify a lack of freeway space, one can still use the vertical measurements obtained with these dentures and compare them directly with those of the reduced vertical dimension when the patient occludes on the recording rims. Where there is excessive freeway space, it is advisable to correct this on the old dentures by adding a resin onlay as described previously, so that when the occlusal vertical dimension for the new dentures is determined it is possible to refer directly to the modified old dentures.

Shaping the Upper Record Block

When replacing an old complete upper denture which has provided several years of satisfactory wear, it is important to carve the record block so that its shape is the same as the old denture. Particular attention should be paid to the following:

(a) shape of the dental arch and its relationship to the underlying ridge,
(b) width of the occlusal table,
(c) labial contour,
(d) level and orientation of the occlusal plane.

The shape of the arch and the width of the occlusal table control the amount of tongue space within the confines of the upper denture. As the tongue is accustomed to functioning within a given space, a reduced space on the replacement denture is liable to induce speech difficulties, problems when manipulating a bolus of food, a sore tongue and a general difficulty in adapting to the new shape in the mouth. The well-accepted shape of the old denture is conveniently maintained by first assessing the overbite–overjet relationship of the buccal and labial segments on the old dentures. The upper recording rim is then carved until, on occluding with the old denture in the mouth, the same relationship is produced. This procedure establishes the overall width of the dental arch. The palatal aspect of the recording rim is then adjusted to produce an occlusal table which is similar in width to that of the old denture (Figure 7.5).

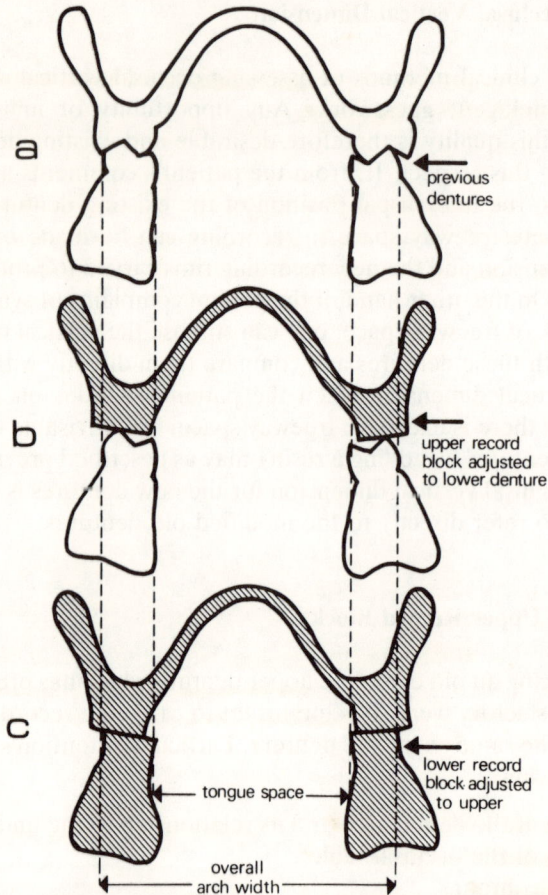

Figure 7.5   Procedure for reproducing the overall arch width and the tongue space on replacement dentures: (a), (b) and (c) illustrate the consecutive stages of the procedure

The support of the upper lip is controlled by the labial contour of the upper record block and, subsequently, the upper denture. In the event of a patient being satisfied with the appearance of a previous denture, it is obviously important that the same amount of lip support is produced by the replacement.

The labial contour is the product of three factors:

(a) the position of the incisal edge in the horizontal plane,
(b) the position of the incisal edge in the vertical plane,
(c) the inclination of the labial surface of the record rim.

The first two factors can be controlled accurately if the incisal relationship on the previous dentures is copied, by following the method of shaping the upper rim as previously described. An alternative and most effective way of establishing the position of the incisal edge in the vertical plane is to measure the distance on the existing denture between the incisive papilla and the incisal edge with calipers (Figure 7.6). The calipers are carefully removed, placed in a similar position on the record block and a line scratched in the wax rim. It is essential to ensure, before making this measurement, that the inclination of the labial surface of the record rim is identical to that of the previous denture, otherwise the measurements on the denture and rim will be made in different planes and will therefore not be comparable. An alternative technique is to use a specially designed gauge (Figure 7.7). With the denture resting on the table of the gauge, and the locating needle positioned in the concavity produced by the incisive papilla, the relationship of the central incisors in both horizontal and vertical planes can be read on the scales attached to the gauge. The record rim is then shaped and the relationship of its mid-line to the incisive papilla checked on the gauge.

Shaping the Lower Record Block

It is essential that adequate tongue space is provided within the confines of the lower denture so that the functional movements of the tongue help rather than hinder the stability of the prosthesis. To maintain such a space when replacing a well-tolerated lower denture, the following points must be borne in mind while shaping the lower rim:

(a) shape of the dental arch and its relationship to the underlying ridge,
(b) width of the occlusal table,
(c) height of the occlusal plane.

The method of shaping the upper record block has already been described. Continuing this process allows one to transfer the characteristics of the arch width and occlusal width of the old lower denture to the rim (Figure 7.5).

If the replacement dentures are being made to a similar occlusal vertical dimension as the old denture, and the height of the upper rim has been correctly established, the correct height of the occlusal plane will be determined automatically once the lower rim is married to the upper rim.

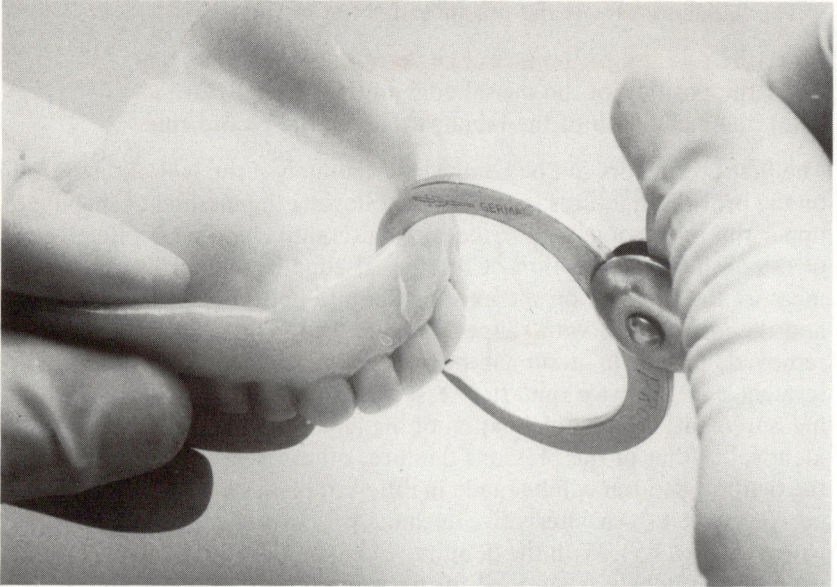

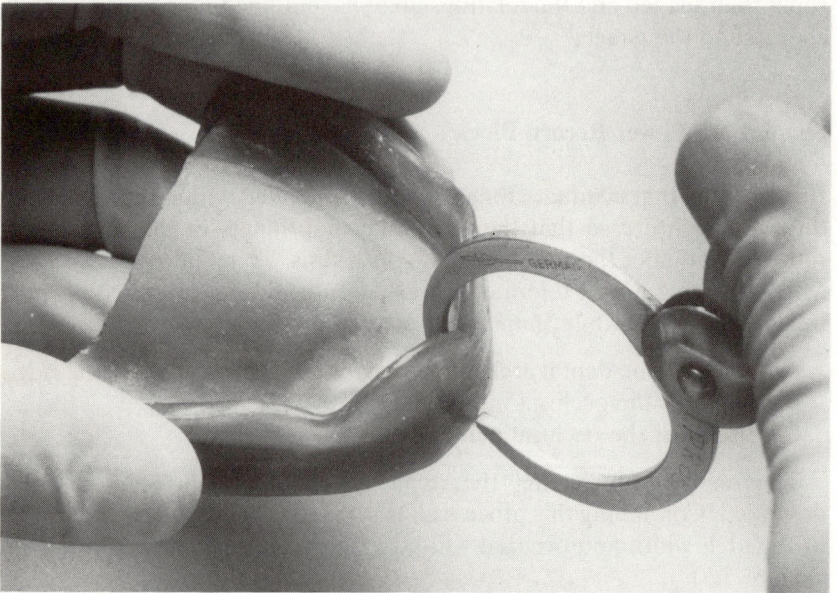

Figure 7.6   Establishing the incisal level. *Top*: Measurement of old denture with calipers. *Bottom*: Transfer of measurement to record rim

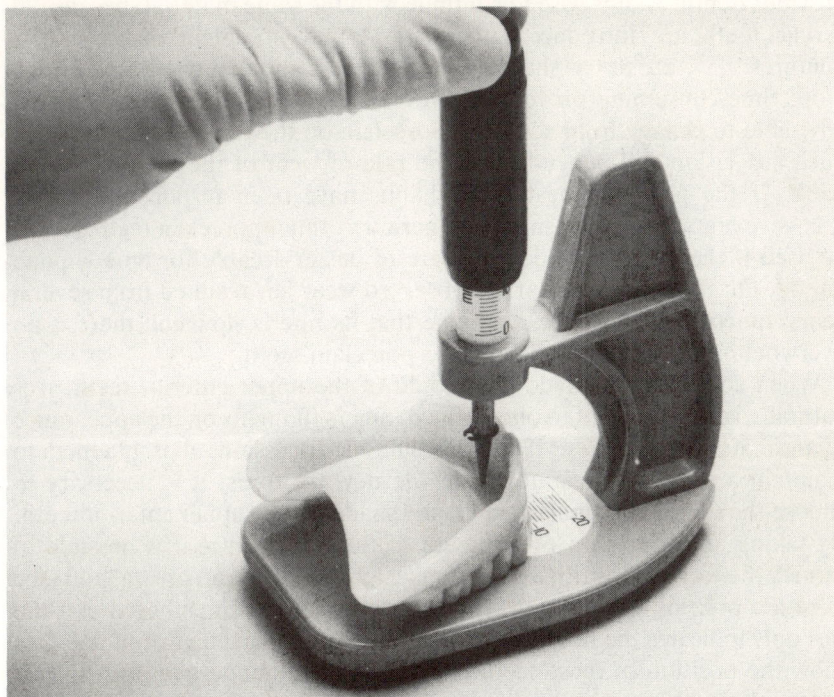

Figure 7.7 The incisal relationship measured in vertical and horizontal planes with an Alma gauge (see text for further details)

On many occasions, however, it is necessary to increase the occlusal vertical dimension to compensate for wear of the old occlusal surfaces. Should the increase be made on the upper or lower rim or shared between both? Each clinical case must be treated on its merits when making such a decision. It is necessary to have a clear idea of the magnitude of change required and to decide whether such an increase, if added to the upper rim, will improve or detract from the appearance of the patient or, if added to the lower rim, will so increase the height of the occlusal plane that the stability of the lower denture will be impaired.

Selecting Artificial Teeth

Unless careful thought is given to this important detail, the time given to the other aspects of denture construction is likely to be wasted. Decisions to be made at this stage are on the choice of material and on the mould and shade of the anterior teeth. If porcelain teeth were used for the patient's previous dentures, it is wise to continue with the same material, because, if acrylic teeth are introduced, the patient may complain that the new dentures ' . . . are not as sharp as the old ones', and that chewing food is a more time-consuming process. However, there are occasions when it is advisable to change from acrylic to porcelain on the replacement denture. Such a decision will depend upon the rate of wear of the existing acrylic teeth. If the patient's masticatory habits have been responsible for an excessive amount of wear in a short period of time, porcelain teeth should be used if the succeeding dentures are to be serviceable for an adequate period. On the other hand, if the observed wear has resulted from several years' function, then one can assume that its rate is slow and there is no overwhelming reason for changing to porcelain teeth.

When choosing the shade and mould of the upper anterior teeth, it is naturally very important to obtain the patient's thoughts on the appearance of the existing dentures. If, as a result of discussion, it is planned to maintain a similar appearance with the new dentures, it is necessary to choose the same, or a similar mould and shade for the upper anterior teeth. By taking an impression of the teeth of the old denture it is possible to furnish the technician with a cast from which he or she can obtain guidance as to the position of the teeth. However, it must be remembered that the cast only indicates the relationship between the artificial teeth and does not show the position of these teeth in relation to the underlying ridge. This latter relationship is obtained by correctly shaping the record rim.

There are occasions, of course, where it is necessary to alter the mould or shade of the existing teeth. For example, the crown length may have been severely reduced by occlusal wear or the colour may have been altered by bleaching or staining. There is no problem if the patient has recognised the deterioration and requests an improvement. However, if the dentist is the first person to notice this state of affairs, he or she must explain and demonstrate the reason for change very carefully. If the ground is well prepared for an alteration in appearance and the patient's full agreement has been obtained, the change will be accepted. It is particularly important to warn the patient that members of the family or close friends may comment on a change in facial appearance or even, tactlessly, enquire whether new dentures have been provided. Such comments are capable of turning the patient against the new dentures unless the ground has been prepared adequately in advance.

Positioning the Posterior Border of the Upper Denture

The dentist may wish to position the posterior border of the upper denture at the vibrating line. However, there may be uncertainty as to whether the patient can tolerate this extension beyond the limit of the previous denture. If, subsequently, the palate of the replacement denture has to be shortened, the post-dam is lost, the border seal broken and the retention of the denture reduced. As an insurance against this eventuality it is wise practice to cut two post-dam lines, one in the position of the old denture and one in the orthodox position. If, after wearing the new denture for a few days, the patient reports that the new position of the posterior border is intolerable, the extension of the palate can be cut back to the old post-dam line without the danger of breaking the continuity of the border seal.

DENTURE COPYING

So far in this chapter, discussion has been restricted to ways in which existing dentures can be used as a guide in the construction of replacements using orthodox clinical procedures. However, none of these methods allows one to copy the shape of the polished surfaces exactly, and it is through the polished surfaces that the oral musculature controls the dentures.

The acquisition of new patterns of muscular activity is dependent on the production of new reflex arcs in the central nervous system. With increasing age, there is progressive loss of the elements of the central nervous system and thus the ability to learn new patterns of muscular behaviour is reduced. An elderly person is therefore likely to have difficulty in controlling a replacement denture whose polished surface is quite unlike the shape of the old one. As more elderly patients are likely to require replacement dentures, it is important to have available a technique for copying the shape of dentures.

Indications for Copying Dentures

The point cannot be overstressed that the correct application of a copying technique depends upon an accurate diagnosis, which itself is dependent upon a careful examination of the three surfaces of the denture. This examination allows one to decide on the adequacy or otherwise of each surface and thus to conclude whether or not a copying technique is a feasible proposition, and, if it is, how best to employ that technique.

In general terms, an assessment of the three surfaces will allow the dentures to be placed into one of the categories shown in Table 7.1.

Category a
This category, where all surfaces are satisfactory, refers to the patient who is perfectly happy with existing dentures but wishes to have the added

Table 7.1

Impression surface	Occlusal surface	Polished surface	Category
√	√	√	a
x	√	√	b
√	x	√	c
x	x	√	d
		x	e
?	?	?	f
?	?	√	g
general deterioration of denture material			h

security of a 'spare set'. The copying technique may be used to satisfy this wish.

Category b
Where an error is found only on the impression surface, the patient's complaint is probably best treated by relining or rebasing the denture (Chapter 14).

Category c
If a patient's complaint can be localised to a small defect on the occlusal surface, treatment may involve simple occlusal adjustment. If the defect is the result of general occlusal wear of posterior teeth, it may be sensible to avoid making new dentures, especially when treating the elderly patient. Instead, the worn teeth can be replaced by new ones which are positioned in the corrected occlusal relationship and ultimately attached to the denture base with cold-curing resin. It should be recognised that the provision of a new denture, using a copying technique, is but only one approach to treatment in this category.

Category d
In cases where there has been progressive deterioration of both the impression and the occlusal surfaces, a copying technique may be the ideal approach when providing new dentures. In this way, the well-accepted polished surface can be accurately retained. This category is perhaps the most common one. The clinical and technical stages required to deal with this situation will be described later in the chapter.

Category e
If it is concluded that a major error exists in the polished surface and that the denture is not positioned in the neutral zone, there is unlikely to be an indication for employing a copying technique. Having said this, a

case can be argued for a modified copy technique in certain circumstances. For example, if a complaint of a loose lower denture is judged to be due to the lower anterior teeth being positioned too far labially, the desired change can be made on the wax replica teeth of the copy denture and the effect of that change judged in the mouth. If the result is a more stable denture, the new well-defined prescription can be passed to the laboratory for the construction of trial dentures.

Category f

Into this category, where there is indecision about the denture design as a whole, can be placed the patient who has experienced problems with many dentures and who is wearing a set which, in effect, is the best of a bad bunch. If the dentist suspects that the problems have been exaggerated by the patient, then he or she may consider that diagnostic modifications should be made to the dentures being worn; it is often better to build on partial success rather than start from scratch. However, there is a risk that if the least unsatisfactory dentures are altered, the end result might be less acceptable and then all is lost. To avoid this danger, it is wise to construct copies on which to carry out the trial modifications which one hopes will prove satisfactory. If the result proves to be unacceptable, then the patient still has the original life-line to hold on to.

Category g

The elderly patient may possess dentures which have given years of successful service but which have subsequently caused trouble because the patient's reducing powers of adaptability can no longer cope with obvious design defects in the impression and occlusal surfaces. For example, the dentures may be underextended and the occlusal surface may have deteriorated as a result of years of function. If the faults are corrected by constructing new dentures, the patient may have great difficulty in adapting to the sudden marked change. An alternative approach is to make the change gradually by incremental additions to the existing dentures (Figure 7.8). Once the final stage has been reached successfully, the dentures will look rather like a patchwork quilt. They can be converted to a new denture by using a copying technique.

Category h

A patient may seek replacements for comfortable and stable dentures which have become unsightly: the denture base material may have deteriorated through the misuse of cleaning agents: although undoubtedly a dying breed, there are still in existence vulcanite dentures which have given years of sterling service but are now past their prime. A copying technique may be the most appropriate way of ensuring that the well-accepted characteristics are faithfully passed on to the replacement dentures.

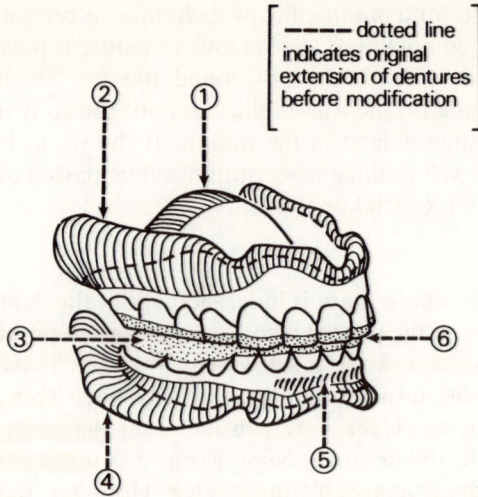

Figure 7.8   Diagram showing examples of diagnostic modifications which may be made to old dentures. (1) Addition to the posterior palatal border to extend the denture to the vibrating line. (2) Modifications to upper buccal flanges to: (a) correct underextension; (b) improve facial seal; (c) produce a form favourable for neuromuscular control of the denture. (3) Posterior occlusal additions to: (a) correct occlusal imbalance; (b) increase occlusal vertical dimension; (c) prevent postural protrusion of the mandible. (4) Extension of lower buccal flange to: (a) improve distribution of occlusal loads to the residual ridge; (b) increase resistance to posterior displacement by contact with the retromolar pad. (5) Hollowing the labial flange to reduce displacement by the mentalis muscle. (6) Additions to the incisal edges to: (a) improve appearance; (b) facilitate speech; (c) allow incision

In addition to these indications, it should be mentioned that the copy technique has the advantage over conventional techniques of allowing a saving in clinical time and possibly in the number of appointments. This can make it a relatively cost-effective technique and one which is particularly suitable for a domiciliary service.

In concluding this section, it should be stressed that a copying technique is but one approach to treatment – albeit a most valuable one. In general terms, the older the patient, the stronger the reasons for using the technique. In fact, this method of treatment may prove to be the only way of realising success for a patient whose powers of adaptation have deteriorated markedly. However, the copy technique must not be regarded by either dentist or technician as a shortcut to denture construction where relatively little care is needed. In fact, unless the decision to use the method is based on a sound diagnosis, and the clinical and technical procedures are undertaken with the greatest care, the course of treatment is highly likely to fail.

Various methods of constructing copy dentures have been described. Each one requires, as the starting point, the existing denture to be invested in an elastic material which is supported adequately in some sort of container. Two differing methods will be described.

Preparation of the Copies

Method 1

The objective of this procedure is to produce a copy of existing dentures in wax and acrylic resin using materials which are readily available in the surgery; thus, the first stage becomes a chairside procedure and not one which relies on laboratory facilities. In principle, the patient's denture is invested in alginate which is supported and contained in a soap box. The soap box is shown in Figure 7.9. A window is cut into its side to provide an exit for sprues. The technique is summarised in Figure 7.10. A variation of this method utilises a specially designed aluminium flask (Figure 7.11). After polymerisation, the copy is removed from the mould and the sprues are cut off. The resulting copy denture has a rigid base together with wax teeth which make the job of the technician so much easier when setting up the trial dentures. Using this technique, it has been shown that accurate copies can be constructed, the maximum dimensional change being -2.12 per cent.

Method 2

This technique uses stock impression trays and silicone putty. First, the occlusal and polished surfaces of the denture are embedded in a mix of silicone putty held in an upper tray. The impression surface is then invested

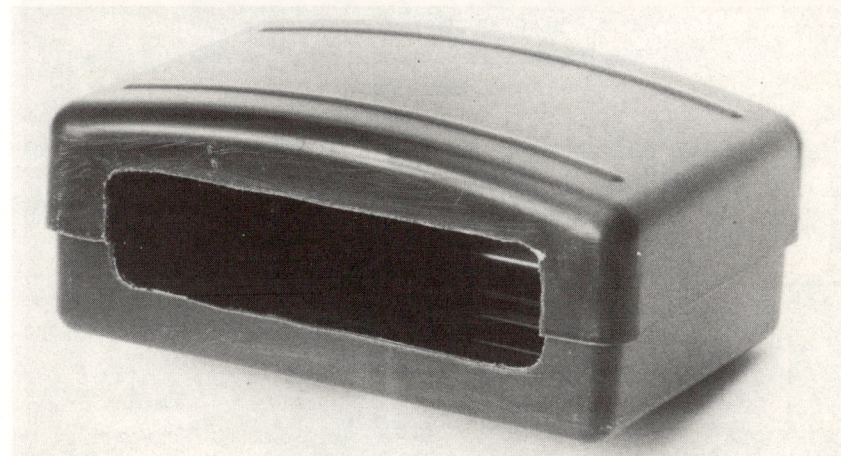

Figure 7.9   Soap box suitable as a container for the copy technique

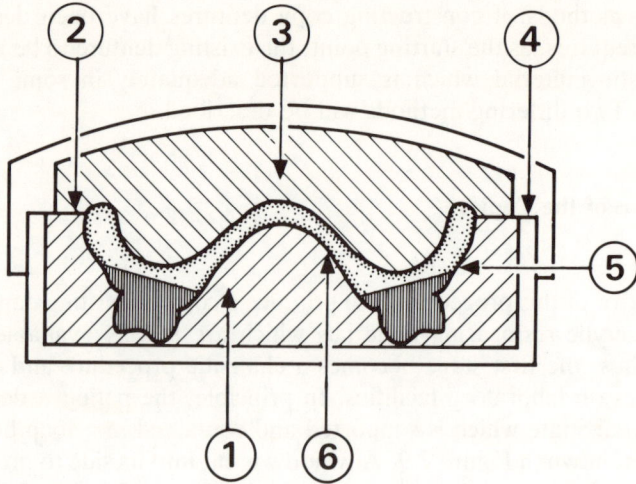

Figure 7.10   Diagrammatic summary of the copy denture technique. (1) First mix of alginate to obtain an impression of polished and occlusal surfaces. Adhesive is not applied to the walls of the container. (2) Alginate is trimmed at the level of the upper border of the box and just below the denture periphery. Petroleum jelly is smeared on the surface of the alginate to facilitate separation of the two halves of the mould. (3) Second mix of alginate to obtain a record of the impression surface. (4) Soap box closed on to stops. Denture removed when alginate set. Sprue channels cut with wax knife into heels of polished surface impression. (5) Wax poured to above level of gingival margin. Mould closed and held together with rubber band. (6) Base poured in a fluid mix of cold-curing acrylic resin

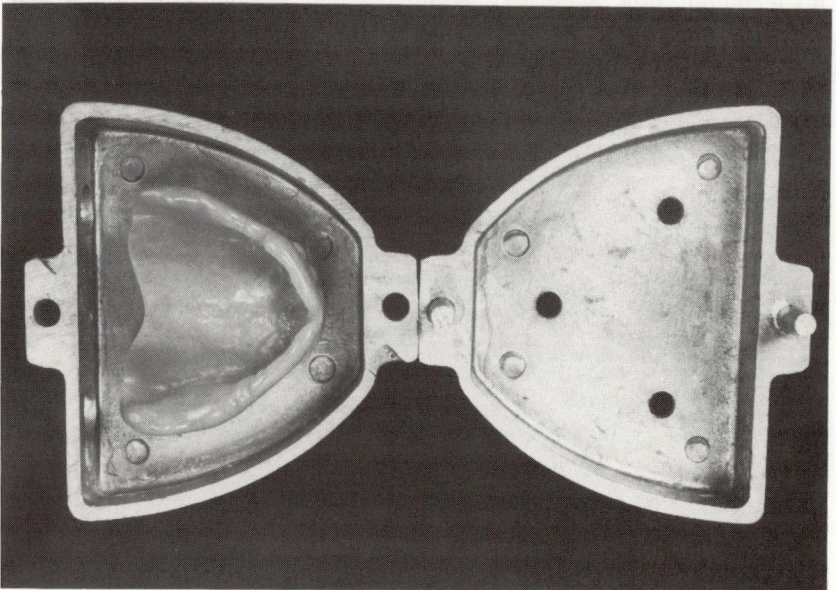

Figure 7.11   Specially designed aluminium flask for the copy technique

in a second mix of putty which is supported on the reverse surface of another tray (Figure 7.12). Once the putty has set, the two impressions are separated and the denture removed. Sprue holes are cut into the heels of the impression. A shellac base is adapted and secured to the putty impression surface, the mould re-assembled and molten wax poured through the sprue holes. The resulting copy consists of wax teeth and 'polished' surfaces on a shellac base.

Modification of the Copy Dentures

As shown in Table 7.1, copy dentures can be modified in numerous ways. Probably the most complex situation arises when impression and occlusal surfaces of upper and lower dentures are to be modified. The various clinical and technical stages are summarised in Table 7.2. It may be possible to undertake more than one clinical stage at the same appointment.

It can be seen from Table 7.2 that the various stages are very similar to those followed when constructing dentures in the conventional manner. If the occlusal surface was not to be altered and the copies could be interdigitated accurately, stage 4 would of course be avoided.

If the copy technique is used with due care, the prescription for the design of the replacement dentures can be made accurately and the

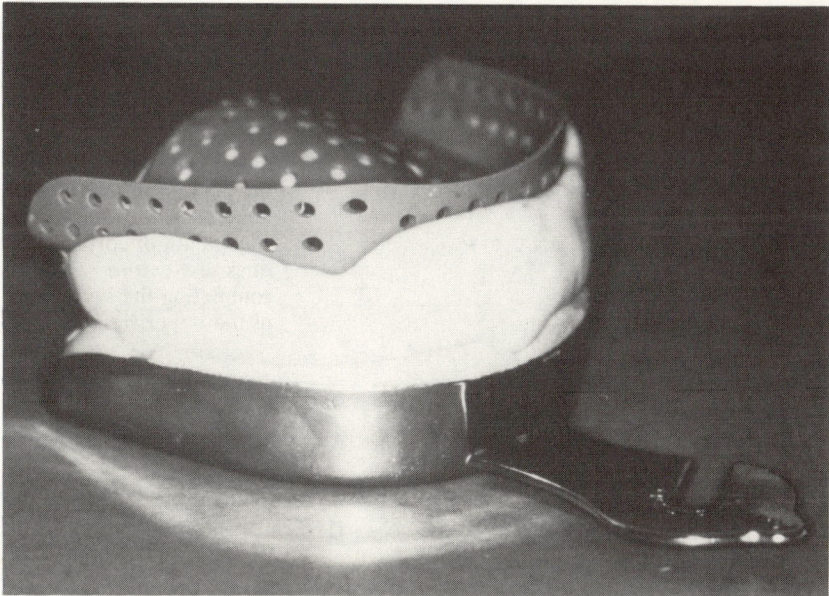

Figure 7.12   Silicone putty mould used for copy method 2 (see text for details)

Table 7.2

Stage	Clinical	Technical	Remarks
1	Diagnosis and treatment plan		List the modifications that will be made to the design of the existing dentures
2	Invest dentures to be copied		
3		Construct copies	Wax teeth on rigid bases
4	Record occlusion, making changes to occlusal vertical dimension, etc. as appropriate		If the impression surface deficiency is such that the copies are unstable in the mouth, border modifications and impressions in a low viscosity silicone should be taken before recording the occlusion (Figure 7.13)
5		Pour casts, articulate copies and make trial dentures	It is important to remove only a few wax teeth at a time so that the remainder act as effective guides to accurate positioning
6	Assess trial dentures: take impressions in low viscosity silicone if not done at stage 4		If impressions were taken at stage 4, sufficient silicone material will still be attached to the bases to ensure acceptable stability of the trial dentures
7		Finish dentures	Remaining cold-curing resin is discarded and the flask packed with heat-curing resin. It will be necessary to lay down a wax palate of correct thickness before completing the investment of the upper trial denture
8	Fit dentures		
9	Recall visit		

laboratory will receive sufficient information such that the decisions made at the treatment planning stage can be carried out effectively.

A final point is worth making. As the lower denture is the more critical of the two, there may be stronger indications for copying it so that such

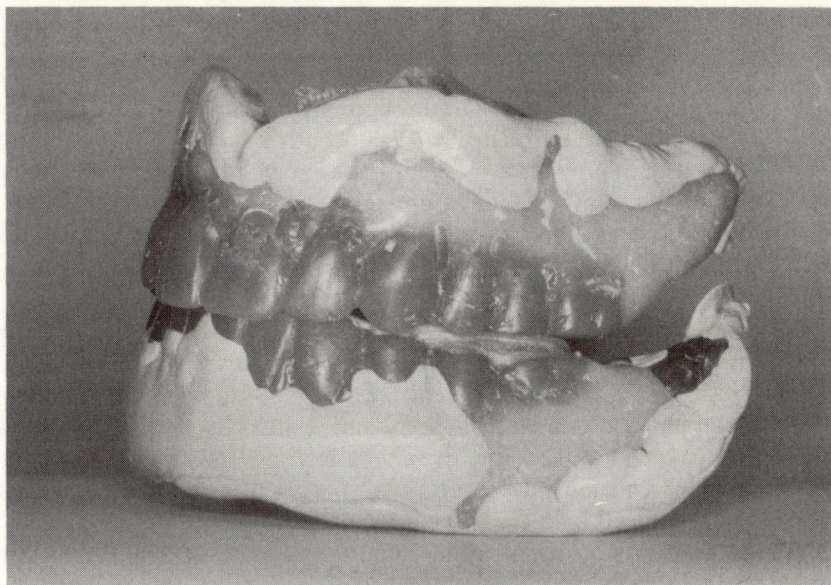

Figure 7.13   Wash impressions taken in the copy dentures at the stage of recording the occlusion

features as the polished surface and the tongue space can be faithfully carried through to the replacement. It will be appreciated that the presence of the lower copy will automatically control the arch shape of the upper denture which is being constructed at the same time, as long as the upper occlusal rim is carved carefully against the lower.

SHORT-TERM RESILIENT LINING MATERIALS

These materials must be differentiated from the group of long-term materials which are discussed on page 259. The short-term materials are placed in existing dentures for the following reasons:

(a) As tissue conditioners when they are applied temporarily to the impression surface of a denture for the purpose of allowing a more equal distribution of load, thus permitting the mucosal tissues to return to their normal shape. In this function, the material should act as a cushion, absorbing the forces of mastication and promoting tissue recovery. Such a material should preferably be soft and elastic.

(b) As a temporary soft reline material to improve the fit of a denture, typically an immediate restoration. If the lining is to be inserted soon after the extraction of teeth, the patient is likely to experience greater comfort if the material is relatively soft. In cases where a reasonable amount of healing has occurred but one still wishes to insert a temporary soft reline, a material with a harder consistency can be selected. In either case, the material should possess a degree of elasticity to allow it to be inserted and removed over undercuts without causing discomfort or resulting in unacceptable dimensional changes.

(c) As a diagnostic aid where the dentist wishes to check the reaction of the patient and the tissues to a change in fit of a denture. If the patient is happy with the change made by the short-term lining material, the dentist has first-hand evidence of the degree of improvement that can be expected if a long-term soft reline is to be inserted. One advantage of this approach is that the information has been obtained by a reversible procedure.

(d) As a functional impression material applied to the impression surface of a denture for the purpose of securing an impression under functional stresses. In this case, the soft material should flow so that it can be moulded by the forces generated by the muscles of mastication and the surrounding oral musculature; thus, the material should be plastic and, having been moulded, should retain its shape when the cast is poured.

Composition

Most materials are supplied in a powder/liquid form. An alternative presentation is in a ready-to-use sheet form which can be found in one product available to the dental profession and in several 'over the counter' products available to the general public. The method of self-treatment is to be discouraged as it is not based on a sound clinical diagnosis and can result in severe tissue destruction. It is essential that traumatised tissue be examined by the dentist and rational, rather than empirical, treatment prescribed.

In the powder/liquid types, the powder consists of poly(ethylmethacrylate) and related copolymers while the liquid is a mixture of an aromatic ester, such as dibutyl phthalate which acts as a plasticiser, and ethyl alcohol. After the powder and liquid have been mixed, the ethyl alcohol causes swelling of the polymer particles and permits penetration by the ester so that a gel is formed. The presence of ethyl alcohol is necessary to initiate this reaction and the amount present in the liquid is related to the particle size and molecular weight of the polymer. If particle size and molecular weight are low, then the ethyl alcohol content can be kept to a minimum. This state of affairs is desirable as large amounts of ethyl alcohol produce an unpleasant taste and sensation in the mouth. Furthermore, when the material is immersed in water, the ethyl alcohol and plasticiser are leached out causing the material to harden and shrink.

Relevant Properties

Certain properties of the setting and the set material are important to the dentist.

The setting material should have sufficient flow to allow it to adapt accurately to the mucosal surface but should not flow so readily that most of it is squeezed out of the denture when the patient occludes on the dentures, leaving too thin a layer that detracts from the cushioning effect. The current range of available materials varies considerably with respect to viscosity and each material can be modified in this respect by altering the powder/liquid ratio, although the scope for altering the ratios is limited. Perhaps the most important point to make is that if one of the less viscous (and thus softer) products is chosen, it is particularly important to instruct the patient to close on the dentures with the lightest possible contact as the material sets so that, ultimately, a thickness of at least 2 mm is created.

From the earlier discussion, it is apparent that the important properties of the set material are:

(a) hardness or softness,
(b) elastic recovery or plastic flow,
(c) dimensional stability.

The properties of the set material alter with time. The longer the powder/liquid types are left in the mouth, the harder they become. However, those with a low alcohol content remain softer for longer and are thus more effective as tissue conditioners. Elasticity increases as the materials age. Some of the powder/liquid materials are elastic from the start and are therefore unsuitable as functional impression materials. Those materials with a low alcohol content exhibit plastic behaviour and good dimensional stability for the first few hours after mixing.

Clinical Implications

Tissue-conditioning Materials
As mentioned earlier, a material for this purpose must be soft and elastic. If such a cushioning layer is applied to the impression surface of an old

Viscosel

denture, it will help to resolve inflammation of the denture-bearing tissues. However, immediately there is some change in shape of the traumatised mucosa, the impression surface of the denture will cease to be accurately adapted and so the rate of healing will be reduced. Of course, if the material remains soft and elastic, its distortion by relatively small forces in the mouth will help it to adapt to the tissues during function. Nevertheless, it is wise practice to change the dressing of tissue-conditioning material after a few days to ensure that the traumatised tissue reverts to a normal state as rapidly as possible. It must be emphasised that a course of tissue conditioning will not be effective unless other traumatic factors, such as an uneven occlusion or border overextension, are corrected before applying the conditioning material to the impression surface of the denture. Needless to say, it is important to ensure that the freeway space of the dentures will allow a sufficient thickness of the material to be inserted.

It is most important to ensure that the tissue-conditioning material is kept clean and that plaque is prevented from collecting on the surface. The significance of denture plaque is considered fully in Chapter 8 while detailed recommendations on cleaning procedures are presented on pages 125 and 244.

Functional Impression Materials

Because many of the functional impression materials exhibit elastic recovery after a few hours, there is the danger that in the time interval between removing the denture from the mouth and making the cast, the impression material will change shape. The following régime is suggested as the best way of achieving optimal results. First, the impression surface and borders of the denture are inspected. Existing undercuts are removed and the border extension is adjusted, if necessary, so that a gap of 1–2 mm is created between the acrylic border and the functional depth of the sulcus. This size of gap allows the functional impression material to be moulded by the sulcus tissues and at the same time provides adequate support to the material when the cast is made. If an undercut ridge is present, it is wise to remove between 2 and 3 mm of the impression surface of the denture in the region of the undercut. This allows for an increased thickness of functional impression material, which has been shown to record the shape of the tissue undercut more accurately. The impression surface of the denture is dried to ensure good adhesion. The impression material is mixed according to the manufacturer's instructions and placed in the denture. After the denture is inserted into the mouth, the patient is instructed to close gently together so that the normal occlusal relationship is maintained. Natural movements of the tongue, cheek and lip musculature are encouraged. After approximately five minutes, the denture is removed and excessive impression material is cut away with a scalpel, care being taken to maintain the full border shape. The functional impression material is applied to the denture approximately one hour before the patient is due to have a meal and the patient is asked to return to the surgery after that meal. If the impression is satisfactory, the denture is removed from the mouth and a cast is made immediately; in this way, the risk of elastic recovery is reduced to a minimum and good results will be obtained from this most useful technique.

Rigid Cold-curing Resins

Recent years have seen the development of a group of useful materials, frequently described as chairside reline materials, which can be used to modify the impression surface of an existing denture. Commonly, these materials consist of a powder containing poly(ethylmethacrylate) together with a liquid, monomeric butylmethacrylate. This formulation allows the materials to be cured in the mouth without the risk of irritating the mucosa. When compared with cold-curing poly(methylmethacrylate), these materials have lower impact strength, rigidity, indentation resistance and glass transition temperature; in addition, they discolour after a few months. Thus, although they can serve a very useful purpose, such as improving the fit of an immediate denture, the surface should be regarded as a temporary one.

BIBLIOGRAPHY

Braden, M. (1970) Tissue conditioners: I. Composition and structure. *Journal of Dental Research*, **49**, 145–8.

Braden, M. (1970) Tissue conditioners: II. Rheological properties. *Journal of Dental Research*, **49**, 496–501.

Braden, M. and Causton, B. E. (1971) Tissue conditioners: III. Water immersion characteristics. *Journal of Dental Research*, **50**, 1544–7.

Campbell, J. (1965) Raising the bite: Inherent aspects of occlusion. *British Dental Journal*, **118**, 187–8.

Davenport, J. C. and Heath, J. R. (1983) The copy denture technique – variables relevant to general dental practice. *British Dental Journal*, **155**, 162–3.

Duthie, N., Lyon, F. F., Sturrock, K. C. and Yemm, R. (1978) A copying technique for replacement of complete dentures. *British Dental Journal*, **144**, 248–52.

Duthie, N. and Yemm, R. (1985) An alternative method for recording the occlusion of the edentulous patient during the construction of replacement dentures. *Journal of Oral Rehabilitation*, **12**, 161–71.

Harrison, A. (1981) Temporary soft lining materials. *British Dental Journal*, **151**, 419–22.

Heath, J. R. and Basker, R. M. (1978) The dimensional variability of duplicate dentures produced in an alginate investment. *British Dental Journal*, **144**, 111–14.

Heath, J. R. and Davenport, J. C. (1982) A modification of the copy denture technique. *British Dental Journal*, **153**, 300–2.

Heath, J. R. and Johnson, A. (1981) The versatility of the copy denture technique. *British Dental Journal*, **150**, 189–93.

McCarthy, J. A. and Moser, J. B. (1978) Undercut reproducibility of functional impression materials (tissue conditioners). *Journal of Oral Rehabilitation*, **5**, 287–92.

Murphy, W. M., Huggett, R., Handley, R. W. and Brooks, S. C. (1986) Rigid cold curing resins for direct use in the oral cavity. *British Dental Journal*, **160**, 391–4.

Murray, I. D. and Wolland, A. W. (1986) New dentures for old. *Dental Practice*, **24**, 1–6.

Newsome, P. R. H., Basker, R. M., Bergman, B. and Glantz, P.-O. (1988) The softness and initial flow of temporary soft lining materials. *Acta Odontologica Scandinavica*, **46**, 9–17.

Osborne, J. (1960) The full lower denture. *British Dental Journal*, **109**, 481–97.

Scher, E. A. and Ritchie, G. M. (1978) Prosthodontic treatment of the elderly by incremental modifications to old dentures. *Quintessence International*, **8**, 47–53.

Watt, D. M. and Lindsay, K. N. (1972) Occlusal pivot appliances. *British Dental Journal*, **132**, 110–12.

Wilson, H. J., Tomlin, H. R. and Osborne, J. (1966) Tissue conditioners and functional impression materials. *British Dental Journal*, **121**, 9–16.

Wilson, H. J., Tomlin, H. R. and Osborne, J. (1969) The assessment of temporary soft materials used in prosthetics. *British Dental Journal*, **126**, 303–6.

8 Preparation of the Mouth

Preparation of the mouth is frequently necessary before dentures are made and may involve the elimination of pathology within the denture-bearing tissues or the creation of a more favourable anatomical situation.

The various conditions requiring treatment may be considered in two sections, those involving the *oral mucosa* and those involving *bone*.

Conditions involving the oral mucosa
    Denture stomatitis
    Inflammatory papillary hyperplasia
    Angular stomatitis (angular cheilitis)
    Denture-induced hyperplasia
    Prominent frena
    Shallow sulci

Conditions involving the bone
    Pathology within the bone
    Sharp and irregular bone
    Undercut ridges
    Prominent maxillary tuberosities
    Tori

CONDITIONS INVOLVING THE ORAL MUCOSA

Denture Stomatitis

The clinical appearance of this condition may vary from a patchy to a diffuse inflammation of the mucosa covered by a denture (Figure 8.1). In spite of the lesion's rather angry appearance the patient rarely complains of soreness, therefore the term 'denture sore mouth' which was formerly used to describe this condition is inappropriate. The condition occurs most commonly in the mucosa of the maxillary denture-bearing area and does

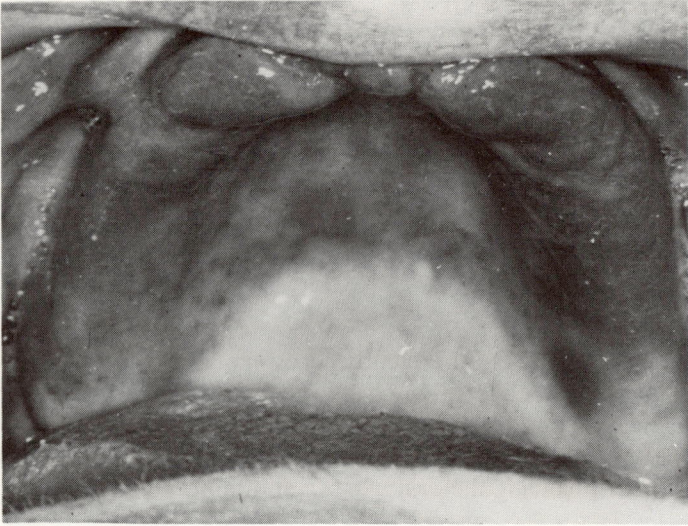

Figure 8.1 Denture stomatitis. The characteristically sharp delineation of the diffuse palatal inflammation by the borders of the denture is seen at the junction of the hard and soft palate where the line separating inflamed from normal corresponds to the posterior border of the denture

not extend beyond the borders of the denture. It may occur alone but is often seen with two associated conditions, inflammatory papillary hyperplasia and angular stomatitis.

Denture stomatitis is a common condition, having been reported in 10–60 per cent of patients wearing complete dentures; it occurs more frequently in females than in males, the ratio being approximately 4:1. Although the cause of this predisposition to denture stomatitis in females is not known, possible explanations include endocrine imbalance, iron deficiency anaemia, vaginal carriage of candida and a higher oral carrier rate of candida. It has been reported that denture stomatitis becomes less common with increasing age.

Aetiology

In 1886, G. V. Black, commenting on the condition we now know as denture stomatitis, stated that 'Fungi grow readily under any plate irrespective of the material of what it is made. They produce acids which if the mouth and palate are not properly cleaned will cause sore mouth.' In 1885, he sampled micro-organisms from under the dentures of patients with this condition and expressed surprise at their abundance. He concluded that plates are not cleaned often enough and that cleanliness is the chief preventive. Thus, well over 100 years ago Black summarised the current views of both the aetiology and management of denture stomatitis which have only relatively recently gained widespread acceptance following extensive research.

Many different factors have been incriminated in the aetiology of denture stomatitis. The current evidence suggests that the most important of these is the presence of micro-organisms in the form of plaque on the impression surface of the denture. The fungus, *Candida albicans* (Figure 8.2), is the organism associated with denture stomatitis which has received the most attention in the literature. This fungus is dimorphic, occurring both as yeast-like blastospores and filamentous pseudohyphae. In denture stomatitis, both forms are usually found in large numbers in plaque on the impression surface of the denture. Although the evidence for a causal relationship between candida and denture stomatitis is strong, a variety of bacteria may also play a part in the condition. It is now widely agreed that denture stomatitis is multifactorial with other possible causes including trauma from dentures, and systemic factors such as immunological deficiencies, deficiencies of vitamin B complex, vitamin C and iron. In addition, a high carbohydrate diet might aggravate the condition by promoting the growth of micro-organisms and increasing the adhesiveness of their cells to the denture surface.

Although a combination of these factors is most commonly responsible for denture stomatitis, it should be remembered that palatal inflammation is a non-specific response to a wide variety of injurious agents. In a small number of patients, a raised level of residual monomer in the denture base (page 273) or self-medication with an irritant preparation will be responsible for the inflammation. A persistent stomatitis can occur in asthmatic

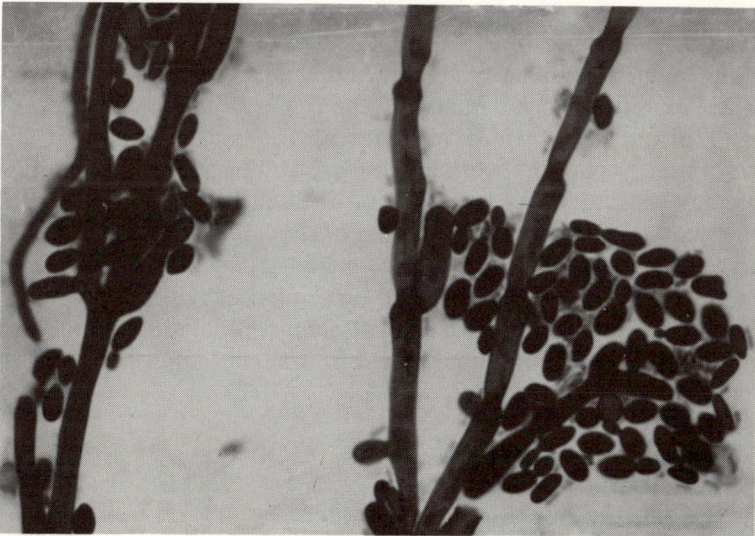

Figure 8.2   Mycelial and yeast forms of *Candida albicans* ($\times$ 1200)

patients who use an inhaler. However, in these instances the clinical signs are usually accompanied by symptoms such as soreness or a burning sensation.

When investigating a patient with denture stomatitis the amount of plaque on the denture should be recorded. This assessment of the quantity and distribution of denture plaque is made easier by applying a disclosing solution to the denture. In those cases where only a little plaque is seen, allowance should be made for the fact that a patient will sometimes have made an effort to clean the dentures in readiness for the visit to the dentist, which is atypical of their normal denture hygiene regimen. As there is no evidence that microbial invasion of the palatal mucosa occurs in denture stomatitis, sampling from this area is not necessary.

In addition to recording denture plaque, the degree of denture trauma should also be assessed. This can be estimated from the relative functional adequacy of the dentures in terms of occlusion and fit, and from evidence of the presence or absence of parafunctional activity.

It should also be noted whether the dentures are worn both day and night, as this will increase the exposure of the mucosa to denture plaque and will extend the period in which the mucosa could be being traumatised. As there is evidence that smoking and a high carbohydrate diet can contribute to the condition, these aspects of the history should also be recorded.

The medical history may provide clues that systemic factors are playing a part. If this is the case, or if the condition subsequently fails to respond to local treatment, appropriate investigations should be arranged.

Treatment

Denture stomatitis should be treated before new dentures are constructed because, as with other inflammatory conditions of the oral mucosa, some swelling of the tissues will have occurred. The consequences of omitting this essential preparatory work are discussed on page 94. Treatment is also important because the mouth may be the source of candida organisms responsible for infection in other parts of the body, such as nail beds, the pharynx and the larynx. In debilitated patients, systemic spread of candida from the mouth can occur with fatal consequences.

The objectives of local treatment of denture stomatitis are to improve denture hygiene and to minimise denture trauma. Appropriate measures include:

(a) denture hygiene instruction,
(b) correction of denture faults,
(c) not wearing the dentures at night.

Denture Hygiene Instruction
The need for meticulous cleaning must be emphasised to the patient and
the methods for carrying it out explained and demonstrated by the dentist
(page 244). Where deposits are heavy and possibly partly calcified, and
where the surface polish of the denture has deteriorated, it is recommended that laboratory cleaning and polishing of the denture is carried out
before home care by the patient is instituted. In addition, the dentures
should be regularly immersed by the patient in a suitable disinfectant. Two
solutions have been shown to be effective in controlling denture plaque:
alkaline hypochlorite and aqueous chlorhexidine gluconate. The former
has been shown to be effective in removing denture plaque while the latter
inhibits its formation. Overnight immersion is necessary if either a
hypochlorite solution containing 0.08 per cent available chlorine or 0.1 per
cent aqueous chlorhexidine gluconate is used. When it is impossible to
persuade a patient to leave the denture out at night, immersion in a
hypochlorite solution containing 0.16 per cent available chlorine for 20
minutes daily or in 2 per cent aqueous chlorhexidine gluconate for
approximately five minutes daily are alternatives. Before immersion, the
denture should be brushed thoroughly to remove most of the plaque and
then, if chlorhexidine is to be used, rinsed carefully to remove any soap, as
this would neutralise the chlorhexidine. Patches of brown staining usually
appear on a denture which has been immersed in chlorhexidine solution.
As a rule, the staining is not severe and can be removed by subsequent
immersion in a hypochlorite cleaner.

NB.

    The presence of a metal denture base complicates matters because the
use of hypochlorite can cause corrosion of the base.

Correction of Denture Faults
An unbalanced occlusion should be corrected by occlusal adjustment or by
the addition of cold-curing acrylic resin to the occlusal surfaces of the
dentures (page 96). Lack of fit in a denture can be corrected by applying a
short-term resilient lining material to the impression surface (page 115).
However, some caution should be exercised in selecting this option as the
presence of a temporary lining will make it more difficult for the patient to
maintain the all-important high level of denture hygiene. It has been
reported that certain of these lining materials exhibit antifungal activity *in
vitro*, but it is very unlikely that this activity is significant *in vivo*.

Leaving the Dentures out at Night
All patients should be strongly advised to leave their dentures out at night;
in some instances, successful treatment will not be possible unless the
patient conforms to this advice. This regime reduces the period the mucosa
is in contact with denture plaque, reduces the intra-oral population of

candida and other organisms, provides an opportunity for prolonged immersion of the dentures in a disinfectant and, for those cases where denture trauma is a contributory factor, reduces the period over which mucosal damage can occur.

An appropriate combination of these simple therapeutic measures will usually effect a cure within two to three weeks if there are no underlying systemic factors. Therefore, if a cure is not achieved in this time, and if persistent local factors cannot be identified, systemic causes should be suspected and the patient referred to a medical practitioner for further investigation.

The antifungal antibiotics, nystatin and amphotericin B, have been advocated for the treatment of denture stomatitis and they have been shown to be effective in the short term. However, they do nothing to modify the oral conditions responsible for the inflammation in the long term. Clinical studies have shown that a rapid relapse usually follows the cessation of antibiotic therapy. There is no difference at one year following start of treatment between patients treated with antibiotics in combination with denture hygiene instruction and correction compared with those treated by denture measures alone. The prescription of nystatin and amphotericin B in the treatment of denture stomatitis is therefore not supported by the available evidence.

Inflammatory Papillary Hyperplasia

This condition, alternatively known as hyperplastic denture stomatitis, involves the palatal mucosa and appears as multiple elevations, usually bright red in colour. It is 'raspberry-like' in appearance and may involve the whole or part of the palate (Figure 8.3). At one time, it was suggested that this condition was premalignant; this is not now considered to be the case. Some believe that the presence of a relief chamber in an upper denture predisposes to this hyperplastic change.

Aetiology
The condition is closely related to the simple atrophic form of denture stomatitis and shares the same aetiology.

Treatment
Treatment may be considered to have two phases: first, the elimination of the mucosal inflammation and second, the surgical or prosthetic management of the hyperplasia.

Treatment of the inflammatory component is the same as that described for denture stomatitis. When this has been successfully carried out, the hyperplastic nodules will still remain, although they will now be pale in

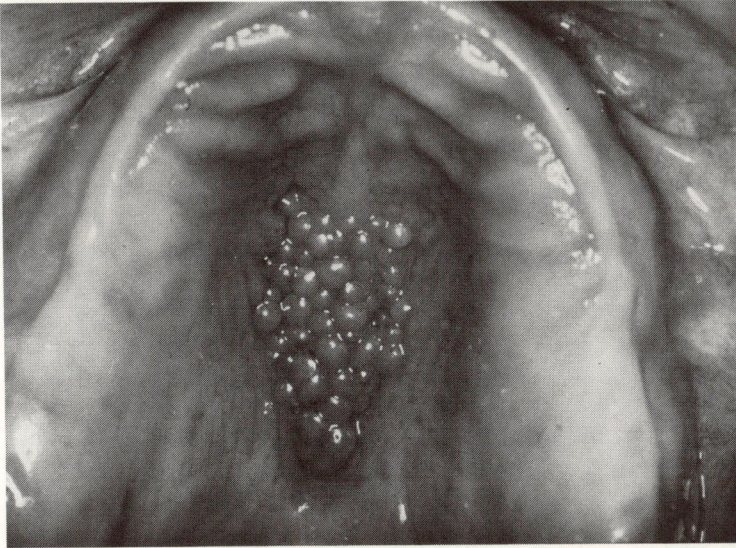

Figure 8.3   Inflammatory papillary hyperplasia of the palate

colour and much reduced in size. A decision then has to be made whether to construct a denture on this foundation or to remove the nodules surgically beforehand. The approach adopted in a particular case will depend on factors such as the size of the nodules, and the patient's age and medical history.

If an acrylic denture is constructed without prior surgical removal of the nodules, sharp spicules of acrylic resin will penetrate the fissures of the lesion (Figure 8.4(a)). As all dentures move to a certain extent during function, these spicules have an abrasive effect on the mucosa and inflammation will recur. To prevent this happening, the spicules should be lightly polished to reduce their sharpness before fitting the denture (Figure 8.4(b)). An alternative approach is to use a stainless steel denture base (Figure 8.4(c)).

Angular Stomatitis

Angular stomatitis, sometimes described as angular cheilitis, is an erythematous, often erosive, non-vesicular skin lesion radiating from the angles of the mouth. It is usually bilateral, frequently painful and is rarely seen except in denture wearers (Figure 8.5). It is more common in females. If left untreated, it can result in unsightly scarring. The majority of patients with angular stomatitis also have an associated denture stomatitis.

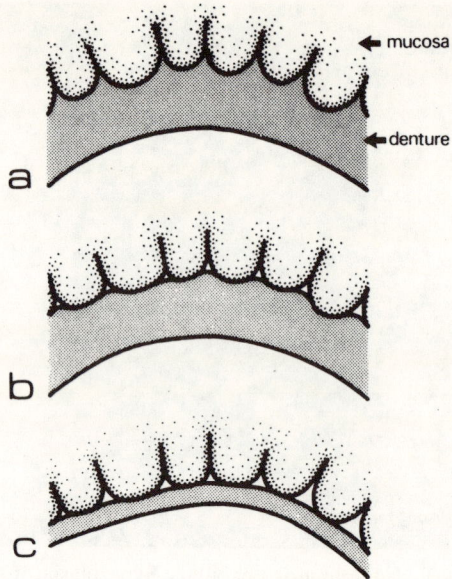

Figure 8.4   The impression surface in inflammatory papillary hyperplasia: (a) sharp spicules of acrylic penetrate the fissures between the hyperplastic papillae if the impression surface is not modified after processing; (b) the spicules of acrylic may be lightly stoned before fitting the denture to reduce the amount of trauma; (c) alternatively, trauma may be reduced by using a stainless steel palate

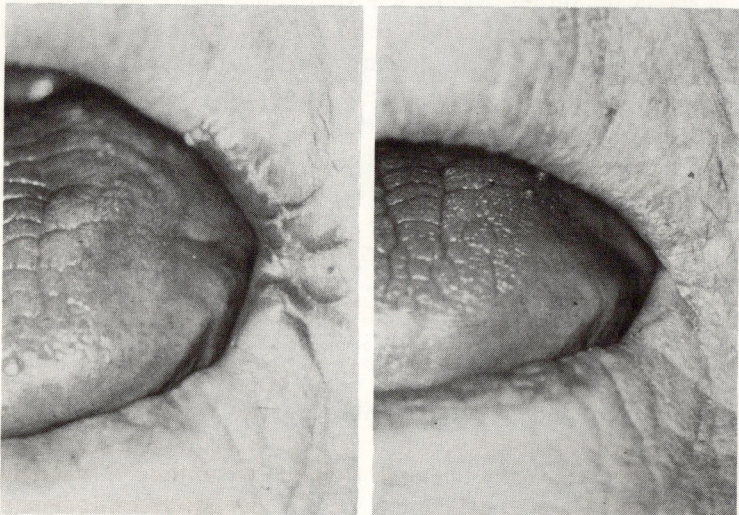

Figure 8.5   Angular stomatitis – clinical appearance. *Left*: Before treatment. *Right*: After two weeks' improved dental hygiene

Aetiology

Common local and systemic factors which may contribute to the development of angular stomatitis are:

Local	Systemic
Maceration of the skin	Iron deficiency
Infection	Vitamin B and C deficiency
Inadequate lip support	

Maceration results from the continuous bathing by saliva of the skin at the corners of the mouth which lowers the resistance of the skin to infection. Maceration is encouraged by the presence of skin creases which may be due to inadequate lip support being provided by the upper denture or to the presence of an excessive freeway space. However, an increased freeway space should never be assumed to be present simply on the evidence of angular stomatitis.

When it is suspected that the skin folds are due to inadequate occlusal vertical dimension or inadequate lip support, the existing dentures may be modified with wax to see whether the correction will eliminate the folds. If so, new dentures should be made accordingly. As an interim measure, the occlusal vertical dimension of the old dentures can be increased by the addition of cold-curing acrylic resin to the occlusal surfaces of the posterior teeth. However, if the modifications have little effect on the folds, it must be accepted that the cause is an irreversible tissue change, such as loss of tissue tone associated with ageing. The persistence of the folds makes treatment more difficult and recurrence of the condition more likely.

Micro-organisms may be carried in the saliva to the lips from intra-oral sites, such as the denture and the dorsum of the tongue. The significance of microbial plaque on the dentures is demonstrated by the observation that if patients with angular stomatitis do not wear their dentures, a complete cure usually results in two weeks even though all dental support to the lips has been lost. *Candida albicans* is frequently isolated from the lesion of angular stomatitis where denture stomatitis is also present. However, if angular stomatitis occurs alone, *Staphylococcus aureus* is recovered from the lesion twice as often as candida. In such cases, the nose may be the source of secondary infection with carriage on the fingers being the method of transmission.

Treatment

The treatment of angular stomatitis in the first instance involves the elimination of local infection and the reduction of the intra-oral population of micro-organisms. General measures include denture hygiene instruction and immersion of the dentures in a hypochlorite denture cleaner, as described for denture stomatitis. In many cases, such simple measures will effect a cure in about two weeks. Improved denture hygiene may be supplemented where necessary by prescribing one of the broad spectrum agents, such as miconazole oral gel or a tetracycline/nystatin ointment, which are active against both fungi and bacteria. It is not advisable however to prescribe one of the many compound skin preparations which contain steroids, as topical steroids have been shown to be by far the commonest cause of peri-oral dermatitis and may therefore aggravate the condition.

If specific antimicrobial therapy is to be employed, a swab from the angles of the lips should be cultured to allow identification of the responsible organisms. If the cultures are positive for candida organisms, amphotericin B lozenges (10 mg) or nystatin pastilles (100 000 units) may be sucked four times a day. These preparations are of value in the treatment of angular stomatitis because candida organisms not only grow in large numbers on the denture but also proliferate on the dorsum of the tongue. Both reservoirs could be contributing to the high salivary count predisposing to the angular stomatitis.

If swabs from the lesion indicate that a bacterial infection is present, benefit may be gained from the topical application of a tetracycline ointment or miconazole gel. Treatment should be continued for two to four weeks. Failure to respond to local measures suggests that systemic factors are playing a part and that further investigations are required.

A suggested interrelation between the local causative factors leading to denture stomatitis, angular stomatitis and inflammatory papillary hyperplasia is shown in Figure 8.6.

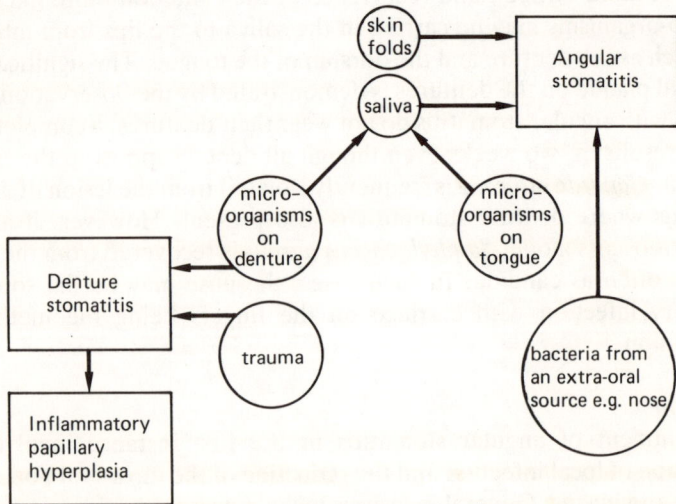

Figure 8.6 Diagram showing a suggested interrelationship between the local causative factors leading to denture stomatitis, angular stomatitis and inflammatory papillary hyperplasia

Denture-induced Hyperplasia

Denture-induced hyperplasia takes the form of single or multiple flaps of fibrous tissue related to the border of a denture (Figure 8.7). The condition is more commonly seen in the lower jaw than in the upper.

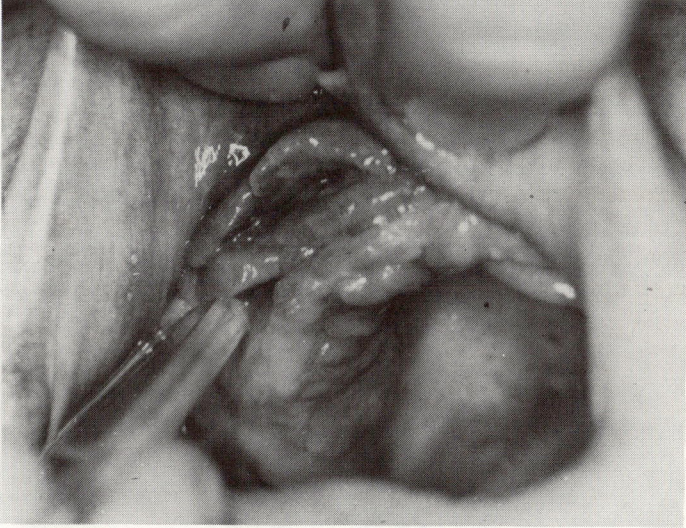

Figure 8.7   Denture-induced hyperplasia – two flaps of fibrous tissue situated in the upper labial sulcus

Aetiology
The primary cause of this condition is overextension of the denture border which may be the result of alveolar ridge resorption and consequent sinkage of the denture. Trauma from the denture border may also occur if excessive tipping, due to an unbalanced occlusion, causes the border to dig into the sulcus tissues. The majority of patients will seek treatment to relieve pain caused by pressure on the mucosa before the lesion becomes hyperplastic. However, there remains a group with a high pain threshold who are not aware of the tissue damage and therefore continue to wear the offending denture.

Treatment
The hyperplastic tissue diminishes in size if the denture is not worn for a period of time or if the flange is cut away from the affected area. In some cases, the degree of resolution is sufficient to allow satisfactory dentures to be made without the necessity for surgical intervention. If, however, the size of the residual lesion is too large to allow adequate extension of the denture, surgical removal is indicated.

It must be remembered that denture-induced hyperplasia is the result of chronic irritation, a well-recognised cause of malignancy. Therefore, the excised hyperplastic tissue should routinely be sent for histological examination.

Prominent Frena

These are bands of fibrous tissue whose attachment may be close to the crest of the alveolar ridge. Prominent frena may be found in both jaws labially in the mid-line and buccally in the premolar regions (Figure 8.8). In order to accommodate this fibrous tissue, it is necessary to make a deep notch in the denture flange. The stress concentrations which are set up at the apex of the notch predispose to fracture of the denture base (page 263). In addition, there may be difficulty in achieving an efficient border seal. Excision of a prominent frenum may be necessary in extreme cases.

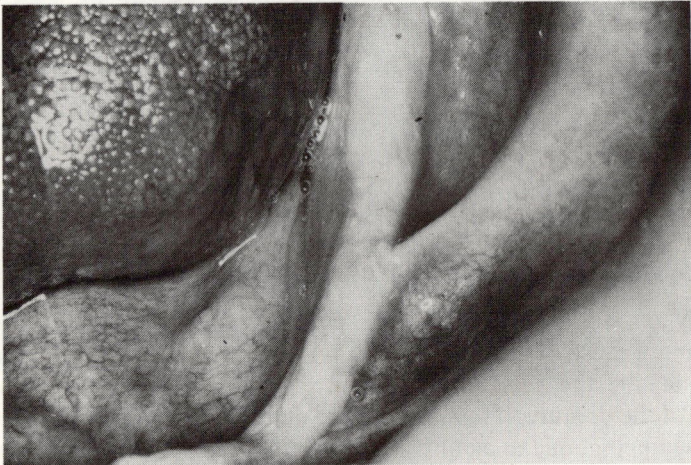

Figure 8.8   A prominent frenum attached to the crest of the ridge in the lower left premolar region

Shallow Sulci

The problems created by a shallow sulcus are two-fold: the dentures may be unstable and the load distribution will be unfavourable. This latter problem occurs predominantly in the lower jaw. Where problems of pain or instability have not been solved by prosthetic means, surgical deepening of the sulci may be undertaken in appropriate cases. Additional possibilities are to augment the resorbed ridge with bone or bone substitutes, or to insert implants

It is important to appreciate that those patients who have the greatest need for surgical improvement of the denture-supporting tissues are often those who are the least suitable candidates. This is because the advanced alveolar resorption which commonly creates the need also limits what surgical intervention can achieve. In addition, the need for improved denture stability tends to occur in the older age groups where ill health and general frailty can make the patient poorly prepared to cope with the trauma associated with even relatively minor oral surgical procedures. Therefore, the surgical approaches to problems of denture stability do not provide an easy answer and should be adopted with caution for carefully selected patients; they should only be used if it is certain that conventional prosthetic treatment cannot provide a solution. With this thought in mind, it is pertinent to report the conclusion of one study which showed that the need for a surgical approach in a group of patients complaining about problems of denture stability was reduced by 43 per cent simply by the provision of satisfactory dentures.

Surgical procedures designed to enhance denture stability, function and comfort are numerous. They include alveolotomy and alveolectomy for immediate replacement dentures, frenectomy, the reduction of undercuts and enlarged tuberosities, the removal of bony prominences such as tori and mylohyoid ridges, transposition of the mental nerve, and sulcus deepening and ridge augmentation using either bone or bone substitutes such as hydroxyapatite. For details of techniques the reader is referred to specialist texts on the subject.

Implants

Implants have had a chequered history and have been surrounded by controversy. A multiplicity of designs and principles have been introduced over the years with little or no scientific evaluation. This, together with frequent failures of treatment, has resulted in many types of implant falling into disrepute.

One of the more successful early implant systems which should be mentioned in relation to denture stability is the subperiosteal implant. This consists of a cobalt–chromium framework, or substructure, which rests on the surface of the bone and is covered by mucoperiosteum. It carries four posts which penetrate the mucoperiosteum in the canine and first molar regions. On to these posts is fitted the metal superstructure which consists of thimbles and joining bars embedded within the denture. This type of implant requires a two-stage surgical procedure: one to obtain the impression of the bone surface and the other to fit the substructure. After the implant has been fitted, epithelium gradually grows down the posts and around the framework, essentially exteriorising it. Gradual failure of the implant therefore occurs, although the process is a slow one; a perhaps cynical interpretation of the situation is that the implant is successful because the elderly patient succumbs first.

Over the last 25 years or so, intra-osseus titanium implants developed by Bränemark have been subjected to controlled scientific study and have been found to have a success rate of around 95 per cent. Bränemark's original work has been replicated in many other centres around the world and the reliability of the technique confirmed. The technique involves the placement of up to six implants, or fixtures, in the edentulous jaw followed by a period of several months in which the fixtures are completely buried. During this time, an intimate relationship develops between the alveolar bone and the implant which is described as osseo-integration. The implants are then uncovered and the superstructure, which may be a bar to which the denture will clip, is attached to provide support and retention for the denture. Alternatively, a denture can be supported and retained by stud attachments which themselves are fixed to the implants (Figure 8.9). As a result of the success of the Bränemark system, there has been an explosion of interest in implants. A large number of alternative designs of implant have recently been marketed. Some follow Bränemark's principles closely while others differ in various ways – for example, by omitting the buried period and loading the implants with the dentures as soon as the implants

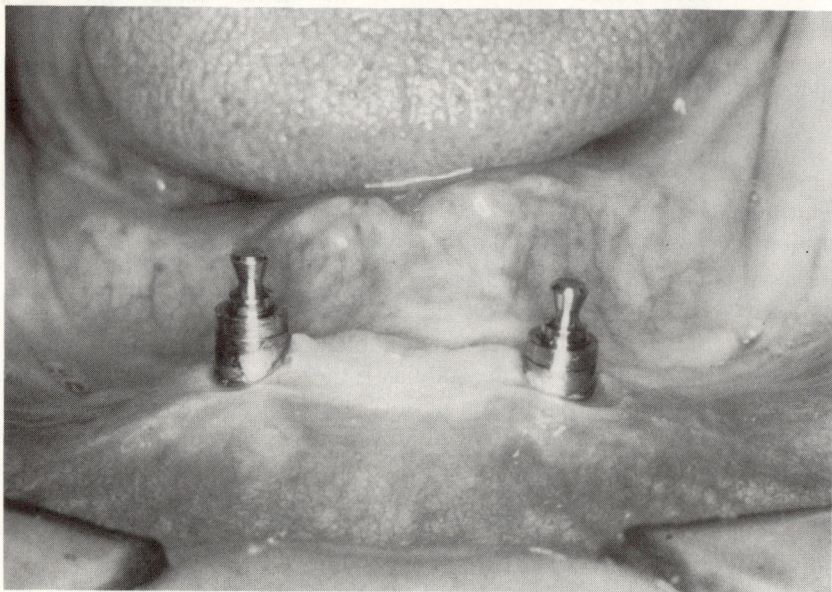

Figure 8.9   Titanium osseo-integrated implants carrying stud attachments which will support and retain a lower denture

have been inserted, or by using different implant materials such as ceramics. In the latter instance, a form of ankylosis is claimed through chemical bonding of bone to the implant surface. An example of this approach is the hydroxylapatite-coated implant. Some of the new designs have been introduced in a less controlled fashion than in Bränemark's original study so that accurate assessment of their relative success will, in some cases, be difficult.

CONDITIONS INVOLVING THE BONE

Pathology within the Bone

The presence of a sinus, a localised swelling or an irregularity in ridge shape leads one to suspect the existence of pathology within the bone. Such clinical evidence necessitates the taking of radiographs to confirm or refute the suspicion.

Whether or not full-mouth radiographs should be taken routinely is debatable. The hazards associated with exposure to X-rays should always be borne in mind. However, the dosage required to carry out a full-mouth radiographic investigation of an edentulous patient can be kept to a minimum by using pantomographic radiography. The dosage in this case is about one-quarter of that received when taking an equivalent series of intra-oral radiographs. Radiographic surveys have revealed the presence of such items as unerupted teeth, retained roots and dental cysts in 30–40 per cent of edentulous patients. One should qualify this finding with the knowledge that only a small percentage of such patients require surgical treatment. For example, if an unerupted tooth is deeply embedded in healthy bone with no associated pathology evident, future complications are unlikely. Surgical removal is not only therefore unnecessary but would involve a considerable loss of alveolar bone. On the other hand, a tooth or tooth fragment lying close to the surface should always be removed because the pressure from a denture is likely to induce resorption of the overlying bone so that the tooth or fragment is exposed to the oral cavity (Figure 8.10).

Sharp and Irregular Bone

Where sharp spicules of bone are present on the crest of a ridge which is covered by thin atrophic mucosa, pain may be produced by pressure from a denture. One reason for the presence of the sharp spicules is that insufficient care was taken when the teeth were extracted, such as the

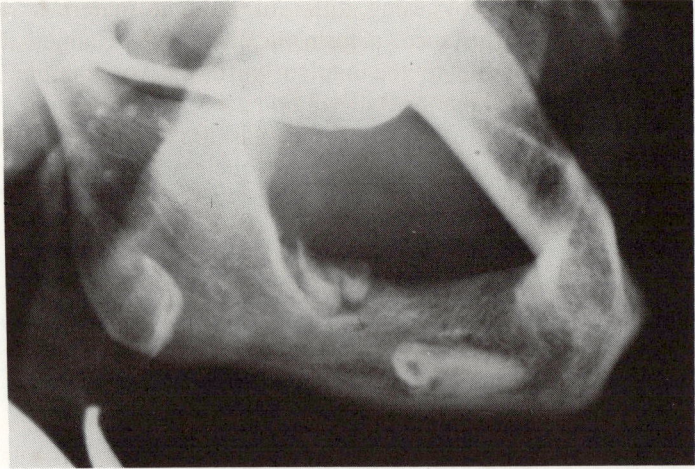

Figure 8.10   A radiograph showing a tooth deeply embedded in bone and a root on the surface. Before making complete dentures, removal of the root is essential: the tooth however should be left undisturbed

failure to compress the sockets adequately. Another possible reason is irregular bone resorption resulting from previous periodontal disease. The most common areas for these spicules to occur is in the lower anterior region (Figure 8.11).

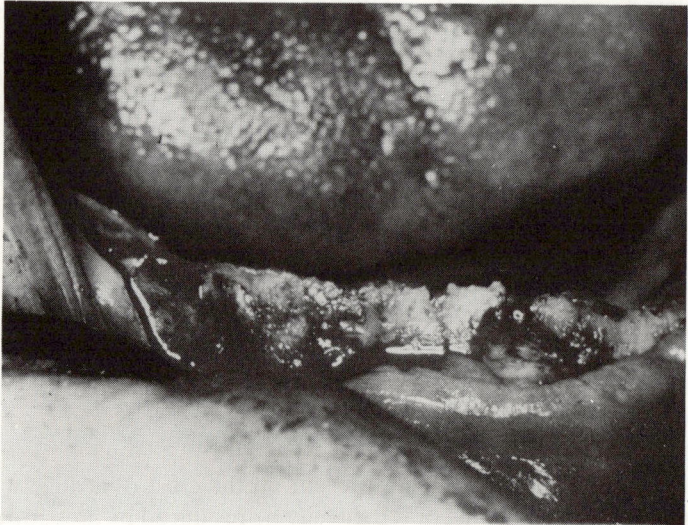

Figure 8.11   A sharp, irregular bony ridge is revealed following reflection of the mucoperiosteum

In some cases, the insertion of a short-term resilient lining material into an existing denture is sufficient to relieve the symptoms; if this occurs, the material can be replaced by a permanent soft-lining material of either silicone rubber or soft acrylic resin.

Frequently, however, it is necessary to smooth the bone surgically. A conservative approach to bone removal is recommended, as in many cases excessive resorption has already occurred and little ridge remains.

Another condition of the bone which may cause discomfort to the patient is the presence of a prominent or sharp-mylohyoid ridge. When the alveolar process is fully developed, the mylohyoid ridge is far down in the lingual sulcus, but when the teeth are lost and the associated alveolar process is resorbed the ridge comes to lie within the denture-bearing area. As the mylohyoid ridge, however, remains functional as a muscle attachment, it is not resorbed and therefore becomes progressively more prominent with increasing age. Thus, discomfort may be caused by a denture exerting pressure on the thin layer of mucosa covering this sharp bony ridge. In some cases, the insertion of a soft lining into the denture gives comfort, but in extreme cases surgery may be necessary. This approach to treatment is also useful in dealing with the similar problems posed by prominent genial tubercles.

Undercut Ridges

If ridges are grossly undercut, insertion of a denture may be impossible without extensive cutting back of the flange and consequent loss of retention (Figure 8.12). To avoid this problem, surgical reduction of the undercut may be necessary. In some instances, the reduction can be carried out unilaterally so as to allow the denture to be rotated into position (Figure 4.9).

Prominent Maxillary Tuberosities

These may be composed of either fibrous tissue or bone and may be so large as to eliminate virtually the interalveolar space. In extreme cases, it is impossible for fully extended denture bases to be accommodated without surgical reduction of the offending tuberosities.

If the enlarged tuberosities consist mainly of fibrous tissue, it may be advisable to use a mucostatic impression technique in order to avoid their distortion.

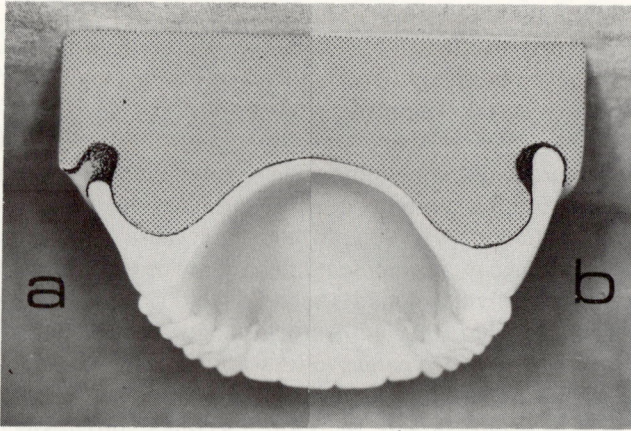

Figure 8.12 If bilateral bony undercuts are not treated, a denture can be fitted only if the flange is extensively cut back (a), or by ensuring that a fully extended flange does not enter the undercut area (b)

Tori

Mandibular tori usually occur bilaterally on the lingual aspect of the mandible, frequently in the premolar region, and are situated close to the mucosal reflection in the lingual sulcus (Figure 8.13). Their presence may make it difficult to provide comfortable dentures as the border of the denture readily traumatises the mucosa overlying the bony protuberances. In such instances, surgical removal of the tori may be necessary.

The presence of a palatine torus which is covered by a thin layer of mucosa may lead to problems of discomfort, instability and mid-line fracture of the upper denture (Figure 8.13). These difficulties are discussed further on page 179. When the palatine torus is very large, or even undercut, surgical removal is indicated.

BIBLIOGRAPHY

Abelson, D. C. (1985) Denture plaque and denture cleansers. *Gerodontics*, **1**, 202–6.

Albrektsson, T., Zarb, G., Worthington, P. and Eriksson, A. R. (1986) The long-term efficacy of currently used dental implants: a review and proposed criteria of success. *International Journal of Oral and Maxillofacial Implants*, **1**, 11–25.

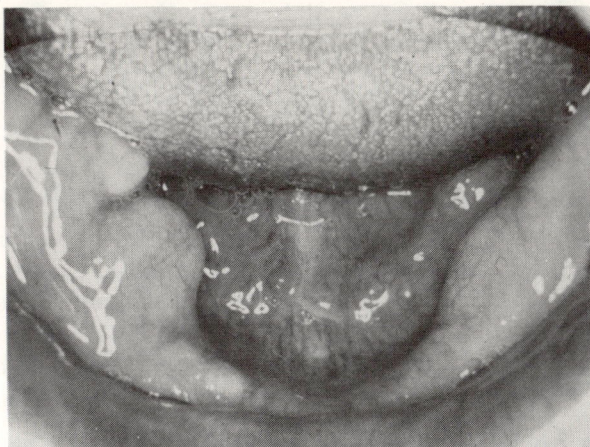

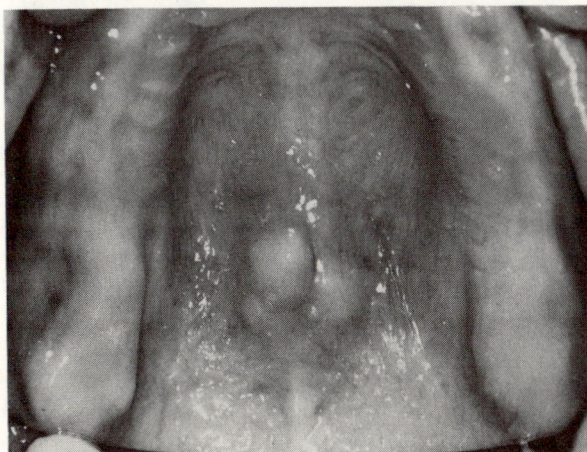

Figure 8.13 Prominent tori. *Top*: Bilateral mandibular tori situated lingually in left and right premolar areas. *Bottom*: A palatine torus

Arendorf, T. M. and Walker, D. M. (1979) Oral candidal populations in health and disease. *British Dental Journal*, **147**, 267–72.

Arendorf, T. M. and Walker, D. M. (1987) Denture stomatitis; a review. *Journal of Oral Rehabilitation*, **14**, 217–27.

Bastian, R. J. (1982) Denture stomatitis. In: *Biocompatibility of Dental Materials*, Vol. 4. D. C. Smith and D. F. Williams (eds). CRC Press, Florida. Chapter 7, 135–50.

Bergendal, T. (1982) Status and treatment of denture stomatitis patients – a 1 year follow-up study. *Scandinavian Journal of Dental Research*, **90**, 227–38.

Bergendal, T., Hiemdahl, A. and Isacsson, G. (1980) Surgery in the treatment of denture-related inflammatory papillary hyperplasia of the palate. *International Journal of Oral Surgery*, **9**, 312–19.

Black, G. V. (1885) Sore mouth under plates. *Dental Items of Interest*, **7**, 492.

Bränemark, P.-I., Zarb, G. A., Albrektsson, T. (eds) (1985) *Tissue Integrated Prostheses*. Quintessence, Chicago/London.

Brook, I. M. and Lamb, D. J. (1987) Treatment of denture-induced hyperplasia. *Dental Update*, **14**, 288–95.

Brown, D. (1988) Resilient soft liners and tissue conditioners. *British Dental Journal*, **164**, 357–60.

Budtz-Jørgensen, E. (1974) The significance of *Candida albicans* in denture stomatitis. *Scandinavian Journal of Dental Research*, **82**, 151–90.

Budtz-Jørgensen, E. (1981) Oral mucosal lesions associated with the wearing of removable dentures. *Journal of Oral Pathology*, **10**, 65–80.

Cawson, R. A. (1963) Denture sore mouth and angular cheilitis. *British Dental Journal*, **115**, 441–9.

Davenport, J. C. (1970) The oral distribution of Candida in denture stomatitis. *British Dental Journal*, **129**, 151–6.

Davenport, J. C. (1972) The denture surface. *British Dental Journal*, **133**, 101–5.

Hobo, S., Ichida, E. and Garcia, L. T. (1989) *Osseointegration and Occlusal Rehabilitation*. Quintessence, Tokyo.

Hopkins, R. (1987) *A Colour Atlas of Pre-prosthetic Surgery*. Wolfe, London.

Hopkins, R., Stafford, G. D. and Gregory, M. C. (1980) Preprosthetic surgery of the edentulous mandible. *British Dental Journal*, **148**, 183–8.

Keur, J. J., Campbell, J. P. S., McCarthy, J. F. and Ralph, W. J. (1987) Radiological findings in 1135 edentulous patients. *Journal of Oral Rehabilitation*, **14**, 183–91.

Lamey, P. J. and Lewis, M. A. O. (1989) Oral medicine in practice: angular cheilitis. *British Dental Journal*, **187**, 15–18.

MacFarlane, T. W. and Helnarska, S. J. (1976) The microbiology of angular cheilitis. *British Dental Journal*, **140**, 403–6.

Moore, T. C., Smith, D. E. and Kenny, G. E. (1984) Sanitization of dentures by several denture hygiene methods. *Journal of Prosthetic Dentistry*, **52**, 158–63.

O'Driscoll, P. M. (1965) Papillary hyperplasia of the palate. *British Dental Journal*, **118**, 77–80.

Olsen, I. (1974) Denture stomatitis – occurrence and distribution of fungi. *Acta Odontologica Scandinavica*, **32**, 329–33.

Ralph, J. P. and Stenhouse, D. (1972) Denture-induced hyperplasia of the oral soft tissues. *British Dental Journal*, **132**, 68–70.

Samaranayake, L. P. (1986) Nutritional factors and oral candidosis. *Journal of Oral Pathology,* **15**, 61–5.

Samaranayake, L. P. and MacFarlane, T. W. (1981) A retrospective study of patients with recurrent chronic atrophic candidosis. *Oral Surgery, Oral Medicine and Oral Pathology*, **52**, 150–3.

Theilade, E. and Budtz-Jørgensen, E. (1988) Predominant cultivable microflora on removable dentures in patients with denture-induced stomatitis. *Oral Microbiology and Immunology*, **3**, 8–13.

Smith, J. M. and Sheiham, A. (1979) How dental conditions handicap the elderly. *Community Dentistry and Oral Epidemiology*, **7**, 305–10.

Williamson, J. J. (1972) Diurnal variation of *Candida albicans* counts in saliva. *Australian Dental Journal*, **17**, 54–60.

9 Impressions

A denture is constructed on a cast of the denture-bearing tissues. Before this cast can be made, an impression, or negative likeness, of these tissues is obtained. The impression material, which is held against the tissues and supported by an impression tray, exhibits plastic flow in the initial stages and then subsequently hardens or sets. Either plaster of Paris or model stone is then poured into the impression to form the cast, or positive likeness, of the denture-bearing tissues.

If maximum accuracy of the casts is to be achieved, a two-stage impression procedure is required. First, preliminary impressions are taken using stock 'off the peg' impression trays and second, the more accurate working impressions are taken using special trays which have been 'tailor made' for a particular patient on casts obtained from the preliminary impressions.

THE DENTURE-BEARING AREAS

The surface anatomy of the denture-bearing areas is illustrated in Figures 9.1 and 9.2.

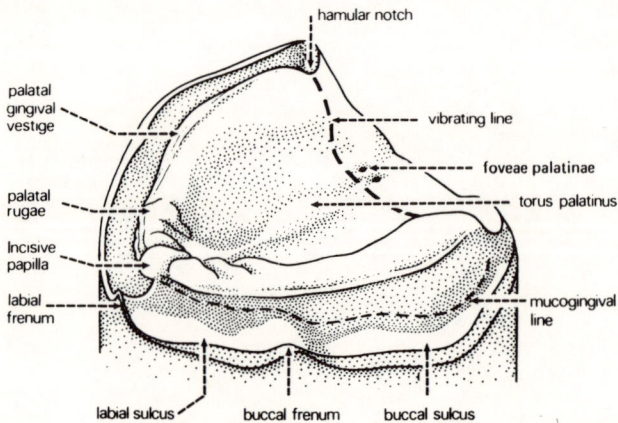

Figure 9.1   Surface anatomy of the upper denture-bearing area. The vibrating line indicates the normal posterior extension of the upper denture.

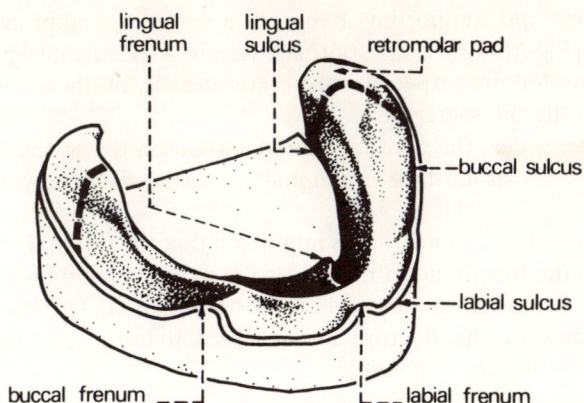

Figure 9.2 Surface anatomy of the lower denture-bearing area. The heavy dotted line indicates the normal posterior extension of the lower denture

The upper denture is normally extended posteriorly to the vibrating line which is the junction between the moving tissues of the soft palate and the static tissues anteriorly (Figure 9.3). Two small depressions in the mucosal surface, the foveae palatinae, common collecting ducts from minor salivary glands, are often seen in this region and are therefore a useful landmark for this junction.

The fibrous band running along the residual ridge is the vestige of the palatal gingivae and, like the incisive papilla, remains relatively constant in position following extraction of the natural teeth. These two structures can therefore be used as landmarks allowing teeth and flanges on complete dentures to be placed in positions similar to those of their natural

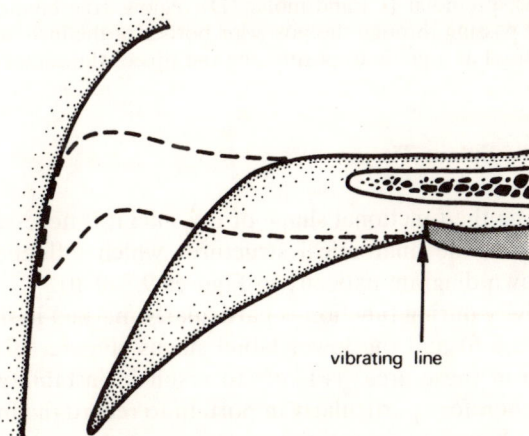

Figure 9.3 Longitudinal section through the palate showing correct relationship of the posterior border of the upper denture to the junction between the moving and static tissues (vibrating line)

predecessors and supporting bone, if a biometric approach is to be employed (Figure 9.4). This approach requires specific design features to be incorporated into special trays – for details of these the reader is referred to the bibliography.

In the lower jaw, the denture should extend on to the retromolar pads. These pads act as buttresses helping to resist distal movement of the denture.

As explained in Chapter 4, it is important that the borders of the denture conform to the functional form of the sulci so that a good facial seal can be produced and maximum physical retention obtained. The broad coverage of the tissues by the denture also ensures that the occlusal loads are distributed as widely as possible.

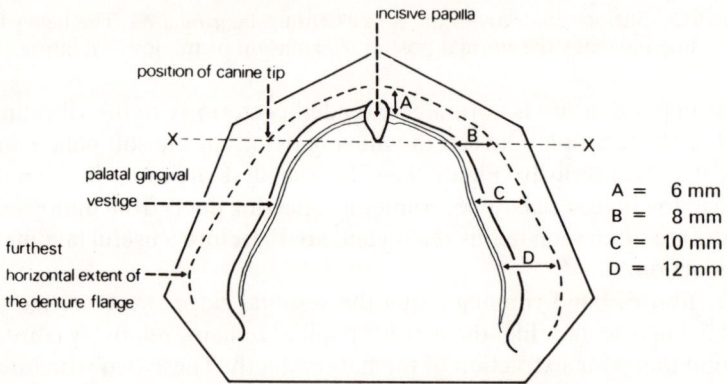

Figure 9.4   Diagram of the upper arch showing average distances from the palatal gingival vestige of the furthest horizontal extent of the denture flange in the incisal (A), canine (B), premolar (C) and molar (D) regions (the biometric approach). The line (X/X) passing through the posterior border of the incisive papilla can be used as a guide to positioning the tips of the canines

Anatomy of the Sulcus Tissues

When recording the functional shape of the sulci it is necessary to have an understanding of the anatomical structures which influence this shape. These are shown diagrammatically in Figures 9.5–9.10.

Muscle activity during function is particularly marked in the floor of the mouth (Figure 9.6) and the lower labial sulcus (Figure 9.7). Even slight overextension in these areas is likely to result in instability of the lower denture. It is therefore particularly important to record the functional form of the sulcus when the associated muscles are contracted.

The area of strong muscle activity in the lower labial sulcus is bounded distally on each side by the modiolus, a decussation of muscle fibres at the

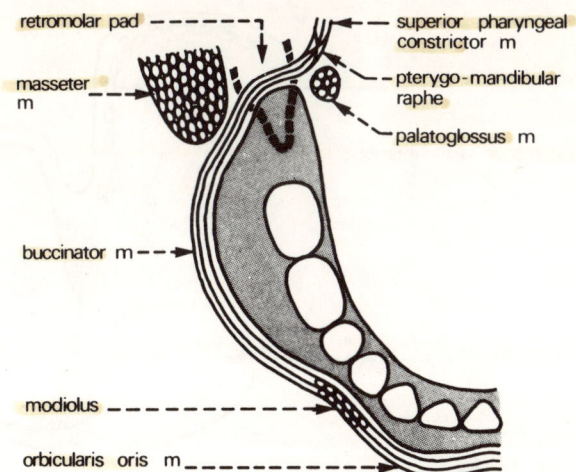

Figure 9.5   The buccal and distal anatomical relations of the lower denture

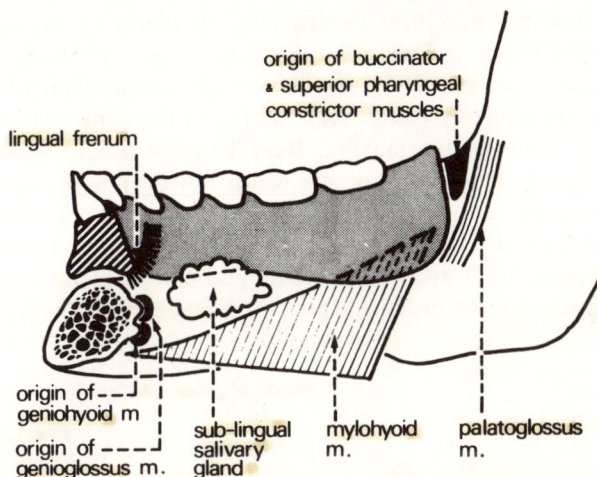

Figure 9.6   The lingual anatomical relations of the lower denture

corner of the mouth (Figure 9.8). Narrowing of the lower denture base related to the modiolus is usually necessary to avoid displacement. The muscles contributing to the modiolus are able to move or fix the corner of the mouth in any required position during function. For example, approximation of the modiolus to the buccal surface of the denture closes the buccal sulci anteriorly during mastication, so helping to contain the bolus of food as it is being crushed between the posterior teeth.

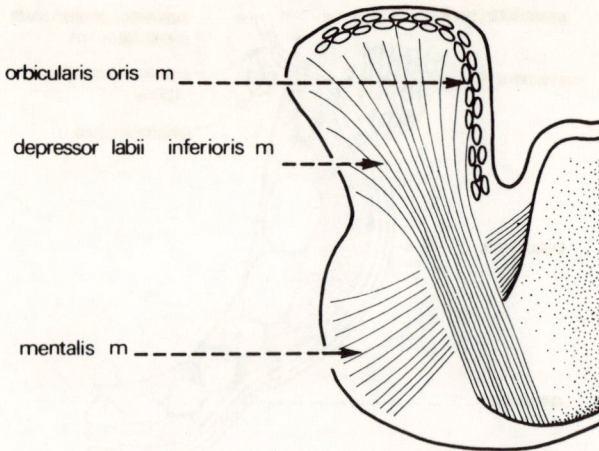

Figure 9.7   Section through the lower lip showing the muscles which influence the shape of the labial sulcus

The anatomical structures determining the form of the sulcus in the upper jaw are shown in Figure 9.9. Particular care must be taken to avoid vertical overextension in the first molar region as mucosal injury may result from a sandwiching of the soft tissues between the denture border and the zygomatic process of the maxilla. Buccal to the tuberosities, the sulcus often reaches its deepest point; its width however is reduced when the mouth is opened because of the close proximity of the coronoid process of the mandible. If the buccal flanges of the eventual denture are too wide posteriorly, they will either restrict mandibular opening or will be displaced by the coronoid process. Thus, the borders of the impression in this

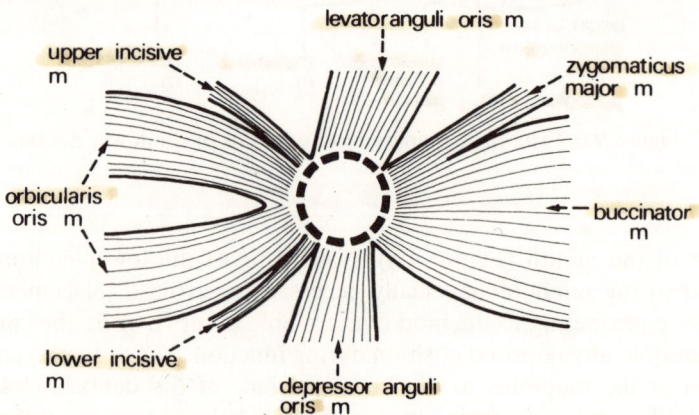

Figure 9.8   The muscles contributing to the modiolus (dotted circle)

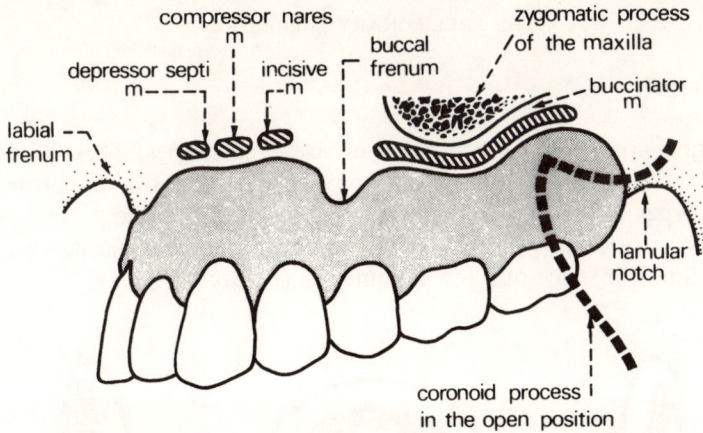

Figure 9.9   The buccal anatomical relations of the upper denture

region should be moulded to the correct width by the patient moving the mandible from side to side when the mouth is open.

A certain amount of lateral displacement of the buccinator muscle by the denture in other areas can occur without causing instability of the denture, and, in fact, is desirable as it will increase physical retention by improving the facial seal (Figure 9.10).

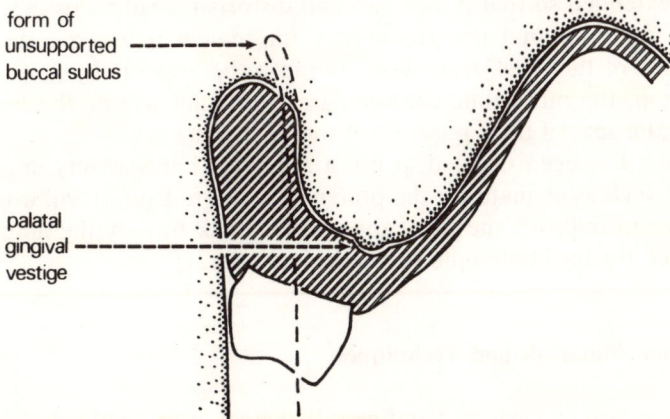

Figure 9.10   Lateral displacement of the buccinator muscle by the denture to improve facial seal

THE PRELIMINARY IMPRESSION

Stock Trays

Stock trays are available in a range of sizes and shapes. These trays are constructed in metal or plastic and may be perforated or unperforated. Certain types of plastic trays are intended to be disposable.

Ideally, a stock tray should cover the entire denture-bearing area and allow a uniform space of a few millimetres (Figure 9.11).

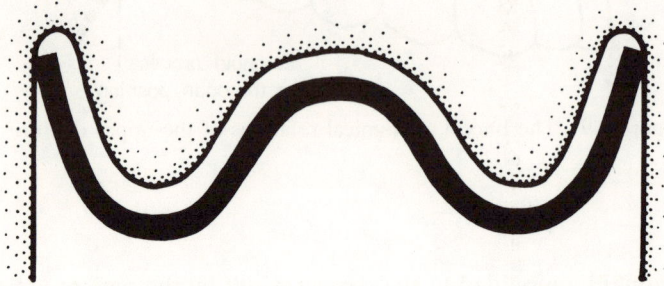

Figure 9.11   The ideal relationship of a stock tray to the sulci and denture-bearing mucosa

However, as the range of sizes and shapes of stock trays is limited and the shape of the denture-bearing areas so varied, the fit of the tray is often less than perfect. The tray may be too wide or too narrow; it may not cover the denture-bearing tissues posteriorly; the tray flange may be under-extended, finishing short of the mucosal reflection in the sulcus, or may be overextended so that it digs into and distorts the sulcus tissues.

It is important that the preliminary impression is as accurate as the limitations of the stock tray allow, because the greater the faults in this impression, the more time consuming and difficult will be the modifications of the special trays required at the next visit.

When it has been decided to use a relatively low viscosity impression material such as alginate for the preliminary impression, it will usually be necessary to improve the fit of the chosen stock tray by the addition of greenstick tracing compound or wax (Figure 9.12).

Impression Materials and Techniques

As even a correctly selected and modified stock tray is unlikely to have a perfect relationship to the denture-bearing tissues, it is preferable for the chosen impression material to have a relatively high viscosity as this allows

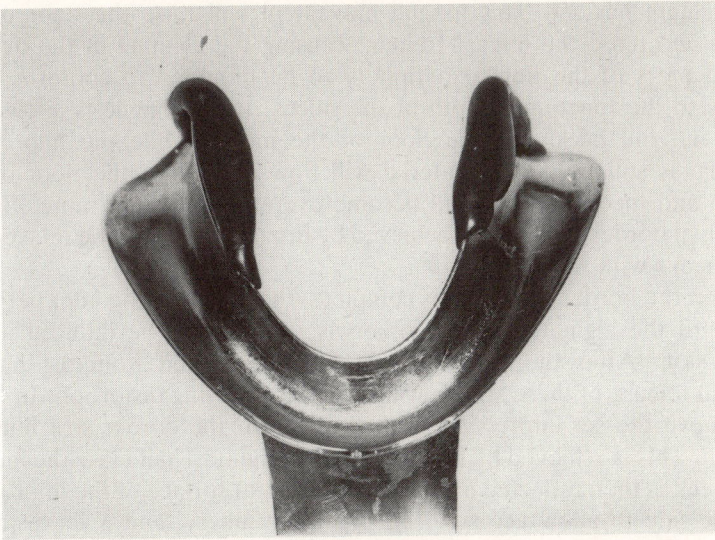

Figure 9.12   Stock trays are frequently underextended in the lingual pouches. Correct extension has been achieved with greenstick tracing compound

it to compensate better for the shortcomings in fit and extension of the stock tray.

Alginate

Alginates vary considerably in their viscosity. A high viscosity type is preferable for preliminary impressions. The limitations of alginates, which are discussed later in this chapter, are not so critical for preliminary impressions as they are for working impressions, because the degree of accuracy required for the preliminary cast on which the special tray is constructed is not as great as that needed for the master cast on which the denture will be made.

Alginate does not adhere to the tray surface and so retention should be provided by using a perforated tray or an adhesive. Perforations allow alginate to flow through and 'rivet' the body of the impression to the tray. If adhesive is used, it should be applied thinly to the entire inner surface of the tray and also carried over the peripheries to include a few millimetres of the outer surface. Time should be allowed after application of the adhesive for it to become tacky. To ensure that the optimum properties of the alginate are realised, the manufacturer's recommendations regarding the powder:water ratio, working time and setting time should be adhered to and great care taken to spatulate the alginate thoroughly.

When taking the lower impression, the patient is asked to raise the tongue to contact the upper lip and to sweep the tongue to touch each cheek in turn before returning to maintain contact with the upper lip until the alginate has set. This tongue movement will raise the floor of the mouth and tense the lingual frenum, causing the alginate in the overextended parts of the lingual periphery to be moulded to conform more closely to the functional depth of the sulcus. If the tongue is allowed to relax and fall back into the floor of the mouth while the impression material is still fluid, the material will flow down into the floor of the mouth and the impression will become overextended once more. Buccal and labial border moulding is achieved by firm stretching of the relaxed lips and cheeks with the fingers.

When the border moulding is complete, the tray must be kept perfectly still until the alginate has set, otherwise strains will be induced in the impression. After the impression has been removed from the mouth, gradual release of these strains will take place causing distortion. In order to remove the set impression from the mouth, the border seal must be broken. This is achieved by first asking the patient to half close the mouth; the cheek is then reflected away from the buccal surface of the impression on one side to allow access of air to the periphery, and a sharp jerk is applied to the tray handle. If the impression is removed slowly, distortion of the alginate is likely to occur. Saliva should be removed from the impression surface by rinsing briefly under a cold tap. Excess water is shaken off and the impression carefully inspected.

If the sulci buccal to the maxillary tuberosities are deep, air may be trapped as the loaded impression tray is inserted. To overcome this problem, these areas should be prepacked with alginate before seating the tray. The tray is first loaded and placed to one side; with the cheek reflected and the patient's mouth half closed, alginate is placed into the buccal sulcus with a spatula or finger. The loaded tray is inserted into the mouth, positioned over the ridge and seated using sufficient pressure to cause the alginate to flow and record the shape of the tissues. Excess alginate will flow into the sulci producing an overextended impression. This overextension must be corrected by carrying out border moulding.

All the denture-bearing area should have been recorded by the completed impression. The surface of the impression should be smooth and show evidence of having been moulded by the tissues (Figure 9.13). The border areas should be rounded and include impressions of the frenal attachments.

The main disadvantage of alginate is its dimensional instability when set. If water is left on the surface of the impression, absorption (imbibition) will take place causing the alginate to swell. If the impression is left in a dry atmosphere, loss of water (syneresis) will occur with consequent shrinkage of the alginate. Thus, a satisfactory impression must be rinsed, disinfected, covered as soon as possible with a damp napkin and placed in a plastic bag. Casts should be poured within 10 minutes of taking the impressions. While the impression is waiting to be poured, it must not be allowed to rest on the

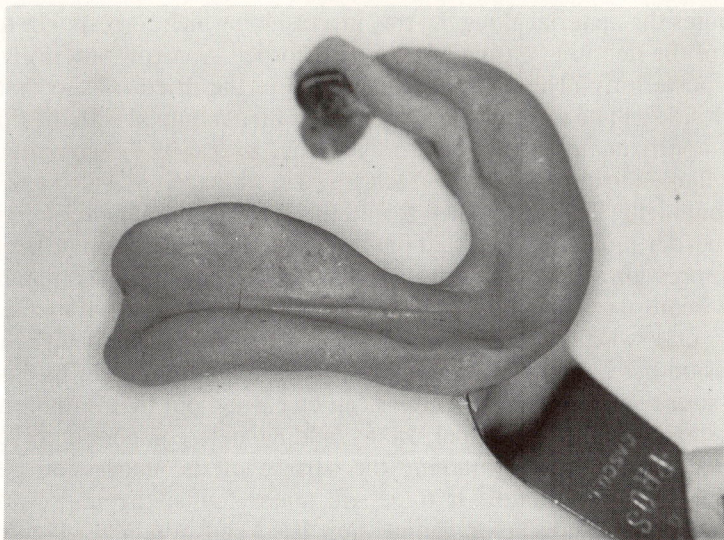

Figure 9.13   A lower impression in alginate showing a border which has been moulded by the adjacent tissues. Correct extension in the lingual pouches has been achieved by suitable extension of the tray (Figure 9.12)

surplus alginate which has flowed over the posterior border of the tray, otherwise distortion is likely to occur.

The dentist must indicate to the technician the type of special tray required for the next appointment. It is essential at this and subsequent clinical stages that written instructions to the technician are clear and comprehensive. Where it is practicable, a discussion with the technician is worth while.

Impression Compound

This is a thermoplastic material which softens when heated in a water-bath to temperatures between 55 °C and 70 °C. The high viscosity of the material and the fact that it becomes rigid when chilled makes it unnecessary to correct any underextensions of a stock tray prior to taking the impression. The compound readily makes up any underextension unaided by additions to the tray.

As the impression compound softens in the water-bath, a portion of sufficient size to take the planned impression is kneaded with the fingers by folding the material inwards from the periphery of the mass to the centre. This produces a smooth, crease-free, surface on one side of the compound; it also improves flow and helps to give the material a uniform consistency.

The lower impression is usually obtained first. The portion of compound is formed into a cylinder and then extended to the length of the tray by pulling on either end. This creates a dumbbell-shaped specimen which distributes the material along the tray in a fashion which corresponds to the width of the denture-bearing area to be recorded – narrow anteriorly and broad posteriorly. The compound is placed in the dried tray so that the smooth side will be towards the tissues and is then moulded with the fingers to the approximate shape of the ridge. The surface of the compound is lightly flamed to improve its flow, tempered in warm water and coated with petroleum jelly. The tray is then seated firmly in the mouth and supported while border moulding is carried out as described for the alginate preliminary impression. However, in this instance, as the impression compound is more viscous than alginate, the moulding must be executed with increased vigour, otherwise overextension of the impression will occur. When the impression has hardened, it is removed from the mouth and inspected. If minor faults are present, corrections can be carried out by trimming away excess material with a scalpel, or by adding new compound to repair deficiencies and then resoftening the surface of the impression before reseating it in the mouth. If there are major faults, the impression is retaken. Once a satisfactory impression has been obtained, it must be thoroughly chilled in cold water.

The impression for the upper jaw is obtained by placing a golf-ball sized portion of softened compound into the centre of a dried tray and preforming it with the fingers to the shape of the ridge and palate. The procedure then is as described for the lower impression.

The completed satisfactory impressions (Figure 9.14) are disinfected before being sent to the laboratory with a clear, comprehensive request for the types of special tray required for the working impressions.

THE WORKING IMPRESSION

Mucostatic and Mucodisplacive Impression Techniques

The dentist's goal when taking working impressions is to record as accurately as possible the shape of the mucosa overlying the alveolar ridges and hard palate together with the functional depth and width of the sulci. There is some disagreement however as to the best method of achieving this goal.

The mucosa overlying the alveolar ridges and hard palate is not of uniform thickness. Consequently, if the dentist uses a mucostatic technique which applies minimal pressure to the tissues, and therefore records their resting shape, there is a possibility that the subsequent distribution of occlusal loads by the finished dentures will be uneven (Figure 9.15). However, as the impression surface of the denture conforms closely to the

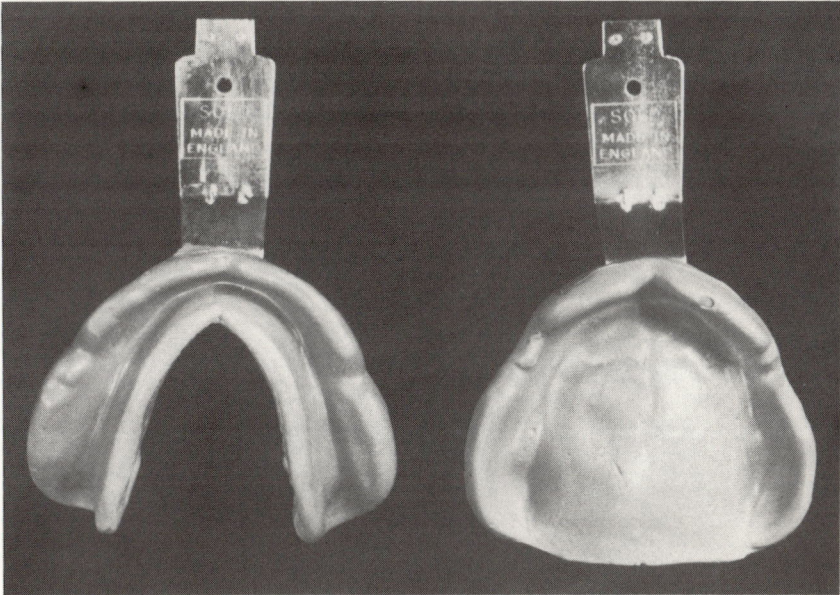

Figure 9.14   Upper and lower impressions taken in impression compound

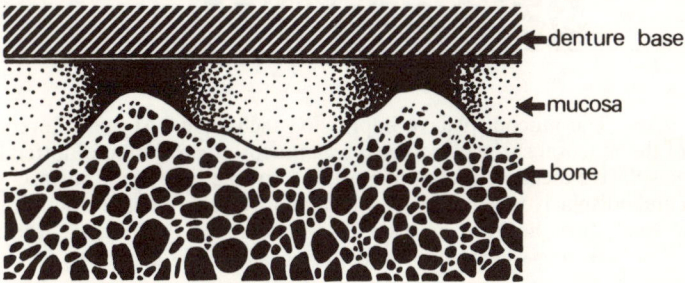

Figure 9.15   Occlusal loads transmitted by the denture to the mucosa will tend to be greatest (dark areas) where the mucosa is thinnest

surface of the underlying mucosa, both when the denture is under load and when it is not, physical retention will be optimal.

The alternative approach, a mucodisplacive technique, is to apply pressure to the mucosa during the impression-taking procedure so that the shape of the tissues under load is recorded. This approach may have the advantage that occlusal loads are more evenly dispersed over the tissues, but has the disadvantage that the physical retention of the denture when the teeth are apart may be less than that using a mucostatic impression technique (Figure 9.16).

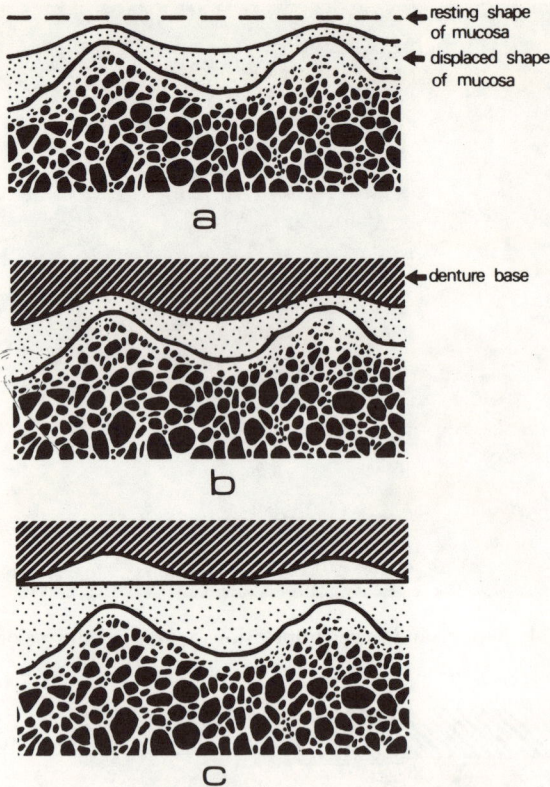

resting shape
of mucosa

displaced shape
of mucosa

a

denture base

b

c

Figure 9.16   The mucodisplacive impression technique: (a) the difference in the shape of the mucosal surface produced by a mucostatic technique (dotted line) and a mucodisplacive technique (continuous line); (b) the impression surface, obtained using a mucodisplacive technique, fits the mucosa closely when the denture is under occlusal load; (c) when the occlusal load is removed the mucosa returns to its resting shape and the denture ceases to fit accurately

Should the mucosa therefore be recorded in its resting state or in its displaced state? In most cases, it will be found that the best results may be most simply obtained by using a mucostatic technique. Pressure on the tissues is reduced as far as possible by using an impression material of low viscosity. Impression plaster, zinc oxide–eugenol paste and low viscosity alginates are examples of suitable materials.

In some patients, a moderate variation in mucosal compressibility may be present and a mucostatic impression, particularly in the case of the lower jaw, results in a denture which distributes the occlusal loads unevenly with consequent mucosal injury and associated discomfort. In this situation, it may be advisable to record the shape of the mucosa in a displaced state by using an impression material of high viscosity. The load applied during the impression-taking procedure should be the same as that occurring during function. A method which fulfils these requirements is known as a functional impression technique and is described on page 118.

Special Trays

In order to avoid permanent distortion of an elastic impression material as it is withdrawn from undercut areas, an adequate thickness of the material is required. The special tray should therefore be constructed on the preliminary cast after a spacer of appropriate thickness has been applied (Figure 9.17).

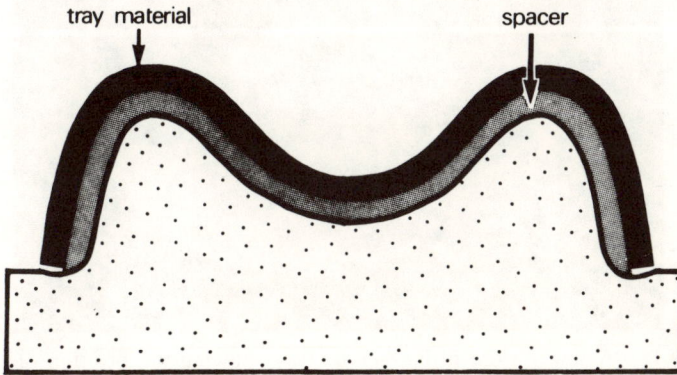

Figure 9.17   A spaced special tray is constructed by adapting the tray material over a spacer which has been applied to the cast

Alginate is the most commonly used elastic impression material for edentulous patients and requires a spacer of about 3 mm. Either cold-curing acrylic resin or aluminium-filled shellac can be used for the construction of this type of tray. Acrylic resin has the advantage of greater rigidity and better dimensional stability than shellac. Problems with the latter material are particularly likely to occur when greenstick tracing compound is used for trimming, as the heat will soften the shellac and allow stress relief. Very thorough chilling of the shellac tray is required after completion of border moulding if this combination of materials is used.

Zinc oxide–eugenol paste is used in thin section and therefore a close-fitting tray is required; cold-curing acrylic resin is indicated for this type of tray, especially in the lower jaw where the denture-bearing area in the anterior region may be quite narrow. The special tray will therefore be thin at this point and, if made of shellac, would distort or fracture during the impression-taking procedure.

A lower acrylic close-fitting tray should have stub handles in the premolar regions to act as finger rests (Figure 9.18). These rests keep the fingers, which stabilise the tray and support the impression, well clear of critical border areas of the impression while it sets. If this is not done, inaccuracies will result from the fingers restricting the border-moulding movements of the soft tissues and displacing excess impression material into the sulci.

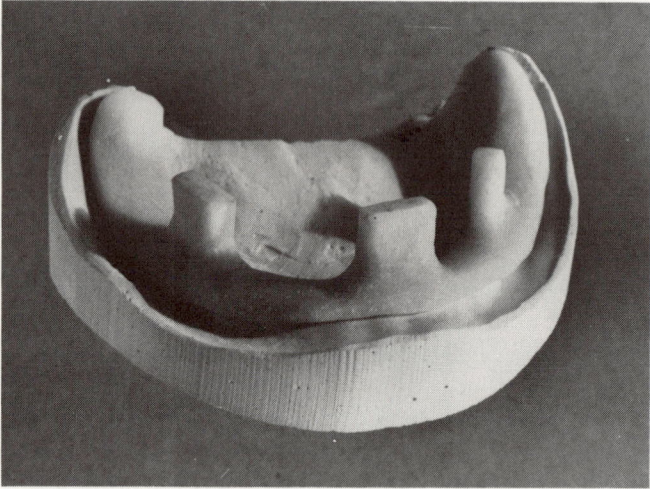

Figure 9.18   A lower close-fitting acrylic tray showing the position of the stub handles

Checking the Special Tray

As a special tray is made on a cast poured from a relatively inaccurate preliminary impression, it will usually be found on checking the tray in the mouth that the periphery does not conform accurately to the shape of the sulcus tissues in all areas. Both overextension and underextension may be present; the former must be corrected by reducing the height of the flange by the appropriate amount and the latter by adding a border-trimming material to the tray to correct the deficiency. Any additions to the tray must be carefully border-moulded by movement of the soft tissues. If overextension of the special tray is not corrected, the sulcus tissues will be stretched and the working impression will be overextended. If this fault is not recognised before the denture is finished, the overextended flange will injure the tissues; in addition, elastic recoil of the displaced sulcus tissues will cause instability of the denture.

If an underextended tray is not corrected, there are two possible sequelae. First, the impression material may not be carried to the full depth of the sulcus and the finished denture will therefore be underextended. The second possibility is that the impression material reaches the full functional depth of the sulcus but is not supported by the underextended tray. When the cast is poured, the weight of the artificial stone will distort the unsupported part of an elastic impression material resulting in a denture which is an inaccurate fit (Figure 9.19).

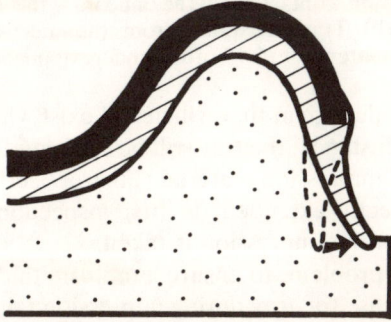

Figure 9.19   Distortion of unsupported elastic impression material by the artificial stone

Border-trimming Materials

There is a variety of materials available for the correction of under-extended impression trays, such as greenstick tracing compound, high viscosity elastomers and cold-curing poly(butylmethacrylate) resin.

Greenstick tracing compound has the advantage over the other types of border-trimming material in that it allows the tray borders to be progressively developed until they are correct. Modifications can be readily made as the material is thermoplastic. The setting of the other materials, on the other hand, is by an irreversible chemical reaction and requires a 'one shot' approach; thus, if the border trimming is deficient at the first attempt the procedure may have to be repeated.

Impression Material and Techniques

Alginate

This material is elastic when set and is therefore indicated where bony undercuts are present.

Whereas high viscosity alginates are indicated for the preliminary impression, they are not recommended for working impressions as they readily cause mucosal displacement, particularly in the border areas.

If an unmodified special tray is tried in the mouth to check its border extension, it will be seated in contact with the underlying mucosa (Figure 9.20(a)). In this position, the borders of the tray bear a different

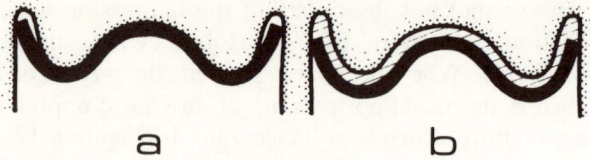

NB

Figure 9.20   (a) Tray in contact with the mucosa – the border appears to be correctly extended. (b) Tray separated from the mucosa by the impression material – tray border underextended

relationship to the sulcus than that which will exist when the impression is taken. In this latter instance, the tray will be separated from the mucosa by a few millimetres of impression material (Figure 9.20(b)). A border which appears to be correctly extended on first inspection may therefore be underextended when the impression is taken.

To overcome this problem, to ensure a uniform thickness of impression material and to stabilise the tray during impression taking, stops should be placed in the tray prior to checking and correcting the borders. These stops are made of greenstick tracing compound. In the lower tray, they are placed in the incisal region and over the retromolar pads, and in the upper tray in the incisal and post-dam regions (Figure 9.21). While the compound is still soft, the tray is seated in the mouth so that the stops are moulded to the ridge tissues providing a space between the tray and the mucosa of 2–3 mm. The border extension of the tray may then be checked. This may be done visually in most areas with the exception of the lingual sulcus, where the tongue obscures the view in the posterior regions, the lingual

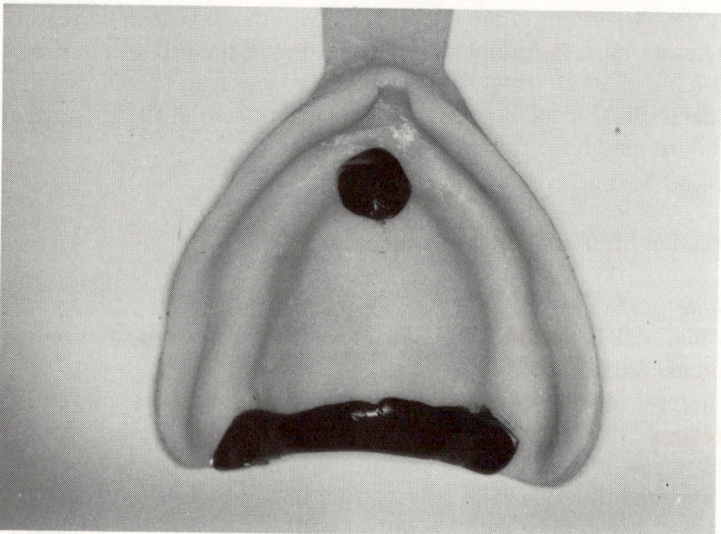

Figure 9.21   An upper-spaced tray showing the position of stops

pouches. Overextension in these regions is present if the tray is displaced upwards when the patient raises the tongue to contact the upper lip. However, as underextension is the more common fault, it is wise to assume its presence if overextension cannot be demonstrated.

If the border is overextended, corrections are made. Underextension may be corrected by adding one of the border-trimming materials. In order to obtain the best possible recording of the lingual sulcus, it is essential to train the patient to make the following tongue movements before making additions lingually to the lower tray. The tip of the tongue is placed in one cheek and then swept round anteriorly to the other cheek. This procedure should be repeated two or three times before the tongue is finally raised to contact the upper lip. The tongue should not be protruded further than the lip as such a movement is rarely used in normal function and only results in an excessive reduction in depth of the lingual flange of the eventual denture. The technique for using greenstick tracing compound is summarised in Figure 9.22. The tracing compound should be applied to one area of the tray border at a time and moulded in the mouth before the next addition is made. If adequate moulding has not been achieved at the first attempt, the overextended compound may be resoftened by using a fine flame and the border moulding repeated. When the adjustment is com-

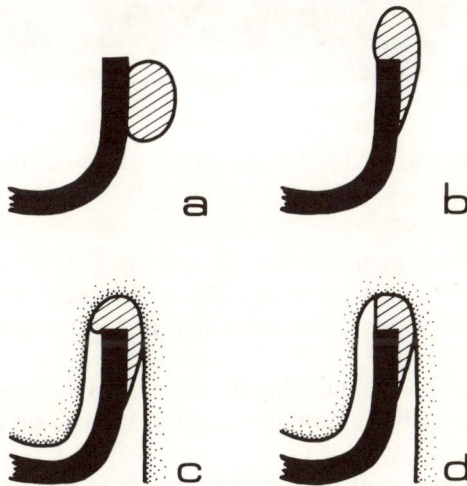

Figure 9.22 A method of applying greenstick tracing compound for correction of underextension: (a) the tracing compound is softened and placed on the outer surface of the tray – sufficient bulk of material should be used to allow a broad area of attachment and to retain heat so that there is an adequate working time for border moulding; (b) the compound is tempered in warm water and moulded with the fingers to produce a flange; (c) border moulding is carried out and then the tray is chilled in cold water; (d) finally, the space between the tracing compound and the alveolar ridge is re-established by removing material with a wax knife

plete, the tracing compound is chilled in cold water. The finished result is shown in Figure 9.23.

With any impression technique, what should be remembered is that common areas of underextension of the upper denture are the posterior border and around the tuberosities, while the lower denture is often underextended in the regions of the retromolar pads and lingual pouches. Whatever technique is used, the greatest care must be taken to ensure that the impression includes these vital areas.

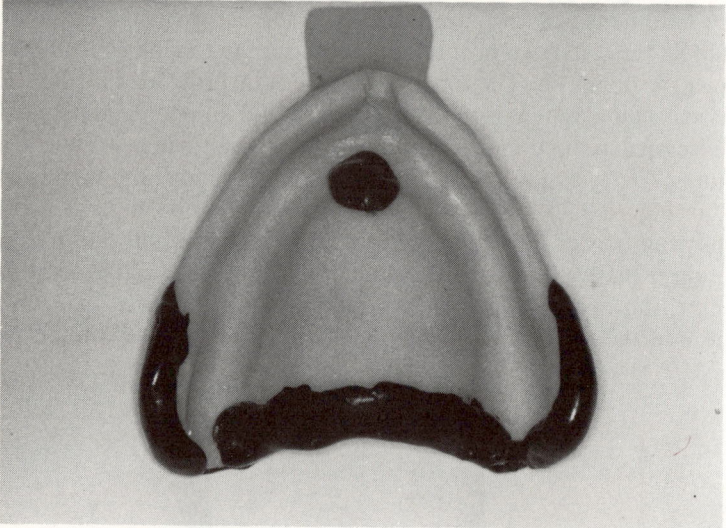

Figure 9.23   Upper tray modified by addition of greenstick tracing compound in underextended areas

If biometric guides, mentioned briefly on page 144, are being followed in the design of a denture, greenstick should be used to extend the tray flanges laterally to support the cheek and lips in the positions shown in Figure 9.4.

The procedures for manipulating the alginate and obtaining the impression are the same as those described for the alginate preliminary impression (page 149).

Figure 9.24 shows a satisfactory impression in which the borders are rounded and well defined. The compound stop shows through the alginate to indicate that the tray has been correctly positioned. It is, of course, important that the shape of the borders is reproduced on the cast. A useful guide is given to the technician by drawing a line on the alginate with indelible pencil 3–4 mm beyond the border of the impression (Figure 9.25). This line is transferred to the cast material and acts as a landmark, preventing overtrimming of the cast which would result in loss of information concerning the functional width of the sulcus (Figure 9.26).

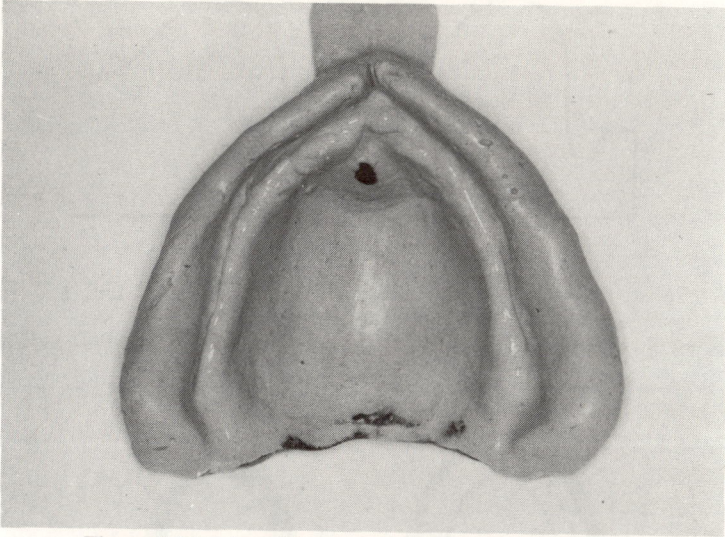

Figure 9.24 A satisfactory upper alginate impression

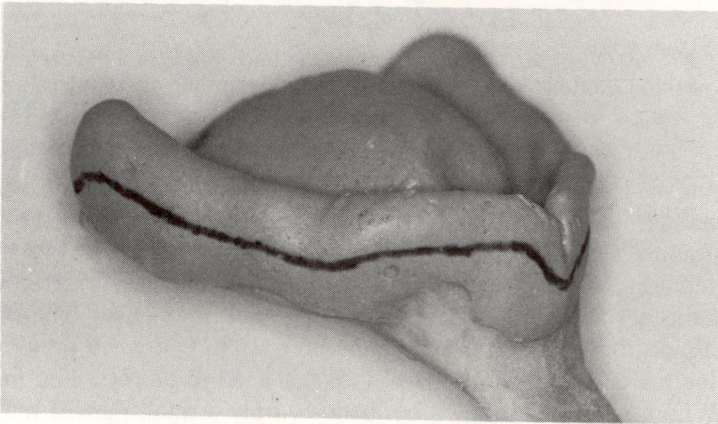

Figure 9.25 An alginate impression showing the position of the indelible pencil line placed as a guide to subsequent trimming of the cast

Zinc Oxide–Eugenol Paste

This material is rigid when set and is dimensionally stable. It is therefore to be preferred to alginate in all cases where there are no bony undercuts. Other advantages of this material accrue from the fact that it is used in a close-fitting tray; the overall bulk of the impression is kept to a minimum and so is better tolerated by the patient; where a sulcus is narrow it is easier to avoid displacement of the buccal mucosa by using a close-fitting rather than a spaced tray (Figure 9.27); if a spaced tray is used to take an impression of a flat lower ridge, it is often very difficult to prevent the mucosa of the floor of the mouth from being trapped beneath the tray.

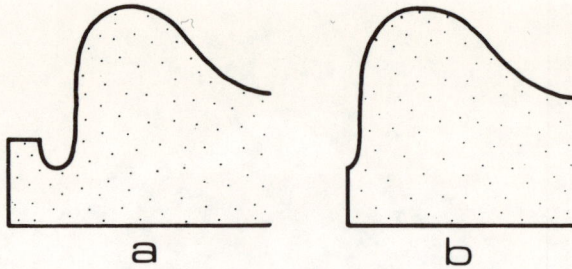

Figure 9.26   Cross-section through (a) a correctly trimmed cast and (b) an overtrimmed cast

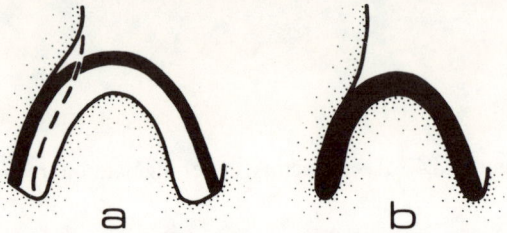

Figure 9.27   (a) A spaced tray may displace the buccal mucosa laterally from its normal position (dotted line). (b) A more accurate recording of the sulcus width is possible with a close-fitting tray

As zinc oxide–eugenol paste is used in a thin film, stops are not added to the special trays. Instead, the borders should be checked with the trays held in contact with the mucosa. Overextension of acrylic trays may be corrected using an acrylic bur while underextension may be corrected using any of the border-trimming materials mentioned previously. The procedure differs from that described for spaced trays in that when the border-trimming material has set, a space does not need to be recreated in that area. Where additions have to be made to only a small part of the tray border, greenstick tracing compound is recommended. When a full border-moulding technique is preferred, greenstick tracing compound can again be used or, alternatively, some saving in chairside time may be gained by adopting the following procedure.

The tray is adjusted so that the border is underextended by 1–2 mm along its entire length. Cold-curing poly(butylmethacrylate) border-trimming material is applied to the tray. In the case of the lower tray, this is most conveniently achieved by filling the entire tray, while in the case of the upper tray the material is added as a thin beading to the border and post-dam region (Figure 9.28). The tray is inserted immediately and border moulding carried out. When the tray is removed from the mouth, it can be placed in hot water to hasten polymerisation of the resin. The impression

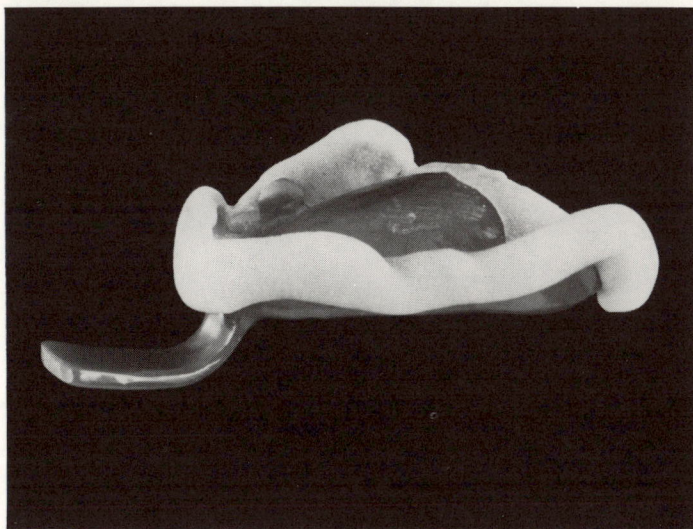

Figure 9.28 An upper close-fitting acrylic special tray with an acrylic border-trimming material added to the borders and post-dam region

surface of the tray should be checked to see if any undercuts are present. If so, they must be removed with an acrylic bur, otherwise when the cast is eventually poured it will lock into these undercut areas and will be damaged when the impression is removed. The tray is then dried and a zinc oxide–eugenol paste impression taken; adhesive is not required for this material. As a guide to the technician when trimming the casts, the width of sulcus to be retained can be indicated by marking the impression with an indelible pencil or by applying a strip of soft wax (Figure 9.29). The completed impression must be disinfected before being sent to the laboratory.

Impression Plaster
This material is rigid when set and is therefore best suited to cases where there are no bony undercuts. It is dimensionally stable. If small bony undercuts are present, plaster may still be used because the material which has entered the undercut area will break off when the impression is removed from the mouth. A spaced special tray should be used so that these fragments are large enough to be relocated accurately and attached to the main part of the impression. Impression plaster has a low viscosity when mixed and is therefore a good material to use when it is important to reduce mucosal displacement to a minimum. However, it is difficult to obtain a satisfactory lower impression in patients who salivate profusely because the saliva mixes with the plaster and a rough, friable surface is produced.

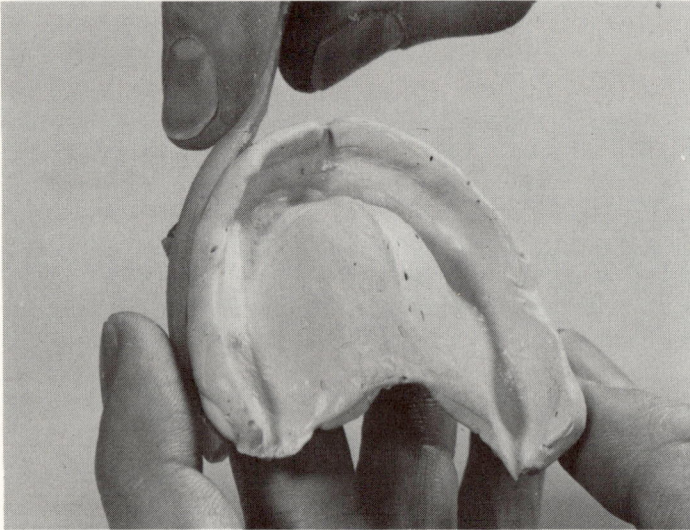

Figure 9.29   An upper zinc oxide–eugenol working impression to which a beading of soft wax is being added to indicate to the technician the depth of the sulcus to be retained on the cast

A measure of powder is sprinkled gradually into a measure of water and then left for a short time to absorb the water before being gently spatulated to a smooth, creamy consistency. The spaced special tray, to which stops have been added, is loaded and then gently puddled, or vibrated, into place in the mouth until it is resting on the stops. Border moulding is completed and the tray supported until the initial set of the plaster has occurred. The point of setting can be monitored by the clinician holding a little of the excess plaster in the hand and testing its consistency from time to time. When the specimen breaks cleanly, it is time to remove the impression. If it is left beyond this stage, the increasing strength of the plaster will make the impression difficult and uncomfortable to remove if the ridges are undercut. The patient should keep the mouth open until the completed impression has been inspected to see if any significant parts have broken off. If they have, they must be carefully recovered from the mouth with tweezers and re-attached to the impression with sticky wax. The limit of model trimming is then indicated on the impression with an indelible pencil, or wax beading (Figure 9.30), and the impression disinfected before being sent to the laboratory.

Elastomers
The elastomers include the polysulphide, polyether, condensation-cured and addition-cured silicone impression materials. They have good elastic recovery and dimensional stability but are relatively expensive, particularly

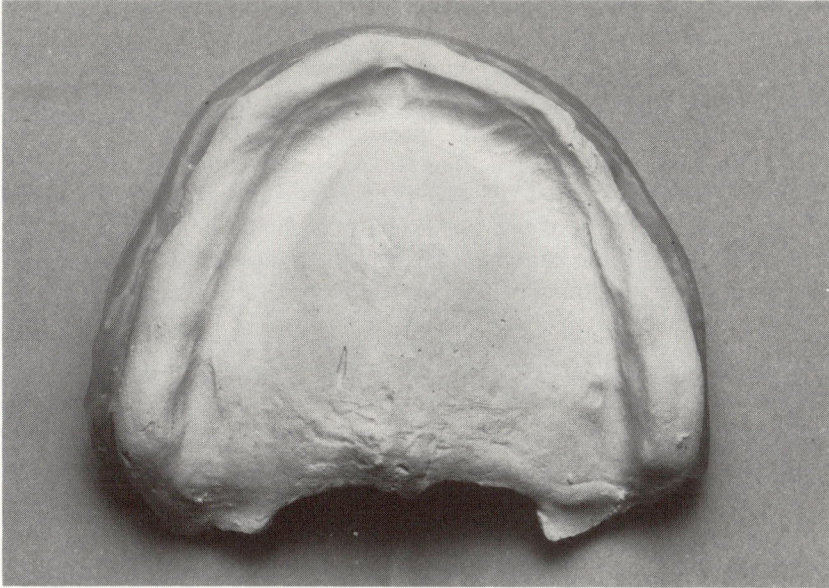

Figure 9.30   Upper impression taken in impression plaster with wax beading added

the addition-cured silicones. In spite of a modest cost penalty compared with alginate and zinc oxide–eugenol impression paste, the condensation-cured silicone materials are becoming increasingly popular for complete-denture impressions. Their wide range of viscosities from heavy-bodied putties to light-bodied perfecting pastes creates a versatile group of materials suitable for a wide variety of clinical applications. These range from the use of putties for border trimming to perfecting pastes for wash impressions. They are clean and easy to handle and have a wide range of working and setting times suitable for most techniques. For example, some materials with an extended setting time are suitable for functional impressions of both the denture-bearing mucosa and the neutral zone. Other materials with short setting times allow a rapid clinical technique and improved patient comfort. The low viscosity silicone materials are suitable alternatives to zinc oxide–eugenol paste for patients with dry mouths, as the latter material can adhere to and irritate the dry mucosa.

Instructions to the Technician

When a satisfactory working impression has been obtained, appropriate instructions to the technician must be carefully considered and recorded on the laboratory prescription. These will include directing the technician's attention to any special requirements for pouring the impression, such as limiting cast trimming to a pencil line or wax beading on the impression. It is worth emphasising in this context that the best prescription for the eventual denture border is an accurately trimmed cast which has been produced from a carefully taken impression (Figure 9.31).

In addition to giving instructions for producing the cast, the clinician must indicate the materials of which the record blocks are to be made. Normally, these consist of wax rims on bases of shellac or acrylic resin. The relative merits of these base materials and the indications for their use are discussed at the beginning of the next chapter.

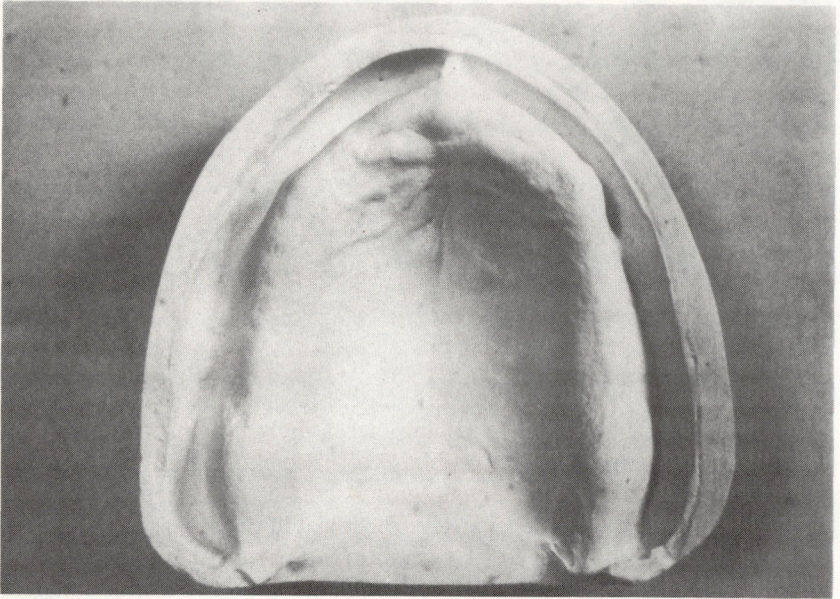

Figure 9.31   Upper cast with the full depth and width of sulci carefully maintained

BIBLIOGRAPHY

Basker, R. M. and Spence, D. (1976) Some properties and clinical uses of a border trimming material. *British Dental Journal*, **140**, 138–42.

Lawson, W. A. (1978) Current concepts and practice in complete dentures. Impressions: principles and practice. *Journal of Dentistry*, **6**, 43–58.

Matthews, E., McIntyre, H., Wain, E. A. and Bates, J. F. (1961) The full denture problem: the Manchester viewpoint. (The impression surface, E. A. Wain). *British Dental Journal*, **111**, 401–18.

Nairn, R. I. (1964) The posterior lingual area of the complete lower denture. *Dental Practitioner and Dental Record*, **15**, 123–30.

Schwarz, W. D. and Braden, M. (1973) Outlining the denture-bearing area: an alternative material. *Journal of Dentistry*, **1**, 179–80.

Shannon, J. L. (1972) The mentalis muscle in relation to edentulous mandibles. *Journal of Prosthetic Dentistry*, **27**, 477–84.

Watt, D. M. (1978) Tooth positions on complete dentures. *Journal of Dentistry*, **6**, 147–60.

Watt, D. M. and MacGregor, A. R. (1976) *Designing Complete Dentures*, W. B. Saunders Co., Philadelphia.

Wilson, H. J. (1966) Elastomeric impression materials. Part 1: The setting material. *British Dental Journal*, **121**, 277–83.

Wilson, H. J. (1966) Elastomeric impression materials. Part 2: The set material. *British Dental Journal*, **121**, 322–8.

Wilson, H. J. (1966) Some properties of alginate impression materials relevant to clinical practice. *British Dental Journal*, **121**, 463–7.

10 Recording Jaw Relations – Clinical Procedures

This chapter describes clinical procedures for recording the jaw relationship of an edentulous patient who has no previous dentures. It is necessary to modify the basic approach when constructing replacement dentures; these modifications are described in Chapter 7.

RECORDING THE REST VERTICAL DIMENSION

In the absence of natural or artificial teeth, it is necessary to determine the rest vertical dimension which will subsequently be used as a point of reference from which the occlusal vertical dimension of the dentures will be derived. Determining the rest vertical dimension is one of the more difficult tasks in dentistry, as indicated by the large number of denture problems which can be attributed to errors in this dimension.

To reduce the chance of error, the first priority is to ensure that the patient is completely relaxed. The patient should sit in a comfortable upright position. External stimuli should be reduced to a minimal level as disturbing noises or a bright light shining in the patient's eyes are likely to increase activity of the mandibular musculature and thus reduce the rest vertical dimension. By adopting a calm unhurried manner, the dentist avoids transmitting a feeling of anxiety to the patient. Relaxation may be further promoted if the patient's eyes are closed, although it is important that the dentist explains what is to be done at the time, otherwise this exercise may achieve quite the opposite effect and induce a state of apprehension. Other ways of coaxing the mandible into the rest position include asking the patient to swallow or to make the sound 'm' before relaxing.

Before making a recording of the rest vertical dimension, the dentist must be satisfied that the patient is truly relaxed. Visual assessment of facial features assists the dentist in judging the progressive development of this state of mind; a measurement should not be made if there are signs of tenseness around the lips, the skin of the chin or around the eyes.

The rest vertical dimension is measured as the distance between two selected points, one related to the upper jaw and one to the lower jaw. Two methods are commonly used to make this measurement, the Willis gauge and the two-dot technique (Figure 10.1). It is most important to appreciate the inherent inaccuracies of both measuring methods and not to rely on the evidence of only one reading. Above all, it should be borne in mind that all clinical methods of measuring the rest vertical dimension are based to a greater or lesser extent on intelligent guesswork.

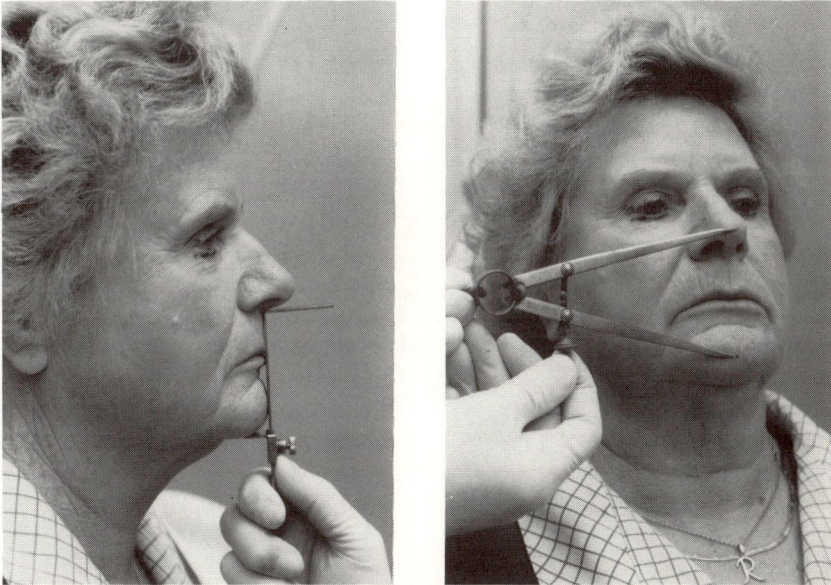

Figure 10.1 Two methods of measuring the rest vertical dimension and the occlusal vertical dimension. *Left*: The Willis gauge. *Right*: The two-dot technique; the distance between the dots is measured with a pair of dividers

In the case of the Willis gauge, three points require attention:

(a) the position of the fixed arm under the nose,
(b) the position of the sliding arm under the chin,
(c) the vertical orientation of the gauge.

If the patient has a well-defined nasolabial angle, the *fixed arm* can be positioned with reasonable accuracy. If the nasolabial angle is obtuse, a small mark may be made on the skin of the upper lip and the fixed arm placed in relation to it (Figure 10.2).

The *sliding arm* should be moved so that it is just touching the undersurface of the chin. If undue pressure is applied to the skin, the position of the mandible will alter. Further inaccuracy arises as it will not be possible to achieve the same degree of compression on subsequent measurements. Inaccuracies may be introduced if the shape of the chin prevents positive location of the sliding arm. This is less likely if the gauge has been previously modified by reducing the length of the arm and modifying its angle (Figure 10.3).

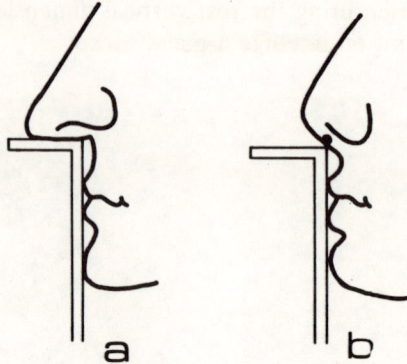

Figure 10.2   (a) The shape of the nasolabial angle allows the fixed arm of the Willis gauge to be accurately located. (b) A location mark may be used where the nasolabial angle is obtuse

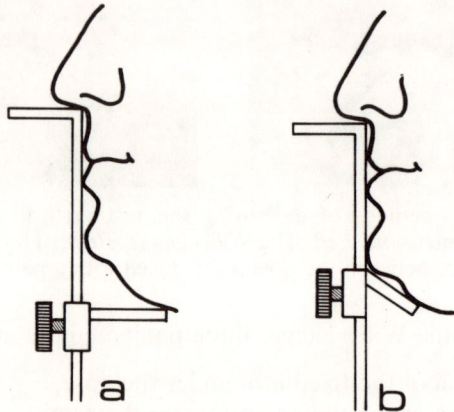

Figure 10.3   (a) Shape of the chin prevents positive location of the sliding arm of the Willis gauge. (b) Sliding arm modified to allow more accurate positioning

The *vertical orientation* of the gauge should be such that the handle is just contacting the skin of the chin in the mental region and that its long axis is in line with the long axis of the face, so that the variation in vertical orientation of the gauge can be kept to a minimum during successive measurements (Figure 10.4). This is difficult to achieve with facial profiles associated with full lips or a severe skeletal class 2 jaw relationship (Chapter 11).

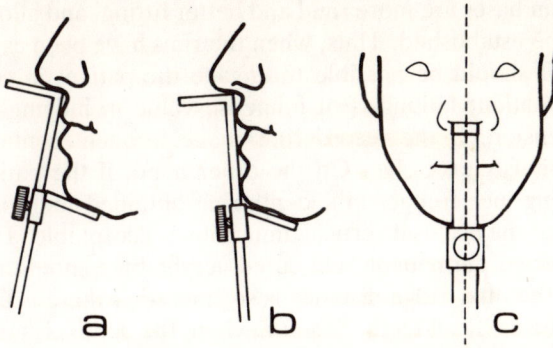

Figure 10.4   (a) Incorrect, and (b) and (c) correct positioning and orientation of the Willis gauge

If the two-dot technique is used, the dot related to the upper jaw is best placed on the tip of the nose and not on the philtrum of the upper lip. The rest vertical dimension is then measured by dividers. This technique has been shown to be particularly subject to error. The cause is usually movement of the dot on the chin due to an inability by the patient to thoroughly relax the muscles of facial expression. A particular complication is that an increase in vertical dimension will not necessarily be associated with a corresponding increase in the distance between the dots. This is because, as the mandible moves further from the maxilla, there is a tendency for the patient to retain a lip seal. The extra muscular effort needed by the lips to achieve this seal pulls the dot on the chin upwards. However, in spite of these limitations, the technique remains a useful one to have in reserve for certain types of facial profile and for bearded patients.

THE RECORD BLOCKS

It is essential that the wax record rims should be placed on well-fitting rigid bases. A non-rigid wax base is likely to change shape during the recording procedure and thus prevent accurate location both in the mouth and subsequently on the casts. Heat-cured acrylic resin, cold-curing acrylic resin and shellac are materials commonly used for the bases. If heat-cured acrylic resin is used, it is common practice for this to become the eventual permanent denture base on which the artificial teeth are processed. In general, it is considered that shellac bases have adequate strength and retention provided they are removed frequently from the mouth, chilled and not subjected to high occlusal forces.

Acrylic resin bases are more rigid and better fitting, and allow maximum retention to be established. Thus, when the rims have been carved to their final shape, it should be possible to engage the patient in conversation. Observing a patient talking is of immense value in judging the occlusal vertical dimension. If the record rims make frequent contact, then the height is obviously excessive. On the other hand, if the patient can talk without making such contacts, the dentist has obtained additional evidence to indicate that the occlusal vertical dimension is acceptable. There are two instances where a permanent heat-cured acrylic base should not be used. First, where the inter-ridge distance is so small that there is little room in which to fit the artificial teeth. Second, where the dentist is uncertain as to the amount of palatal coverage the patient can tolerate. Because the decision on positioning the posterior border has to be taken at the working impression stage, before the heat-cured base is constructed, it is safer to order a shellac base so that modifications can be made in the light of the patient's reactions when the upper record block is placed in the mouth.

There are obviously no such complications in the lower jaw and so a heat-cured acrylic base can be used more frequently. Thus, benefit can be gained from the dual advantages of strength and accuracy of fit which are especially pertinent to problems associated with the smaller denture-bearing area.

Before starting to carve the rims, the record blocks should be placed in the mouth and checked for comfort and retention. A painful sensation may disturb normal mandibular movement, while lack of retention will either force the patient to actively control the blocks, encouraging altered movement patterns, or invoke such a feeling of insecurity that relaxation is not achieved.

THE POST-DAM

The physical forces of retention are created and maintained in the labial and buccal sulci by the intimate contact between the flange of the denture and the mucosa. Obviously, this valve-like seal cannot be produced at the posterior border of the upper denture and so the close adaptation has to be achieved by other means.

A groove is cut into the master cast where the posterior border is to be placed; when the permanent denture base is processed on the master cast, a ridge is consequently created. This projection, the post-dam, compresses the palatal mucosa once the denture is placed in the mouth and thus creates a border seal. At the same time, the polished surface of the denture can be bevelled in this region so that the edge of the denture is not so noticeable to the patient's tongue (Figure 10.5). Because the successful retention of an

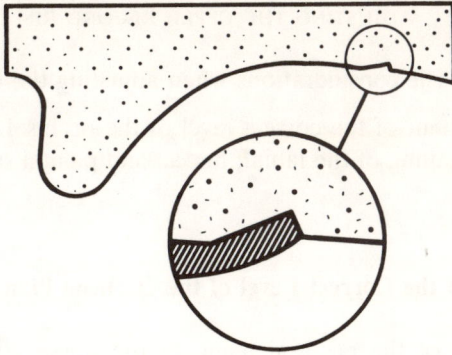

Figure 10.5 The post-dam region of an upper denture. *Inset*: The bevelled polished surface allows the denture to merge with the mucosa

upper record block, as well as the eventual denture, depends upon a post-dam, it is good practice to cut the groove into the cast and then adapt the shellac baseplate into the groove. All this should be carried out before starting to carve the record rim to its correct shape.

The dentist, not the technician, should be responsible for positioning and cutting the post-dam because only he or she can make the two important assessments:

(a) the position of the post-dam,
(b) the depth of the post-dam.

The orthodox position of the post-dam is at the junction of the moving tissues of the soft palate and the static tissues anteriorly. It should extend laterally to the mucosa overlying the hamular notches. If the border of the denture is taken further posteriorly, the patient may well complain of nausea. Furthermore, the continual movement of the soft palate against the posterior border of the denture will result in inflammation and, perhaps, ulceration of the mucous membrane. If the post-dam is placed anteriorly to the junction, it terminates on relatively incompressible tissue. It is then impossible to achieve a reasonable depth to the post-dam and, as a result, the peripheral seal is less efficient.

The depth to which a post-dam can be cut depends upon the compressibility of the mucosa, which may vary across the extent of the posterior border. For example, the mucosa in the mid-line is bound tightly to the underlying periosteum, while along the lateral wall of the palate there is much greater compressibility. Such variation is detected clinically and the depth of the post-dam modified accordingly.

There are two basic considerations when adjusting the upper record rim:

(a) establishment of the correct level of the occlusal plane,
(b) correct shaping of the labial, buccal and palatal surfaces of the wax rim.

Establishment of the Correct Level of the Occlusal Plane

The orientation of the occlusal plane of the upper rim is conveniently judged by using a Fox's occlusal plane indicator (Figure 10.6) or a disposable wooden tongue spatula. The intra-oral part of the instrument rests on the occlusal surface of the record rim while the extra-oral extension allows the clinician to judge the relationship of the plane to the facial guide-lines.

The rim is adjusted so that the occlusal plane is parallel to the interpupillary line, or, alternatively, at right angles to the long axis of the patient's face. A satisfactory guide-line to anteroposterior orientation is the ala-tragal line to which the plane is made parallel (Figure 10.6). If the

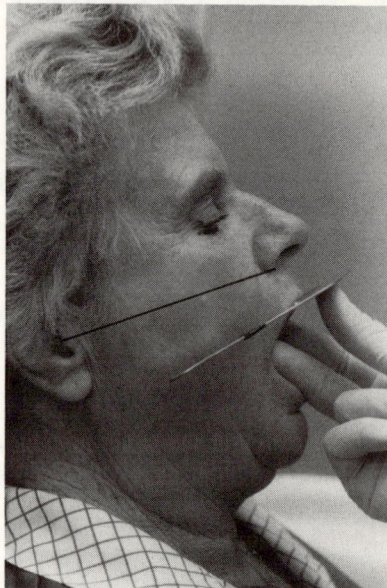

Figure 10.6 A Fox's occlusal plane indicator; the intra-oral portion is held against the occlusal surface of the upper record block; the extra-oral extension allows the clinician to judge the orientation of the occlusal plane with the interpupillary line and with the ala-tragal line. The latter line is superimposed on the figure. It can be seen that, as yet, the orientation of the occlusal plane is not correct

posterior portion of the occlusal plane drops below this line, its inclination is such that, when the dentures occlude, a horizontal component of force encourages the lower denture to slide forwards. In addition, the lower position of the premolar and molar teeth may detract from the aesthetic result.

The incisal level of the upper rim is related to the upper lip, but it is impossible to describe hard and fast rules for determining this relationship. For example, whereas a patient with a long upper lip will show very little of the upper teeth during normal function, the patient with a short upper lip will display more tooth. As a baseline from which to start adjusting the rim, the incisal edges of the upper central incisors can be placed on the same level as the resting lip. As the rim is either reduced or added to, the gross errors in appearance are easy enough to identify. The eventual answer comes as the result of trial and error and by exercising a little visual common sense.

Correct Shaping of the Labial, Buccal and Palatal Surfaces of the Wax Rim

Adequate lip support depends upon the position and inclination of the labial face of the wax rim. As a guide, it is worth bearing in mind that the incisal edges of the upper central incisors can be placed up to 1 cm in front of the centre of the incisive papilla to compensate for the resorption of the alveolar ridge. Once again, an acceptable appearance can be produced by trial and error (Figure 10.7). However, a useful guide-line is that, with the upper lip adequately supported by the record block, the nasolabial angle should be approximately 90°. In fact, the actual angle which is appropriate for a particular patient may deviate from this because of factors such as the nasal profile.

It is, of course, essential that the position of the labial surface is compatible with the stability of the record block. The further forward the rim is placed, the greater will be the displacing force of the lip acting on the labial surface. Also, when the finished denture is worn, the greater will be the displacing force occurring when incising food. It may be necessary to effect a compromise between function and appearance if the prognosis for retention of the upper denture is unfavourable as a result of extensive post-extraction resorption of bone.

The record rim posteriorly should be shaped so that the buccal flange fills the sulcus and slightly displaces the buccal mucosa laterally. This will contribute to retention by achieving an efficient facial seal. The buccal and palatal surfaces of the rim should converge occlusally so that pressure from the cheeks and tongue has a resultant force towards the ridge, thus aiding neuromuscular control. The rim itself will usually be buccal to the crest of the ridge by an amount proportional to the amount of resorption that has

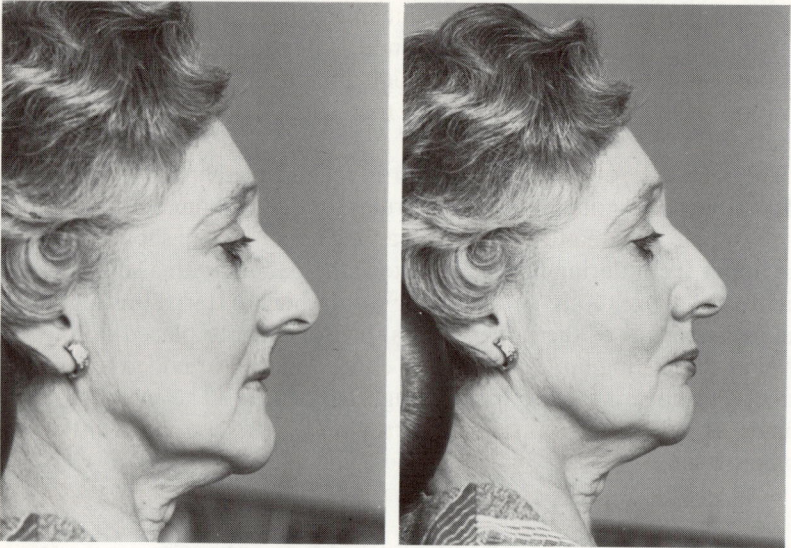

Figure 10.7   *Left*: An upper record block providing inadequate support to the upper lip – the nasolabial angle is obtuse. *Right*: Addition of wax to the labial face of the upper record block providing more support for the upper lip – the nasolabial angle is 90°

occurred. Reference to the biometric guides will help to identify an appropriate position. Care should be taken not to place the rim too far buccally as it will then be outside the neutral zone and increased force from the buccinator muscle will cause displacement. Similarly, it is essential to create adequate space for the tongue by ensuring that the rim is not placed too far lingually and by reducing the width of the rim where necessary by removing wax from the palatal aspect until it corresponds to the width of the artificial teeth which will replace it. If the record block is too bulky, the constriction of the tongue and the resulting abnormal sensory feedback may influence mandibular posture and so lead to inaccuracies in recording the jaw relationship. In addition, speech quality, which can be most valuable in confirming the accuracy of jaw relationship recordings, can only make a contribution to this assessment if the dimensions of the rims are similar to those of the eventual dentures.

ADJUSTING THE LOWER RECORD RIM

The orientation of the occlusal plane has already been established on the upper rim while the overall height of the lower rim will be governed by the existing height of the upper and the need to fit both into the required occlusal vertical dimension. However, the dentist should be prepared to modify the upper occlusal plane if problems arise when shaping the lower. For example, if it becomes increasingly apparent that the lower rim is going to be so high that stability will be poor, or so low that there will be no room for the teeth, then appropriate modifications must be carried out on the upper block.

The first step is to adjust the height of the lower record rim to approximate the required occlusal vertical dimension. The labial, buccal and lingual surfaces of the wax may then be shaped to accommodate the surrounding musculature, because the lower rim will be unstable until it is positioned in the neutral zone. First, it is necessary to ensure that the buccal surface of the wax lies close to the cheek mucosa but that neither buccal nor labial surfaces are placed so far out that they displace the musculature of the lips and cheeks. Second, it is vital to carve the rim on the lingual side to allow adequate tongue space.

When judging the relationship of the rim to the neutral zone, it is important that the tongue takes up a normal resting position forwards in the mouth. Occasionally, the tongue is drawn towards the back of the mouth to adopt a posture which has been aptly described as a 'defensive tongue'. This posture is probably the result of a subconscious wish to guard the pharynx against the foreign body in the mouth. It is impossible to achieve muscular balance with such tongue behaviour and it is necessary, therefore, to coax the tongue to take up its more anterior position before the stability of the record block can be assessed adequately.

Reference was made on page 71 to the change in the mandibular rest position that takes place when a lower denture is inserted into the mouth. The observations are of particular significance at the stage now reached. Once the lower rim has been adapted to the oral musculature and is judged to be an acceptable substitute for the natural teeth and alveolar bone which has been resorbed, it is advisable to recheck the recording of the rest vertical dimension with the lower block in position. If, as may well be the case, the rest vertical dimension is increased, the new reading should be used to calculate the occlusal vertical dimension.

RECORDING THE RETRUDED JAW RELATIONSHIP

If the patient has no dentures to which one can refer, it is acceptable to establish the occlusal vertical dimension approximately 3 mm less than the rest vertical dimension. The freeway space so produced is satisfactory for the vast majority of patients. The next stage is therefore to establish even occlusal contact at the chosen vertical dimension with the mandible in the retruded position. It has been shown that there is least activity in the anterior temporalis, lateral pterygoid and digastric muscles when the patient is in the supine position. It is suggested, therefore, that this position is most suitable for recording the retruded jaw relationship when difficulties are experienced in relaxing the patient or in achieving a constant horizontal jaw relationship. However, it should be remembered that elderly patients may not be comfortable in the supine position and so a more upright position should be adopted.

In addition to placing the patient supine, every effort is made to achieve relaxation, to reduce jaw muscle activity as completely as possible. By adopting a relaxed manner, by gently guiding the mandible and by giving instructions such as 'Close together on your back teeth', the dentist is most likely to encourage the mandible to fall back into its retruded position. An additional procedure which may be of help is to ask the patient to curl the tongue to the back of the mouth and to touch the posterior border of the upper record block. The patient may be assisted in this by placing a small blob of wax in the centre of the posterior border to act as a 'target' indicating to the patient when the tongue is in the correct position.

Initially, the occlusal surface of the lower rim should be thoroughly softened and the patient asked to close together. Closure is stopped when the jaw separation appears to be correct. However, as a means of making the final recording of the retruded position, this method is fraught with danger. Unless the patient is able to close into a surface of equal softness in all areas, there is every chance that contact on a harder portion of wax will compress the underlying mucosa in that area. In addition, contact on the harder wax is likely to initiate an abnormal path of closure. It is necessary therefore to separate the two rims after chilling, cut away the excess wax which has been squeezed out, reinsert the record blocks and check that even occlusal contact has been produced. After any necessary corrections have been carried out, three check lines are drawn with a wax knife from one rim to the other, one in the mid-line and one either side in the premolar regions. These lines enable the blocks to be located outside the mouth to establish whether there is any premature contact on the posterior aspects of the rim. In addition, the check lines allow the clinician to judge whether the patient continues to close in a consistent manner. The patient may be encouraged to make contact in the retruded position if the height of the lower rim is reduced in the incisal region by about 1 mm, to eliminate the possibility of an anterior contact promoting protrusion of the mandible.

Before the rims are finally located, it is wise to check five basic points:

(a) stability,
(b) consistent horizontal jaw relationship,
(c) adequate freeway space,
(d) even occlusal contact,
(e) a pleasing appearance.

If any fault is left uncorrected at this stage, it will re-appear on the trial dentures.

If the final recording of the jaw relationship is made by asking the patient to close firmly on the rims, even occlusal contact of the subsequent teeth will be achieved only under this loading condition. There is the possibility that when initial contact is made under light pressure, uneven occlusal contact will cause the denture base to move. If, on the other hand, the recording is made with the patient exerting only light pressure, the resultant dentures will meet evenly at the initial contact position and will not move subsequently as occlusal pressure is increased. To locate the rims it is therefore advisable to use a recording medium which initially is fluid, thus offering little resistance to closure of the jaws, but which subsequently sets hard so that it cannot be distorted when the casts are mounted on an articulator. A suitable material is a zinc oxide–eugenol occlusal registration paste. This paste, when mixed, remains fluid for a considerable time at room temperature but sets rigidly within about 30 seconds at mouth temperature.

The clinical procedure for using the paste is as follows: two locating notches are cut into the occlusal surface of the upper rim, one either side of the arch in the premolar areas. The occlusal surface of the upper rim is then coated with a thin film of petroleum jelly which acts as a separating medium. The registration paste is applied to the premolar and molar regions of the lower rim and the patient is guided into the retruded position. An alternative method for recording the jaw relationship which allows a very rapid chairside procedure is to reduce the lower rim to two occlusal pillars about 1 cm in length in the second premolar region. These pillars can be quickly adjusted by softening or adding wax to achieve balanced occlusal contact in the retruded jaw relation at the appropriate occlusal vertical dimension. The missing sections of the lower rim are then reconstructed by placing impression plaster into the spaces with a spatula and getting the patient to close into the plaster until the wax pillars occlude with the upper rim (Figure 10.8).

Having recorded the jaw relationship, the following decisions must be made:

(a) the location of a palatal relief chamber, if required,
(b) the choice of artificial teeth.

PALATAL RELIEF

When the upper denture-bearing tissues are palpated, the mucosa covering the ridge is occasionally found to be more compressible than the mucosa in

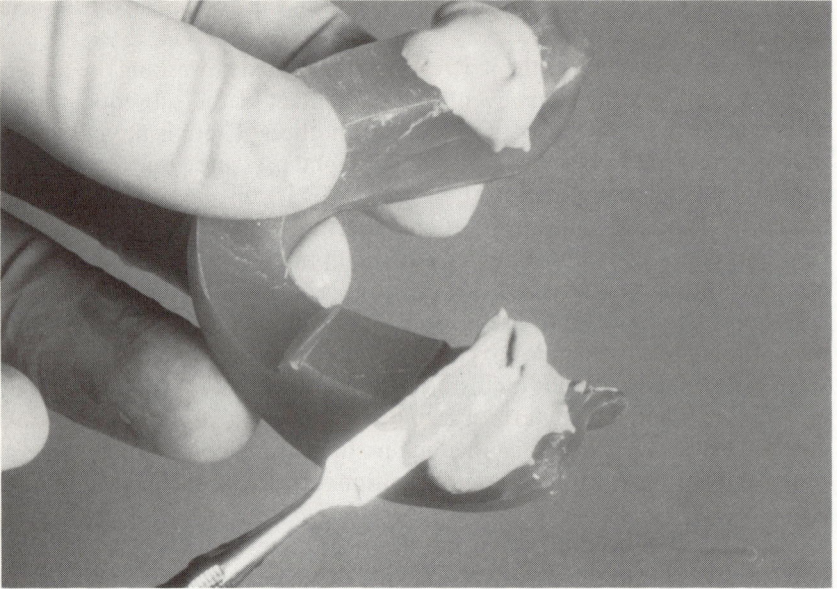

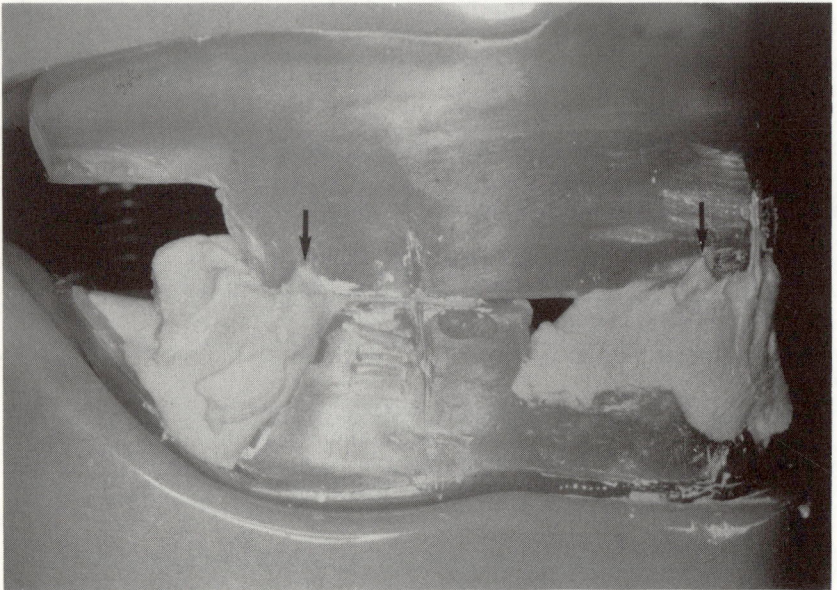

Figure 10.8   *Top*: Lower record block with occlusal contact area restricted to the premolar areas. Impression plaster is being applied to fill the spaces posteriorly. *Bottom*: Completed registration. Note that the impression plaster has filled locating notches (arrows) cut into the upper rim

the middle of the palate. If an impression records these tissues in an undistorted state and a denture is constructed on the resulting cast then, when the denture is fitted, the compressible ridges will offer less support than the centre of the palate so that occlusal contact will result in pivoting and flexing of the denture about the mid-line. Initially, this pivoting may cause loss of border seal or inflammation of the mucosa. Over a long period of time, the continual flexing is likely to produce a fatigue fracture of the acrylic denture base.

There are two ways of avoiding these problems. A more viscous impression material may be used so that the shape of the tissues over the ridge is recorded in a compressed state. Alternatively, if a less viscous impression material is used, a sheet of tin foil, trimmed to correspond to the area of incompressible mucosa, may be cemented to the resulting cast in the mid-line so that when the denture is processed, a relief chamber is created. That part of the denture base overlying the in-compressible mid-line will stand away from the mucosal surface and will only contact the tissues when the ridge mucosa has already been com-pressed.

As the authors favour an impression technique which records the shape of the mucosa with minimal distortion, for reasons discussed on page 152, they prefer to use relief as a means of overcoming the problem of varying compressibility. However, this approach has its drawback because air will be trapped in the relief chamber, so reducing the physical forces of retention. For this reason, it is important that relief is provided only when positively indicated. Although a palatine torus may be present, there is no need to provide palatal relief unless the overlying mucosa is less com-pressible than that over the ridges.

The decision on providing relief belongs to the dentist not the techni-cian. If the clinical situation warrants its inclusion, then the appropriate area should be marked on the cast. If a heat-cured acrylic base is to be used for the upper record block, a decision on palatal relief must be made after the working impression has been taken. The area for relief can be marked on the impression with an indelible pencil.

CHOICE OF TEETH

Just as the overall blueprint for the new dentures is built up stage by stage, so is the necessary information acquired in order to produce a pleasing appearance. Appearance depends upon:

(a) the incisal level,
(b) the amount of lip support provided by the anterior teeth and labial flange,

(c) the occlusal vertical dimension,
(d) colour, shape and size of the artificial teeth,
(e) arrangement of the artificial teeth.

Incisal level, lip support and occlusal vertical dimension are determined by the shape of the record rims. A decision on details of colour, shape and size of the teeth must now be made. With this information, the technician is able to set up the trial dentures. The last stage in creating a pleasing appearance, the arrangement of the teeth within the dental arch, is finalised on the trial dentures; a discussion on this particular topic is contained in Chapter 12.

Colour of Teeth

An appropriate colour of artificial tooth is selected from a shade guide. When making the choice, it is advisable to moisten the teeth with water and hold them just inside the patient's open mouth. The teeth should be viewed in natural rather than artificial light. It can be positively misleading if the teeth are viewed by the patient against a light background, such as a white coat; under these conditions the shade will appear darker. As a result, the patient may be inclined to choose lighter teeth which, when placed in the mouth, would be quite inappropriate.

It is, of course, important that a decision on colour should be influenced by the patient's comments. However, as it is often difficult for the patient to forecast the final result from the appearance of one tooth positioned in the mouth, the dentist should offer guidance on the colour which is likely to be most suitable.

It is impossible to provide hard and fast rules on choice of colour in view of the variation in the natural dentition. However, the following comments are offered as useful guide-lines. The older the patient, the darker the natural teeth become; it is, therefore, appropriate to choose artificial replacements which are in keeping with age. A less artificial appearance is more likely to be obtained if people with dark, swarthy complexions are provided with darker teeth while those with blond hair and pale skins are given lighter teeth.

Shape and Size of Teeth

It is possible to offer only very general guide-lines as to choice of shape and size of artificial teeth in view of the enormous variation found in the natural dentition. One cannot even state categorically that patients with large faces and strong features have large teeth – or vice versa – because jaw size and tooth size have different genetic origins. Nevertheless, when choosing artificial replacements, it is usually more appropriate to decide upon a large tooth shape for those patients with a heavier skeletal make-up. Certainly, providing small teeth for such a person is more likely to suggest artificiality.

Several papers have offered guidance on the choice and arrangement of artificial teeth to reflect the sex, age and personality of the patient. As a generalisation, it is stated that masculinity is associated with 'vigour, boldness and hardness' while femininity, in contrast, is described in terms of 'roundness, softness and smoothness'. Whereas larger and more angular tooth shapes indicate strength, a delicate feeling is suggested by moulds which are rounder and somewhat smaller. A further suggestion is that the shape of the upper anterior teeth should complement the shape of the patient's face. Three basic facial shapes have been described – square, ovoid and tapering – and appropriate tooth moulds have been produced which are an inverted version of these shapes. It should be emphasised that this idea has no scientific basis. However, it forms a useful starting point for selecting teeth in the absence of evidence from previous natural or artificial dentitions.

Two suggestions are offered as guidance when choosing the width of the anterior teeth. First, it has been stated that the overall width of the central incisors is frequently similar to the width of the philtrum of the upper lip. Second, the projection of a line drawn from the inner canthus of the eye to the ala of the nose passes through the upper canine tooth. The crown length of the artificial teeth is governed by the height of the recording rim which has been carved to produce an acceptable incisal level.

The choice of mould for the upper anterior teeth can be made from actual samples of moulds available, or from a printed mould guide. If the dentist has a selection of upper tooth moulds set in conventional tooth arrangements, he or she can position them inside the upper lip. It is preferable to use only half the anterior segment so that the set-up can be rotated in the mouth to follow the shape of the dental arch. The full complement of anterior teeth may be so unlike the shape of the dental arch that the appearance resembles the teeth found in a Christmas cracker, and thus offers little guidance to the dentist and even less to the patient (Figure 10.9).

Having recorded the information on colour and shape of the artificial teeth, it is advisable to ask if the patient remembers any particular characteristic in the arrangement of the natural teeth which could be included in the artificial set-up. For example, the request for a median diastema or for imbricated incisors can be passed to the technician for inclusion in the trial dentures. However, one's common experience is of limited help from this line of questioning. So often, patients remember only gross irregularities which in any case they want modifying in the artificial dentition.

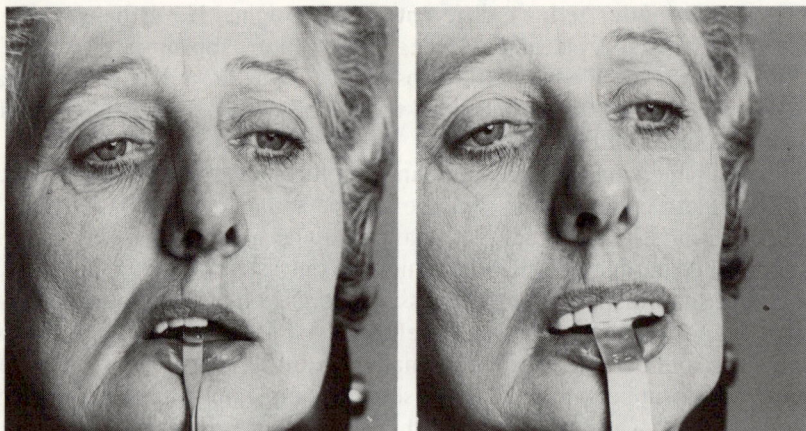

Figure 10.9   Choosing the mould for the anterior teeth. More guidance on the width of the teeth can be gained from trying in 321| only (*left*) rather than a set-up of 321|123 whose arch shape is quite inappropriate for the patient (*right*)

Most of this process of tooth selection and arrangement is a matter of inspired, creative guesswork helped by applying principles of proven clinical value. The uncertainty of this approach underlines the value of pre-extraction records, such as good quality photographs, notes and dental casts. Immediate dentures are also an excellent way of transferring the desirable features of the natural dentition to the artificial one. Whenever possible, records such as these should be used when selecting and arranging artificial teeth rather than falling back on the guide-lines mentioned in this chapter.

Comparison of Acrylic and Porcelain Teeth

As a choice must be made between acrylic and porcelain teeth, it is appropriate to consider their respective qualities at this stage.

Appearance

A very satisfactory appearance can be obtained from both good quality acrylic and porcelain teeth. In the manufacture of both types of teeth, it is possible to produce a satisfactory gradation of colour throughout the length of the crown and to introduce striations and stains to mimic the imperfections of natural teeth. However, the acrylic tooth deteriorates more rapidly in the mouth because of its lower resistance to wear.

Attachment to the Denture Base

The attachment of acrylic teeth to the denture base is by chemical union, while porcelain teeth are retained by means of pins or holes. Under normal circumstances, both methods work perfectly satisfactorily. However, in cases where the inter-ridge distance is small, it may be necessary to reduce the length of the tooth so much that, in the case of porcelain, the retentive element is removed. Under these circumstances, it is obvious that acrylic teeth must be used.

As a denture cools following processing, acrylic resin contracts 20 times more than porcelain. This means that around the necks of porcelain teeth, where contraction is restricted, areas of strain are set up and reduce the resistance of the acrylic to fracture. This does not mean that all dentures with porcelain teeth are prone to fracture. However, the combination of a deep frenal notch in the labial flange area together with areas of strain around adjacent porcelain teeth may initiate fracture of the denture base.

Transmission of Masticatory Forces

Porcelain teeth transmit a greater proportion of the masticatory forces to the underlying mucosa. Thus, the use of porcelain teeth can be a disadvantage in those patients whose denture-bearing tissues are less able to tolerate the higher forces. This is because of the widely differing values in the modulus of elasticity of the two materials, that for porcelain being about nine times greater than the value for acrylic; porcelain is therefore less likely to absorb as much of the transmitted force.

Response to Function

Noise

Porcelain teeth are approximately twice as hard as enamel and 10 times as hard as acrylic; when biting together on porcelain teeth, more noise is made. During normal function, however, this point is of minimal importance. If an even occlusion is produced at the correct occlusal vertical dimension, the teeth will not contact during speech. Furthermore, during mastication, a layer of food separates the two occluding surfaces for much of the time and before the teeth make contact there is always a deceleration. These are the possible reasons for the small percentage of patients who in fact complain of noise from porcelain teeth.

Resistance to Chipping

As acrylic has a lower modulus of elasticity, it will absorb much more energy before fracturing; thus, a sudden impact is more likely to chip porcelain teeth.

Occlusal Wear

The resistance of the two materials to occlusal wear is perhaps the most significant difference between the two types of teeth from a clinical standpoint. As porcelain teeth are so much harder, their occlusal surfaces wear only very slowly. Thus, the established jaw relationship in both horizontal and vertical planes is maintained for much longer. Some people believe that the more rapid wear of acrylic teeth allows the patient to 'grind in' a personal occlusal pattern. This may be a justifiable view in the early stages of wear. However, further deterioration of the occlusal surfaces leads to irregular occlusal contact and loss of the jaw relationship. Another argument put forward in favour of acrylic teeth is that the masticatory forces wear the teeth away rather than cause resorption of the underlying bone. However, anything more than minimal occlusal wear results in an unbalanced occlusion which is itself a potent cause of resorption.

OBTAINING BALANCED OCCLUSAL CONTACT DURING FUNCTION

Balanced occlusion is established when there are simultaneous contacts between opposing artificial teeth on both sides of the dental arches. This term describes a static situation and applies when upper and lower dentures are meeting in any position.

Articulation is the term used to describe the dynamic situation as the mandible moves during function, and is defined as the contact relationship of the upper and lower teeth when moving into and away from the intercuspal position. If, during this movement, there are bilateral, simultaneous, anterior and posterior contact of teeth in central and eccentric positions, balanced articulation has been provided.

The side to which the mandible moves in order to break up a bolus of food is known as the working side. The opposite side of the arch is termed the balancing or non-working side.

If balance exists when dentures occlude, the masticatory forces are transmitted as widely as possible over the denture-bearing tissues. Furthermore, the even contact positively assists in retaining the dentures. In contrast, if the occlusion is unbalanced, the dentures are unstable and the masticatory forces are transmitted to a reduced area of tissue, thus causing inflammation of the mucosa and resorption of the underlying bone.

If the articulation is unbalanced and the mandible returns from an eccentric occlusal position to the intercuspal position, it is likely that the dentures will be displaced by the premature contacts. Of course, the lower denture is more vulnerable in this respect as it is usually less retentive than the upper denture and therefore less able to resist displacing forces. The result of denture movement is, once again, mucosal inflammation and resorption of the underlying bone.

Balanced occlusion and articulation are relevant when a patient is making tooth contact while swallowing saliva, or at the end of the chewing cycle when the bolus of food has been softened and broken down into small enough pieces. At the beginning of the chewing cycle, the teeth are prevented from meeting if the mouthful of food is too large or too hard to allow immediate penetration. Thus, it is unlikely that balanced occlusion has any relevance during this stage of the chewing cycle or during initial incision when the mandible is protruded and the piece of food broken off.

If complete dentures are to be constructed with a balanced articulation, the articulator should be capable of reproducing certain basic characteristics of the patient, namely:

(a) the condylar angle,
(b) the relationship of the maxilla to the condylar axis.

The route taken by the mandibular condyle as it moves forwards and downwards from the glenoid fossa to the articular eminence is known as the condylar path; the angle between the condylar path and the Frankfort plane is the condylar angle (Figure 10.10). The condylar axis is a line between the mandibular condyles close to a hinge axis around which the mandible can rotate without translatory movement.

Examples of three types of articulator commonly employed are shown in Figure 10.11. If complete dentures are constructed on a simple hinge articulator, all that can be produced with certainty is balanced occlusion in the position in which the jaw relationship was recorded. In the case of an adjustable articulator, there is provision for mounting the casts in the anatomically correct position relative to the condylar axis and for adjusting the condylar path to correspond with that of the patient. Lateral and

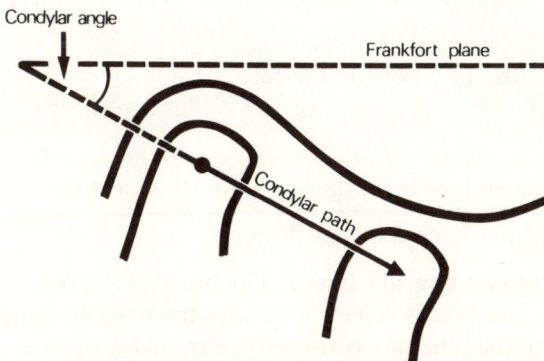

Figure 10.10   Diagrammatic representation of the relationship of the Frankfort plane, the condylar path and the condylar angle

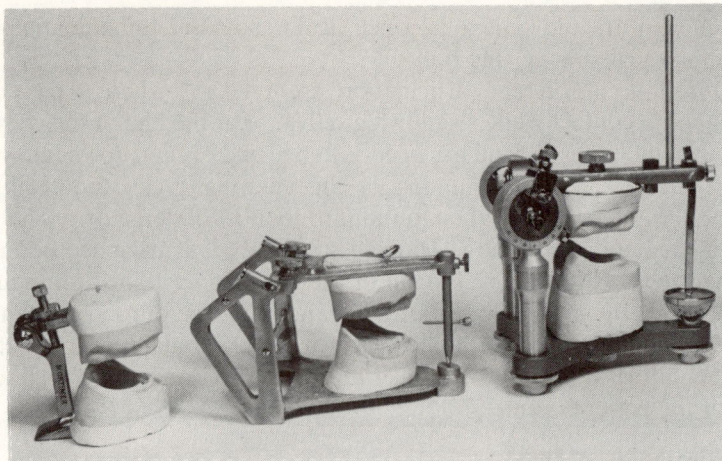

Figure 10.11 Examples of three articulators. *Left*: A simple hinge articulator. *Centre*: An average-movement articulator. *Right*: An adjustable articulator (Dentatus)

protrusive movements of the mandible can therefore be simulated, allowing dentures to be constructed with occlusal balance in eccentric positions. Accurate records are required to adjust this type of articulator; however, the degree of accuracy that can be achieved in the edentulous patient is limited by the inevitable movement of the record blocks on the compressible denture-bearing mucosa. Consequently, it is important when using an adjustable articulator to ensure that the record blocks are as stable as circumstances allow; acrylic bases are to be preferred for this reason.

The relationship of the upper dental arch to the condylar axis is recorded using a face bow (Figure 10.12). The occlusal fork is attached to the upper record rim and the fork's handle is inserted into a clamp on the frame of the face bow. The face bow is then adjusted to achieve three objectives:

(a) to record the location of the condyles,
(b) to centre the face bow on the face,
(c) to record the relationship of the occlusal plane to the Frankfort plane.

With some types of face bow, there is a fourth objective:

(d) to record the inter-condylar distance.

With the type of face bow illustrated in Figure 10.12, condyle location and centring of the face bow is achieved by adjustment of the condylar rods so that their tips contact the skin overlying the condyles and the values on the scales, inscribed on each rod, are equal. The relationship of the occlusal plane to the Frankfort plane is recorded by positioning the orbital pointer

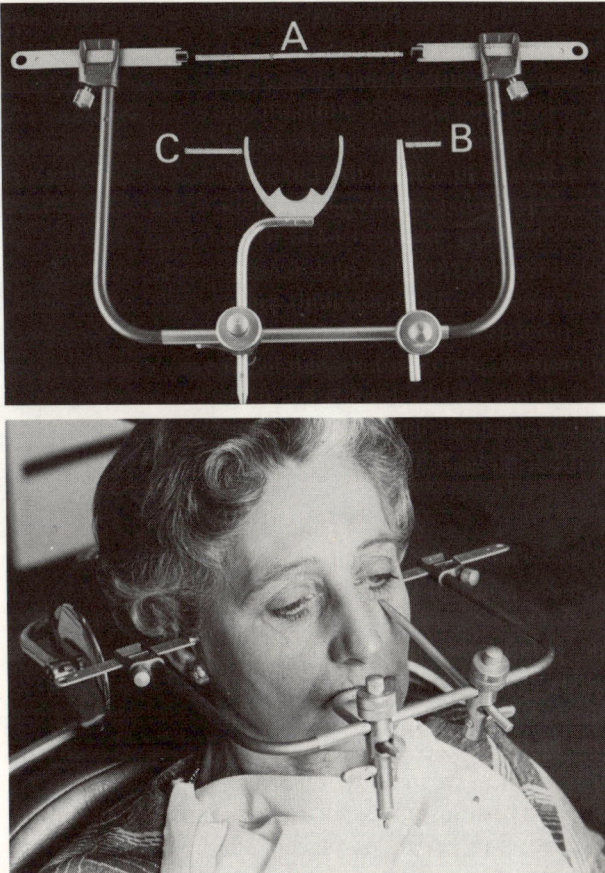

Figure 10.12   *Top*: The Dentatus face bow: (A) condylar rods; (B) orbital pointer; (C) occlusal fork. *Bottom*: Face bow in position on a patient

so that its tip contacts the skin overlying the lowest point on the infra-orbital margin (Figure 10.12).

Once the adjustments have been completed, all the joints of the face bow are fully tightened to form a rigid unit which is then taken to the articulator so that the clinical measurements can be transferred.

The face bow is placed on the Dentatus articulator as shown in Figure 10.13. The condyle rods fit over the axle ends of the articulator and the face bow is centred by moving it until the scales on the condyle rods are once more equal. The face bow is raised or lowered to bring the orbital pointer into contact with the undersurface of the orbital axis plane indicator. The upper cast is then located on the bite fork and plastered to the articulator. After removing the face bow, the lower cast can be mounted in its correct relationship with the upper cast.

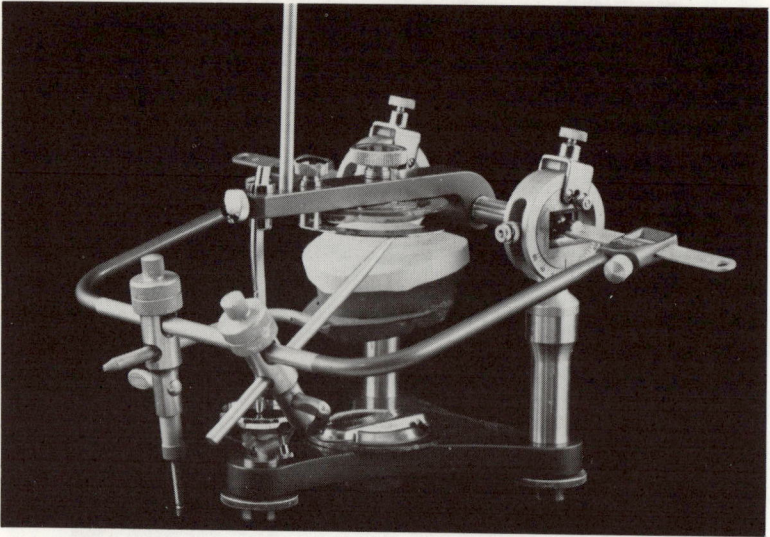

Figure 10.13   Face bow in position on a Dentatus articulator

As shown in Figure 10.14, the condylar tracks on the articulator can be adjusted in two planes, the angle to the horizontal plane (condylar angle) and the angle to the sagittal plane (Bennett angle). When constructing complete dentures, it is acceptable to use an arbitrary value of 15° for the angle to the sagittal plane. A recording of the jaw relationship in protrusion is used to adjust the angle of the condylar track to the horizontal plane. The protrusive record is placed on the lower record rim on the articulator. As the upper rim is seated in the record, the condylar track is caused to rotate. The resulting condylar angle can be read from the scale on the side of the joint assembly.

On the average-movement articulator, the value for the condylar angle and the relationship of the maxilla to the hinge axis are predetermined according to average measurements obtained from many patients. In both adjustable and average-movement articulators, the upper arm moves in the horizontal plane, thus the technician is able to simulate lateral and protrusive movements of the mandible and check that the arrangement of the artificial teeth allows balanced articulation.

In spite of the limitations of the simple hinge articulators, many dentures are made on this instrument and function quite satisfactorily. The likely reason for success is the ability of most patients to adapt to the limitations of the occlusal surface. The patient recognises that certain functional movements cause instability or discomfort and therefore ceases to make them. It will, of course, be apparent that such dentures are likely to fail in those patients whose ability to adapt is more restricted.

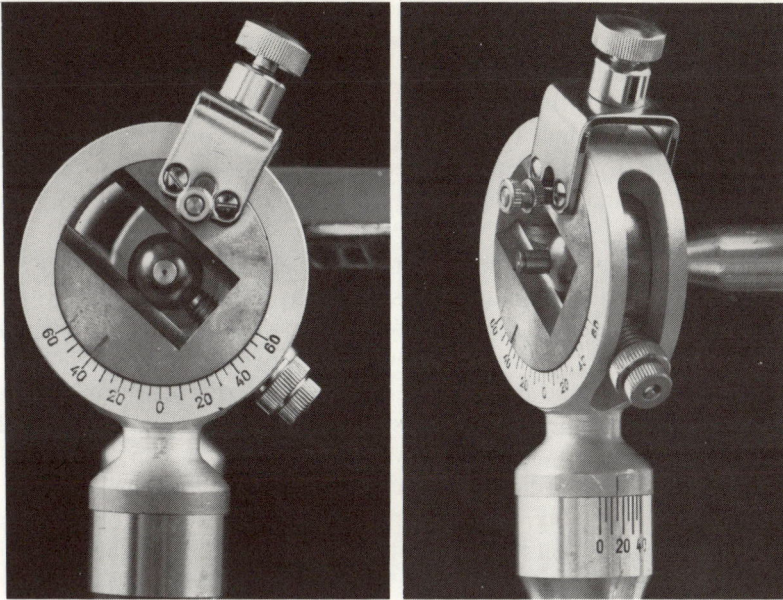

Figure 10.14   *Left*: The condylar angle – the angle of the condylar track to the horizontal plane. *Right*: The Bennett angle – the angle of the condylar track to the sagittal plane

Although the Dentatus articulator is a more complex instrument, there are features of its design which prevent it from reproducing mandibular movement with complete accuracy. For example, when a patient's mandible moves laterally, the head of the condyle on the balancing side moves downwards, forwards and medially along an articular surface whose shape is sigmoid; furthermore, vertical downward movement of the head of the condyle away from the articular surface of the temporal bone is possible. In contrast, the condylar sphere of the articulator moves forwards, downwards and medially along a straight path and is held rigidly in its articular track.

The average-movement articulator may be considered as lying somewhere between the two other instruments. It possesses the same limitations mentioned above, but is less complicated to use than the semi-adjustable articulator and, at the same time, allows a balanced articulation to be produced which will satisfy most patients.

Faced with the alternative techniques just mentioned, which method is most appropriate for the edentulous patient? Is the sophistication of the semi-adjustable articulator justified for all patients or can satisfactory results be obtained with the less complicated instruments?

To help answer these questions, it is logical to consider what actually happens to complete dentures during normal function.

The first point to realise is that although a perfectly balanced articulation may be produced on the articulator when the dentures are fixed rigidly to the underlying casts, the situation is likely to be considerably different in the mouth. Once in the mouth, dentures are placed on a compressible foundation and they inevitably move when occlusal contact is made. Even if the mucosa is firm, there is the possibility of up to 1 mm of movement in the horizontal plane. With increasing compressibility, more movement will of course occur.

The relative stability of the dentures themselves has received considerable attention in the literature. Research has shown quite clearly that, during normal function, complete dentures are remarkably unstable. During incision, the posterior border of an upper denture usually drops. When the bolus of food is transferred to the posterior teeth for chewing, the upper denture commonly slides towards the working side and the balancing side tends to drop. The lower denture is often seen to lift bodily.

The frequency of occlusal contact increases as the bolus of food is broken down; inevitably, the softer the food the easier it is for contact to be made. It appears that most of the tooth contact occurs in the proximity of the retruded position.

The results of the experimental observations may now be applied to the clinical situation and the following conclusions drawn and recommendations made.

(1) Because of the compressibility of the denture foundation and the inevitable movement of the dentures themselves, the apparent precision of a sophisticated adjustable articulator seems to be superfluous. The use of an average-movement articulator makes for simpler technique while at the same time providing the facility to produce an acceptable level of balanced articulation.

(2) As it appears that functional tooth contact occurs in the region of the retruded position, it is usually sufficient to develop an occlusion which minimises the possibility of imbalance in an area 2–3 mm lateral and anterior to this position. The objectives for a functional balanced articulation within this zone are as follows:

(a) In lateral occlusion, there should be even interdigitation on the working side and a balancing contact or contacts on the opposite side (Figure 10.15(a)). It is important to avoid a premature contact or complete lack of contact on the balancing side (Figures 10.15(b) and (c)).

(b) In protrusive occlusion, there should be bilateral balancing contacts on one or more posterior teeth (Figure 10.15(d)). It may be more difficult to produce a balancing contact in some instances where the tooth arrangement appropriate for the patient necessitates a deep vertical overlap (Chapter 11).

However, within the zone in which balance is advantageous, the problem is frequently solved by a slight reduction in height of the lower incisors.

With regard to the choice of posterior teeth, studies into patients' acceptance of cusped or cuspless types have failed to demonstrate a clear-cut preference for one or the other. The use of cuspless teeth results in less well defined occlusal positions but there is no consensus as to whether this lack of precision is advantageous or not. On the positive side, the use of cuspless teeth allows a greater freedom of movement of the mandible in the horizontal plane without creating occlusal interferences. Similarly, it has been argued that cuspless teeth are better able to accommodate positional changes of the dentures relative to the supporting tissues brought about by resorption of alveolar bone. It has been suggested that cuspless teeth are particularly suitable for elderly patients because an increased variation in occlusal contact positions is characteristic of this group. However, others argue that the positive interdigitation offered by cusped teeth helps to reduce the variation and that this can provide functional benefits for the elderly. If it is considered desirable to create a fully balanced articulation, then cusped teeth will facilitate the task.

By applying the principles described in this section, balanced occlusal contact can be achieved on the articulator. However, once the dentures are

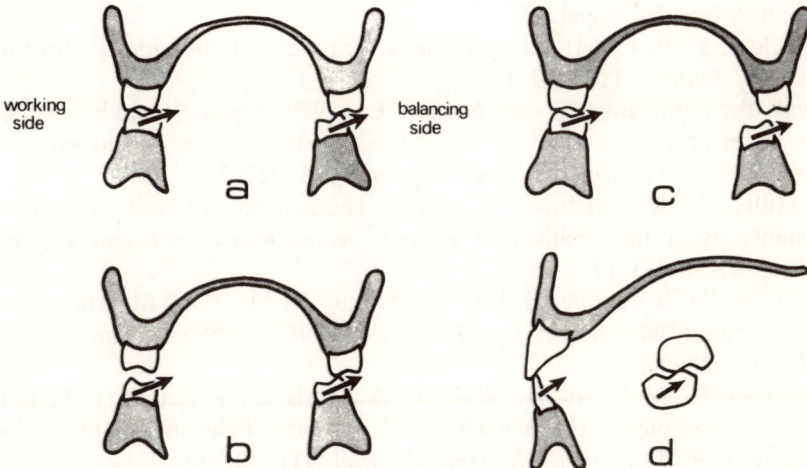

working
side

balancing
side

a

c

b

d

Figure 10.15   (a) Balanced occlusion with contact on the working side (*left*) and on the balancing side (*right*). The arrows indicate the direction of movement of the mandible as it returns to the intercuspal position. (b) A premature contact on the balancing side. (c) A premature contact on the working side. (d) Balancing contact on posterior teeth in protrusion

fitted in the mouth, discrepancies may be seen which necessitate adjustment of the occlusion in order to maintain this balance. The clinical procedures are described in Chapter 13.

BIBLIOGRAPHY

Arstad, T. (1959) The resiliency of the edentulous alveolar ridges. *Odontologisk Tidskrift*, **67**, 508–21.

Brewer, A. A., Reibel, P. R. and Nassif, N. J. (1967) Comparison of zero degree teeth and anatomic teeth on complete dentures. *Journal of Prosthetic Dentistry*, **17**, 28–35.

Brill, N. (1957) Reflexes, registrations, and prosthetic therapy. *Journal of Prosthetic Dentistry*, **7**, 341–60.

Feldmann, E. E. (1971) Tooth contacts in denture occlusion – centric occlusion only. *Dental Clinics of North America*, **15**, 875–87.

Harcourt, J. K. (1974) Accuracy in registration and transfer of prosthetic records. *Australian Dental Journal*, **19**, 182–90.

Helkimo, M., Ingervall, B. and Carlsson, G. E. (1973) Comparison of different methods in active and passive recording of the retruded position of the mandible. *Scandinavian Journal of Dental Research*, **81**, 265–71.

Kobowicz, W. E. and Geering, A. H. (1972) Transfer of maxillomandibular relations to the articulator. In *International Prosthodontic Workshop on Complete Denture Occlusion*, B. R. Land and C. C. Kelsey (eds), Ann Arbor, Michigan.

Liddelow, K. P. (1964) The prosthetic treatment of the elderly. *British Dental Journal*, **117**, 307–18.

Lund, P., Nishiyama, T. and Møller, E. (1970) Postural activity in the muscles of mastication with the subject upright, inclined, and supine. *Scandinavian Journal of Dental Research*, **78**, 417–24.

McMillan, D. R. and Imber, S. (1968) The accuracy of facial measurements using the Willis bite gauge. *Dental Practitioner and Dental Record*, **18**, 213–17.

McMillan, D. R., Barbenel, J. C. and Quinn, D. M. (1969) Measurement of occlusal face height by dividers. *Dental Practitioner and Dental Record*, **20**, 177–9.

Matthews, E., McIntyre, H., Wain, E. A. and Bates, J. F. (1961) The full denture problem: The Manchester Viewpoint. (The articulatory surfaces, J. F. Bates.) *British Dental Journal*, **111**, 401–18.

Nairn, R. I. (1973) Lateral and protrusive occlusions. *Journal of Dentistry*, **1**, 181–7.

Preiskel, H. W. (1967) Anteroposterior jaw relations in complete denture construction. *Dental Practitioner and Dental Record*, **18**, 39–44.

Trapozzano, V. R. (1960) Tests of balanced and imbalanced occlusions. *Journal of Prosthetic Dentistry*, **10**, 476–87.

Tryde, G., McMillan, D. R., Christensen, J. and Brill, N. (1976) The fallacy of facial measurements of occlusal face height in edentulous subjects. *Journal of Oral Rehabilitation*, **3**, 353–8.

Turrell, A. J. W. (1972) Clinical assessment of vertical dimension. *Journal of Prosthetic Dentistry*, **28**, 238–46.

Yurkstas, A. A. and Kapur, K. K. (1964) Factors influencing centric relation records in edentulous mouths. *Journal of Prosthetic Dentistry*, **14**, 1054–65.

11 Dentures and Muscles

Earlier in the book, mention was made of the importance of the muscular control of dentures. Success in this area, as in so many aspects of prosthetic dentistry, is dependent upon a three-person effort: the effort of the dentist in recognising the importance of the concept of muscular control as well as designing and prescribing the shapes of dentures to be compatible with the facial structure; the effort of the dental technician in following the prescription and translating it into correctly designed dentures; and the effort of the patient in, literally, getting to grips with the final product.

In this chapter, we focus primarily on the positioning of incisor teeth but also present a technique for recording the position of the neutral zone.

THE RELEVANCE OF A PATIENT'S NATURAL INCISAL RELATIONSHIP

A consideration of natural and artificial incisal relationships reveals a close similarity between orthodontic and prosthetic knowledge. At first thought, the two specialities might appear to be poles apart as they are concerned largely with patients from opposite ends of the age range. However, a study of the factors which govern the development of the natural occlusion reveals fundamental similarities. Furthermore, it becomes increasingly apparent that prosthetic dentistry can be practised successfully only if orthodontic knowledge is applied to the clinical prosthetic situation.

Development of the Natural Occlusion

As teeth erupt into the oral environment, their position is influenced by the activity and posture of the surrounding muscles, the size, shape and relationship of the jaws, and the occlusal forces produced by tooth contact. The shape and size of the jaws is inherited and, after growth has ceased, cannot be changed other than by surgical intervention; the functional behaviour of the muscles is partly inherited but may also be modified by treatment. It is important to consider the muscles and jaws as one unit because the muscles function from their skeletal origins and insertions.

The position of natural teeth is influenced more by the long-term forces associated with muscle posture than by the short-term forces occurring during function. As the teeth erupt into a mould of muscular tissue created by the lips, cheeks and tongue, they eventually take up positions of stability related to the relaxed posture of these muscles. This situation contrasts with that occurring with complete dentures which are all too readily displaced both by the short-term functional forces and also perhaps by the long-term postural forces. The design of complete dentures, particularly that of the lower denture, has therefore to take muscular displacement into account if stability is to be achieved.

The Prosthetic Problem

When both dentist and dental technician are taught to set up artificial teeth for complete dentures, the first picture is usually that of the Angle's Class I incisal relationship with horizontal overlap of 2 mm and vertical overlap of 2 mm. But for how many edentulous patients does this 'normal' incisal relationship resemble the previous natural dentition? In a survey of English school children aged 11 to 12 years, the percentages for the various dental arch relationships assessed on a modified Angle's classification were as follows:

Class I	44.3 per cent
Class II division 1	27.2 per cent
Class II division 2	17.7 per cent
Class II unclassified	7.3 per cent
Class III	3.5 per cent

Thus, 52.2 per cent of the children possessed a Class II occlusion. Of course, it is possible to correct some of the incisal relationships, but it must be remembered that the success of such treatment depends upon the underlying jaw relationship. The greater the discrepancy in jaw size and relationship, the harder it is to produce an ideal incisal relationship. More significant, therefore, are the results of the survey showing the variation in skeletal pattern:

skeletal Class I	40.8 per cent
skeletal Class II	53.8 per cent
skeletal Class III	5.3 per cent

It must be pointed out that these figures are representative of a group of young adolescents and that further growth of the mandible may reduce the number of those possessing a skeletal Class II pattern. However, it is unlikely that parity will be established between this group and the one possessing a normal jaw relationship.

The results of the surveys suggest that, in the UK, the most common occlusion is a Class II tooth relationship superimposed upon a skeletal Class II jaw relationship. As a result, it may be expected that if all edentulous patients are provided with dentures with a Class I incisal relationship, many such artificial dentitions will be quite unlike the previous natural ones. Some modification of the artificial arrangement is, of course, permissible and even requested by the patient – just as orthodontic treatment can be undertaken to modify a malocclusion where the prognosis is favourable. Of the remainder, the patient will either adapt to the dentures with difficulty or will find them quite intolerable. However, as discussed fully in Chapter 2, the success of prosthetic treatment depends so much upon the adaptability of a patient that if additional demands are made by creating an incisal relationship completely divorced from the natural state the chances of prosthetic treatment succeeding are reduced. In the next few pages, the reasons for possible failure will be discussed, after which ways of preventing failure will be described.

Reasons for Failure of Treatment

To discover why prosthetic treatment may fail as a result of an incorrect incisal relationship, it is logical to consider each group in Angle's classification and ask the questions 'How can a Class I artificial incisal relationship be produced?' and 'What is likely to happen as a result?'

Class I
Figure 11.1 illustrates the tracing from a lateral skull radiograph of a dentate adult subject possessing a Class I incisal relationship. Of course, if complete dentures are constructed with a 'normal' incisal relationship, the artificial occlusion will be similar to the previous natural one, and few problems will be expected.

Class II Division I
In order to produce a Class I incisal relationship it is necessary to modify both the horizontal and vertical overlap. The former may be reduced either by moving the lower incisors labially or the upper incisors palatally, while the latter can be altered by reducing the crown length or increasing the occlusal vertical dimension of the dentures. This last possibility means that the freeway space is doubtless eliminated and so is condemned outright. Complications which are likely to arise when following the other suggestions become apparent when considering the adult patient illustrated in Figure 11.2(a).

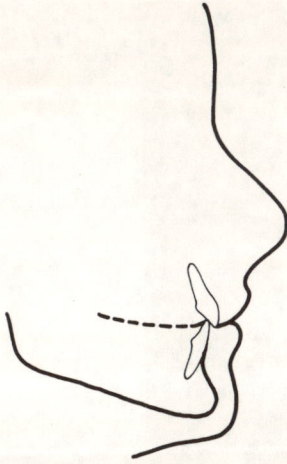

Figure 11.1   Tracing from a lateral skull radiograph of a dentate patient showing a
Class I incisal relationship

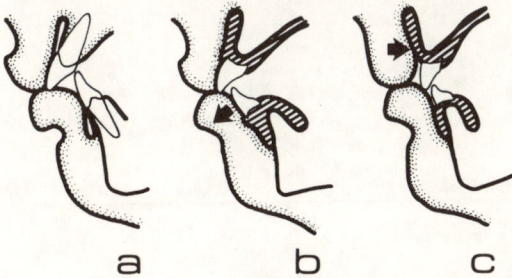

a   b   c

Figure 11.2   (a) Class II division 1 natural incisal relationship. (b) Upper artificial
teeth placed in the same position as the natural ones; lower teeth proclined
forwards. (c) Lower artificial teeth placed in the same position as the natural ones,
although the crown length is reduced; upper teeth moved back

In Figure 11.2(b), the upper artificial teeth are placed in the same
position as the natural ones while the lower teeth are placed further
forwards. The result of this modification is to position the lower labial
segment anterior to the neutral zone. The force exerted by the lower lip is
no longer balanced by that of the tongue and the lower denture becomes
unstable. This error is not an uncommon one and is illustrated by the
clinical case shown in Figure 11.3.

In Figure 11.2(c), the lower incisors are placed in the natural position
and, this time, the upper anterior segment is moved backwards. This
treatment may be quite acceptable if the skeletal relationship is favourable,
just as orthodontic treatment in the natural dentition may successfully
reduce a large horizontal overlap.

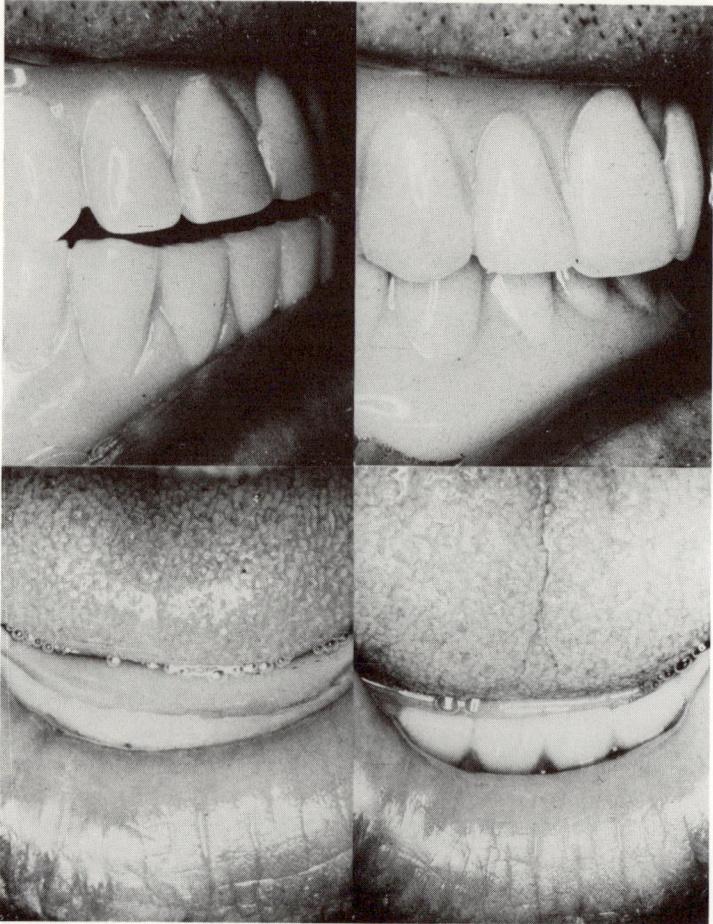

Figure 11.3   *Top left*: The incisal relationship of a patient complaining of a loose lower denture. *Bottom left*: The lower anterior teeth are positioned forwards of the neutral zone. Pressure from the lip results in mobility of the denture. *Bottom right*: Replacement denture with the teeth placed in muscle balance. *Top right*: As a result of this change in incisal position, a Class II division 1 relationship is produced

If the natural horizontal overlap was large, allowing the lower lip to fall behind the upper incisors, a partial reduction in the subsequent dentures may result in a very unsatisfactory 'half-way house' where the lower lip is unable to take up a comfortable position either behind or in front of the incisors. Persistent irritation of the lip by the incisal edge results. In some instances, problems can arise as a result of excessive reduction of the horizontal overlap, effectively converting the patient from a Class II division 1 to a Class I incisal relationship. The dramatic change in appearance that results may be considered disastrous by the patient, as in

Figure 11.4 where the anterior teeth and upper lip almost appear to be strangers. A treatment possibility that can be explored to overcome the problems described in situations of this type is to retrocline the upper incisors rather than move them palatally. This produces a Class II division 2 relationship which reduces the horizontal overlap while retaining a realistic relationship of the necks of the teeth to the underlying ridge.

There is a group of patients possessing a severe skeletal Class II relationship, which is the result of a prominent maxilla rather than an underdeveloped mandible, where treatment can be carried out to correct a horizontal overlap which may be in the region of 10–20 mm. Although a combination of prosthetic treatment and surgical removal of bone from the

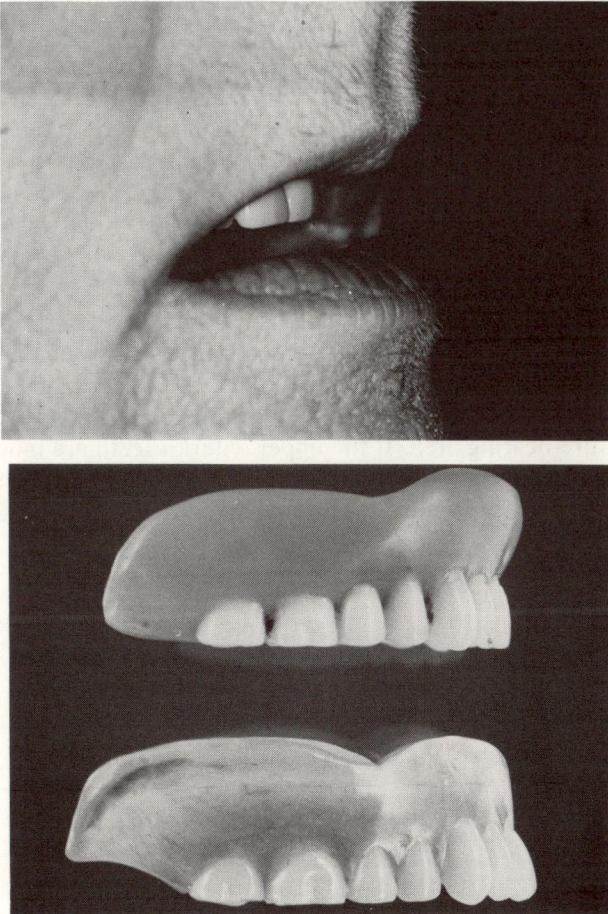

Figure 11.4 *Top*: Unsatisfactory relationship of upper teeth to the upper lip produced by the top denture. *Bottom*: Bottom denture is a replacement with the anterior teeth placed further labially to improve their relationship with the lip

prominent premaxilla may improve the situation, it is frequently impossible to reduce the discrepancy completely and the patient will retain a Class II division 1 incisal relationship with the overlap reduced to perhaps 5–10 mm. Any further reduction may be impossible because the amount of bone to be removed would totally eliminate the alveolar ridge. In addition, it is important to realise that the alveolar bone provides the upper lip with some of its support. If too radical an approach is chosen, the loss of lip support may be such that the change in appearance is anything but acceptable.

Class II Division 2
The vertical overlap can be reduced in the same two ways as mentioned in the last section and, for reasons already stated, any increase in occlusal vertical dimension is deprecated.

The deep vertical overlap shown in Figure 11.5 may be altered by reducing the crown length of the upper artificial teeth. However, the patient with this type of natural incisal relationship rarely complains about the appearance of the teeth and so a change in incisal level is not readily accepted. Fortunately, the situation regarding the lower teeth is not so critical and it is usually possible to reduce the crown length without detriment to appearance.

Class III
Two extremes of skeletal make-up are recognised. In the one the maxilla is small and the Frankfort–mandibular plane is large (Figure 11.6). The prognosis for retention of an upper denture is often poor because of the small denture-bearing area. If the upper anterior teeth are moved labially in order to establish a 'normal' incisal relationship, the force of the upper lip on the labial face of the denture may be so great as to tip the balance

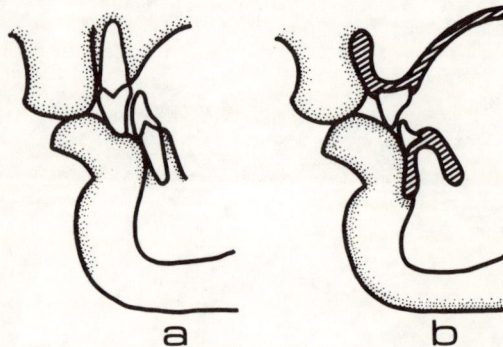

Figure 11.5   (a) Class II division 2 natural incisal relationship. (b) Artificial teeth placed in the same position as the natural ones; the crown length of both the upper and lower teeth has been reduced

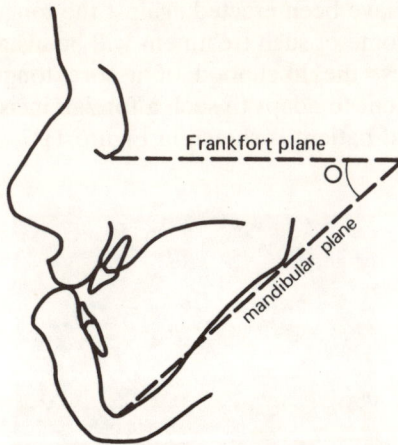

Figure 11.6   A lateral skull tracing from a patient with a skeletal Class III relationship and a large Frankfort–mandibular plane angle

between adequate stability and complete failure. At best, it is advisable to create no more than an edge-to-edge incisal relationship; on occasions, a reverse horizontal overlap must be accepted if a stable upper denture is to be produced.

At the other extreme of skeletal type, the maxilla is developed normally, the mandible is large and the Frankfort–mandibular plane angle is small. Because of favourable palatal shape, the prognosis for retention of an upper denture is usually good and thus some latitude may be allowed in positioning the artificial teeth.

Anterior Open Occlusion

The act of swallowing involves the production of an anterior oral seal which is normally made by the lips meeting and the tongue remaining within the dental arches. However, in some people the seal is made by the tongue thrusting between the upper and lower anterior teeth and contacting the lips. In the majority of cases, this behavioural pattern is adaptive. For example, if the upper incisors are unduly protrusive, the lower lip finds it extremely hard to move around the dental barrier and meet the upper lip; the anterior oral seal is made more economically by the tongue meeting the lower lip. If the dental barrier is removed by orthodontic or prosthetic treatment, the lips are allowed to come together and the tongue returns to more normal function.

There remains a very small number of people, calculated as 0.6 per cent of the population, where the tongue thrust appears to be the result of an innate neuromuscular behavioural pattern. This so-called endogenous tongue thrust is frequently associated with a severe lisp and is resistant to treatment. If artificial teeth are positioned in a Class I relationship, a dental barrier will have been erected against the tongue as it continues to protrude. The outcome of such treatment will be instability of both upper and lower dentures, the likelihood of a sore tongue and a complete inability of the patient to adapt to such a foreign incisal arrangement. An example of a typical patient is shown in Figure 11.7.

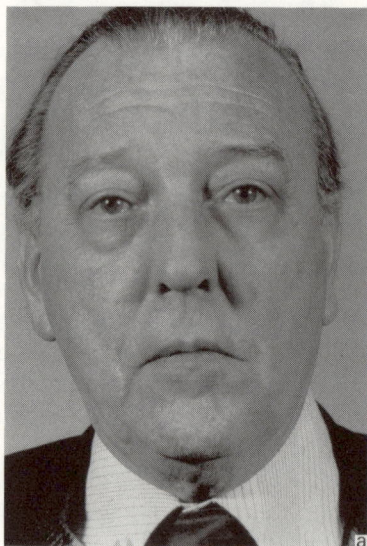

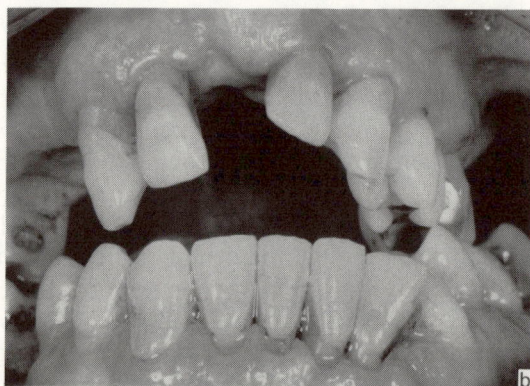

Figure 11.7   *Top*: This dentate patient has a large lower face height. Considerable muscular effort is required to bring the lips together. *Bottom*: The anterior oral seal is normally made between the tongue and the lower lip, resulting in the anterior open occlusion shown here

PREVENTION OF FAILURE

Treatment failure can be prevented if particular care is taken in the assessment of the patient, in the recording technique and in subsequent laboratory procedures.

Assessment of the Patient

The task of assessing the edentulous patient and deciding upon the classification of the previous natural incisal relationship becomes more difficult the longer the patient has been edentulous:

The reasons are as follows:

(a) The patient's own fading memory of the relationship of the natural teeth.

(b) Resorption of the alveolar bone leads to loss of support for the lips and cheeks and consequent changes in the facial features upon which one depends for vital clues.

(c) An alteration in the jaw relationship following loss of teeth will occur through change in mandibular posture. Loss of tooth support allows the mandible to move closer to the maxilla and assume a more protrusive position which might falsely suggest a skeletal Class III relationship (Figure 11.8).

(d) Increased activity of the lower portion of the orbicularis oris and mentalis muscles has been reported in long-term denture wearers. This change in muscle activity may cloud one's judgement when assessing the patient.

Nevertheless, in spite of these difficulties, orthodontic knowledge does allow one to seek for clues in the edentulous patient. In the ideal situation, one observes a picture made up of competent lips, a skeletal Class I jaw relationship and an obtuse labiomental groove.

A patient who possesses a Class II division 1 relationship superimposed upon a skeletal Class II base is relatively easy to diagnose. Typical features to observe are an oval face, a retrusive mandible, an acute labiomental groove and frequently a small lower face height (Figure 11.9).

A patient with a Class II division 2 incisal relationship possesses certain features which are, in the dentate patient, distinctive and may still be clearly seen in the edentulous state (Figure 11.10). These features include a small lower face height, an acute labiomental groove, a small Frankfort–mandibular plane angle, a prominent mental region of the mandible, a square gonial angle and prominent zygoma. It is common for this type of patient to have a less marked skeletal discrepancy than is

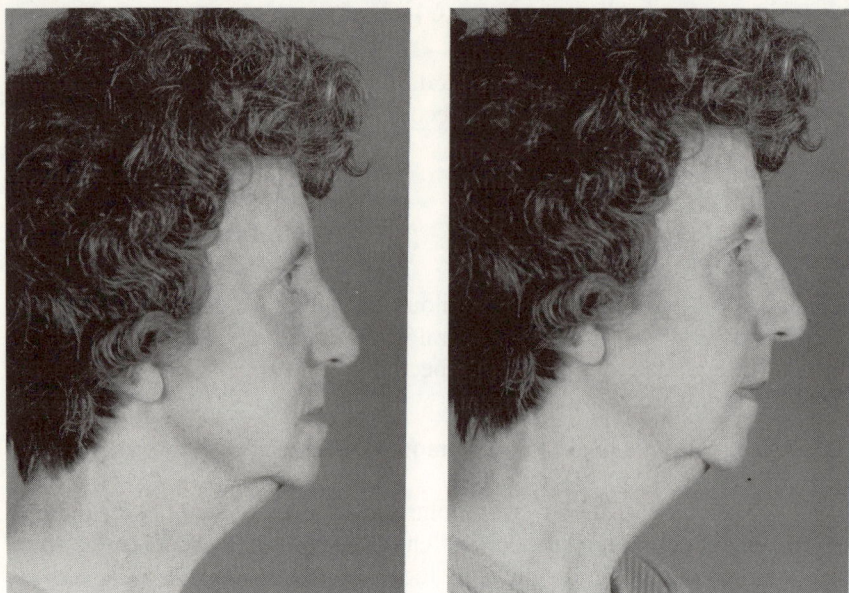

Figure 11.8 *Left*: A patient in occlusion wearing her old dentures which have become badly worn. She appears to have a skeletal Class III jaw relationship. *Right*: The true jaw relationship once the occlusal vertical dimension has been restored with new dentures. The patient, in fact, possesses a skeletal Class II jaw relationship

sometimes seen in the Class II division 1 subject. It is necessary to stress, however, that these features are not necessarily diagnostic outside the UK. For example, such a facial structure is commonly seen in Scandinavia and is not associated with a Class II division 2 incisal relationship.

An edentulous patient who possesses a Class III relationship on one of the two skeletal Class III base types is perhaps the easiest to diagnose. In the first type there may be evidence of the large lower face height, the obtuse Frankfort–mandibular plane angle and the overall length of the face (Figure 11.11). The second type with a normal maxilla and overdeveloped mandible is also readily recognised. In the dentate subject possessing an anterior open occlusion associated with an endogenous tongue thrust, one sees circumoral muscular activity during swallowing and one often hears a characteristic lisp. Neither of these diagnostic clues is reliable in the edentulous patient because the absence of teeth leads to indistinct speech while the absence of lip support results in abnormal muscular behaviour during swallowing. However, a combination of these factors may point the way to the correct assessment. Without doubt, this small group of patients creates considerable problems in assessment and diagnosis.

Reliable information on the degree of lip competence is more likely to be obtained if the patient is encouraged to relax completely and is then

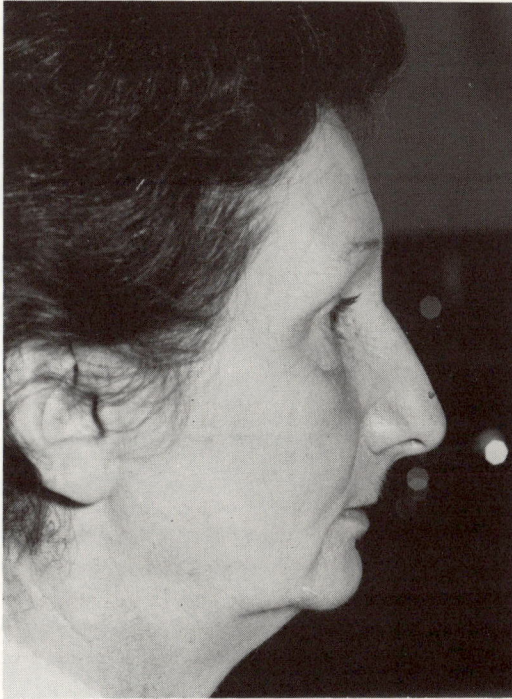

Figure 11.9 An edentulous patient. The retrusive mandible, small lower face height and acute labiomental groove point to the fact that the patient probably possessed a Class II division 1 natural incisal relationship

assessed from a distance. If the patient is seemingly unobserved, there is more likelihood of natural lip activity being encouraged.

Careful Recording Technique

Remembering that one of the objectives of recording the occlusion is to show the technician where the artificial teeth are to be placed, it is vital that the record rims are so shaped that the correct incisal relationship is reproduced. In patients where only a horizontal overlap is required, the procedure is relatively simple. Thus, for the Class I patient the record rims are carved in the conventional manner. To indicate the Class III incisal relationship, it may be found necessary to carve the rims to an edge-to-edge incisal relationship. In the gross skeletal Class III situation, the upper record block may be stable only if a reverse horizontal overlap is produced, thus reducing the muscular force of the lip on the labial face of the upper rim.

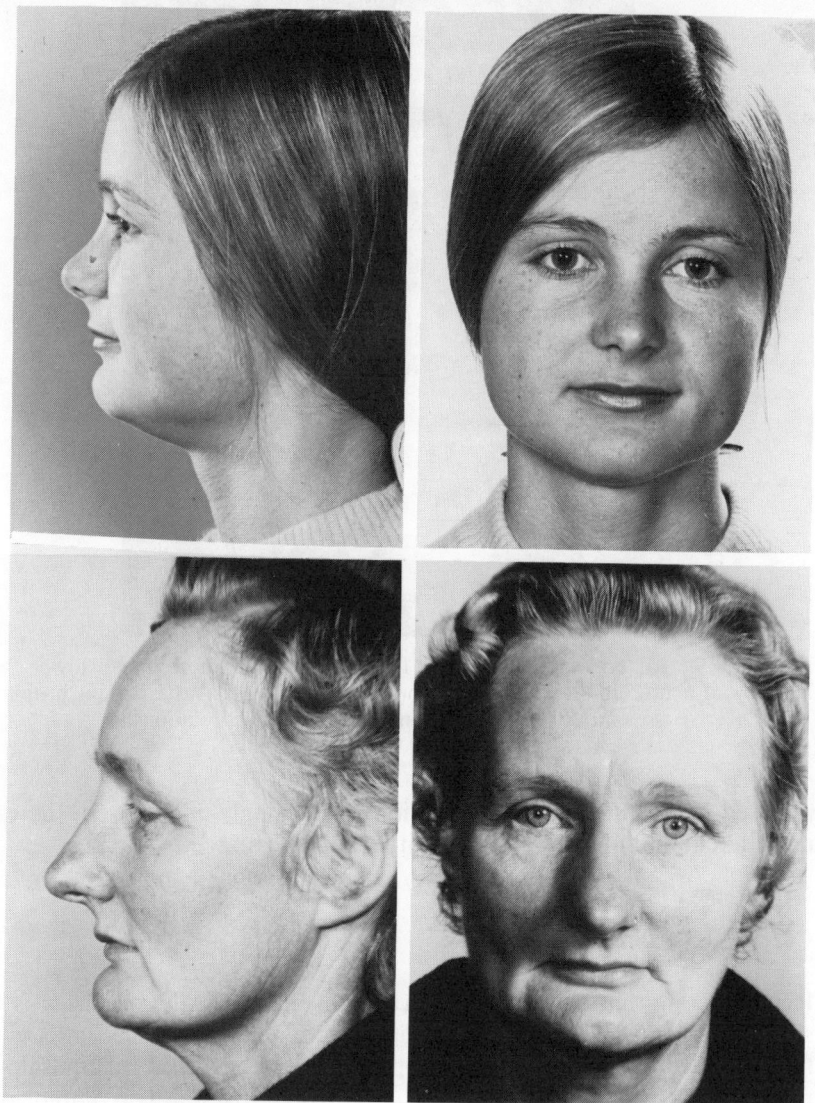

Figure 11.10   The upper pictures are of a dentate subject possessing a Class II division 2 incisal relationship and illustrate the characteristic facial features described in the text. The similar features of the edentulous woman shown in the lower pictures suggest that she once possessed a Class II division 2 natural incisal relationship

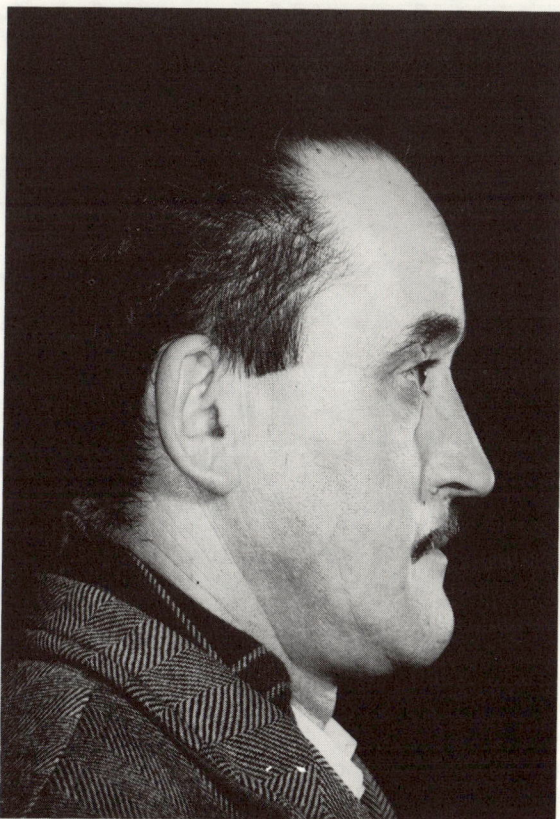

Figure 11.11   An edentulous patient. The combination of large lower face height, obtuse Frankfort–mandibular plane angle and obtuse labiomental groove indicate that he possesses a skeletal Class III jaw relationship

Unnecessary complications arise if one inadvertently reduces the occlusal vertical dimension when recording the occlusion for a skeletal Class III patient. The existing skeletal discrepancy is magnified as the mandible approaches the maxilla with the result that the production of an acceptable incisal relationship becomes increasingly difficult. Thus, the possibility of positioning the labial segment outside the neutral zone is increased (Figure 11.12).

For a Class II patient, a horizontal overlap is automatically produced if the routine objectives of recording the occlusion are satisfied, namely the rims being shaped to provide satisfactory lip support and positioned in the neutral zone to achieve stability. However, difficulties arise where a marked vertical overlap is required. If the incisal level of each rim is adjusted to produce a pleasing appearance and the same height maintained

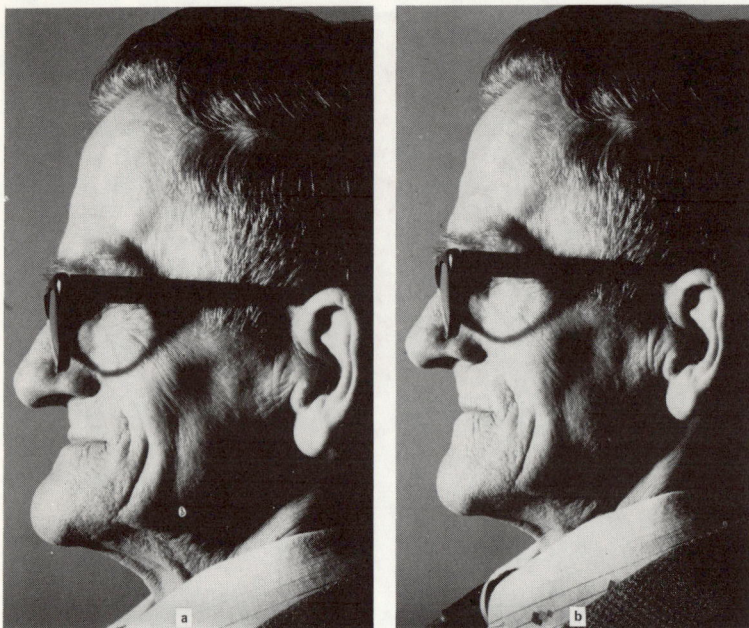

Figure 11.12   Effect of change in occlusal vertical dimension on a skeletal Class III jaw relationship. *Left*: A reduction in occlusal vertical dimension accentuating the Class III jaw relationship. *Right*: Restoration of the occlusal vertical dimension allowing a more acceptable incisal relationship to be produced

over the entire occlusal surface, it is likely that the occlusal vertical dimension will be excessive. The reasons for this become apparent when considering the occlusal plane of the natural dentition shown in Figure 11.13, where it can be seen that the vertical overlap is the product of an unusually steep curve in the occlusal plane. If this curve is reproduced on the record block, then it is possible to provide the technician with the exact information on incisal relationship and height of occlusal plane. One method of achieving this is as follows.

Providing Exact Information on the Class II Division 1 Incisal Relationship
First, the upper rim is carved to indicate the correct position for the incisors; palatally, the rim is reduced in thickness to resemble the size of the natural incisors. The lower rim is then shaped to the neutral zone and to the correct incisal height. The height of the lower rim in the buccal region is reduced so that the correct occlusal vertical dimension is established; when the patient closes together on the rims, the lower labial segment will fit in behind the upper one and so establish the required vertical overlap (Figure 11.14). In some instances, it will be necessary to reduce the height of the upper buccal segments as well in order to gain adequate freeway space.

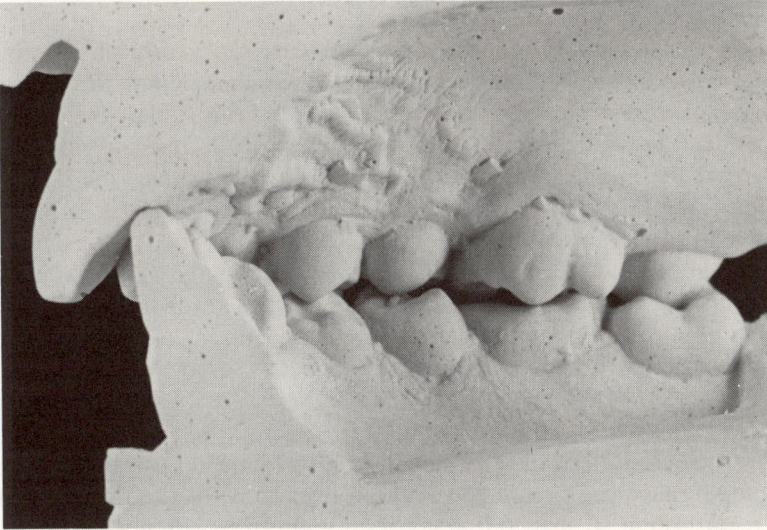

Figure 11.13   A sagittal section through casts of a Class II division 1 incisal relationship. The vertical overlap is the result of a steeply curved occlusal plane

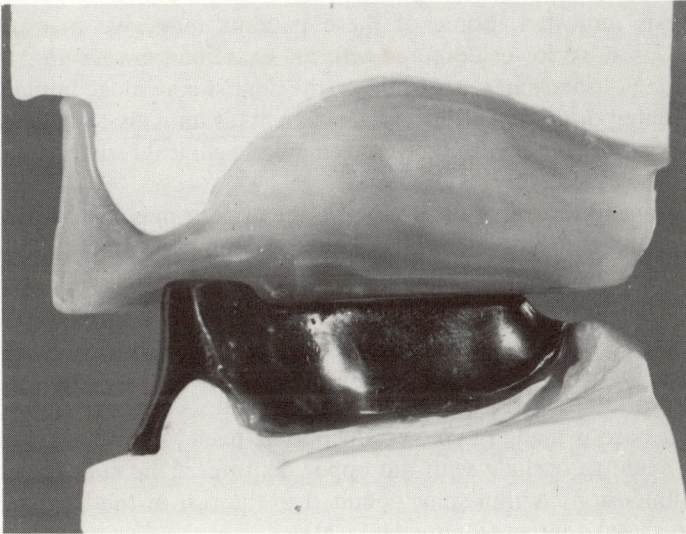

Figure 11.14   Recording the jaw relationship for a patient who possessed a Class II division 1 incisal relationship. Correct incisal levels and the degree of vertical overlap are produced by creating a step on the lower rim

At this stage, a somewhat artificial step has been created between labial and buccal segments of each rim. This abrupt step is softened when the rim is replaced by the artificial teeth but the overall curvature of the occlusal plane, as found in the natural dentition, is retained.

Positioning Lower Anterior Teeth

Placing the lower anterior teeth in muscle balance can be critical, especially if there has been considerable resorption of the mandible and the mentalis muscle is exerting a strong influence. As a general rule, unless the necks of the artificial teeth are placed close to the crest of the residual ridge, it is likely that the muscle activity of the lower lip will displace the denture. Having made this point, it should also be mentioned that it is frequently possible to tilt the incisal aspects of the teeth labially. Such a proclination, if done carefully, will ensure that there is no unsightly gap between the labial surfaces of the teeth and the mucosa of the lower lip, while at the same time ensuring that the incisors are placed in a position of muscle balance between the lower lip and the tongue.

Recording the Neutral Zone

So far, the descriptions of recording the neutral zone in this chapter and in Chapter 10 have been restricted to the conventional method whereby the wax record rim is so shaped that it does not interfere with postural muscle balance and thus is stable. For the vast majority of patients, this technique is perfectly successful.

There are, however, a few patients for whom a functional recording technique is indicated. Some of these patients may give a history of numerous unstable lower dentures with the examination revealing design faults in the polished surface. In others, the dentist may judge initially that the positioning of the labial or buccal segments is unlikely to be achieved with reasonable accuracy. In such cases the basic clinical technique may be modified as follows.

At the stage of recording the occlusion, the upper rim is shaped carefully so that it supports the muscles of the cheeks and upper lip and fulfills all the criteria listed on page 174. The lower rim is trimmed so that a recording of the correct jaw relationship can be made. This stage can be accomplished quickly if the occlusal contact is restricted to a limited area in the premolar–molar region as described on page 179. After the casts have been articulated, the upper trial denture is constructed.

A lower base is made in cold-curing acrylic resin. Molar pillars on the base are made to occlude with the upper denture at the correct occlusal vertical dimension. A thin spine is added to the rest of the base and left clear of occlusal contact (Figure 11.15(a)).

At the stage of recording the position of the neutral zone, checks are made of the upper trial denture and of the occlusal contact with the molar pillars. A mouldable material, such as a short-term resilient lining material, a light-bodied silicone putty or a cold-curing poly(butyl-methacrylate) resin, is applied to the lower base which is then reinserted in the mouth. The bulk of the added material must be carefully judged so that the rim produced does not exceed the anticipated thickness of the finished denture. The patient is instructed alternately to sip water and talk. In this way, the surrounding muscles work at their functional length and shape the recording material (Figure 11.15(b)).

When the material has set, the recording of the denture space is returned to the laboratory where it is seated on the master cast and indices constructed around the polished surface (Figure 11.15(c)). The technician now has a recording of the denture space enabling him or her to position the artificial teeth within its boundaries.

Care in the Laboratory

It is, of course, essential that the technician follows the blueprint of the record blocks when setting up the trial dentures. This is best achieved if only a small portion of the rim is cut away at a time and replaced by artificial teeth. The remaining rim acts as a reliable guide to the overall arch shape. An alternative method is to pour a plaster index over the labial segment of the record rims (Figure 11.16). Subsequently, this index can be used as a guide when positioning the artificial teeth.

SUMMARY

Having read this chapter, the reader may conclude that the construction of complete dentures is to some extent a matter of deduction and guesswork. This is in fact true when one is faced with an edentulous patient and no record of the previous natural dentition. Many methods of obtaining pre-extraction records have been described. Certainly, good quality photographs and occluded casts of the natural dentition provide information as to the incisal relationship. However, the casts do not indicate the all-important relationship of the teeth to the underlying jaw and the surrounding musculature. Ultimately, such information can be obtained only by the recording rims being carved in the mouth.

The best method of transmitting the characteristics of the natural dentition through to the artificial one is undoubtedly by means of immediate dentures. The patient should be advised that these will always be a valuable source of information to a dentist constructing replacement dentures and therefore should never be discarded.

It can be argued that if all edentulous patients possessed their original immediate dentures, the number of prosthetic problems would be reduced considerably. For although many immediate dentures will cease to fit the mouth accurately after a few years, at least the dentist has evidence of tooth selection, tooth position and incisal relationship. Without doubt, some positive evidence is better than no evidence at all.

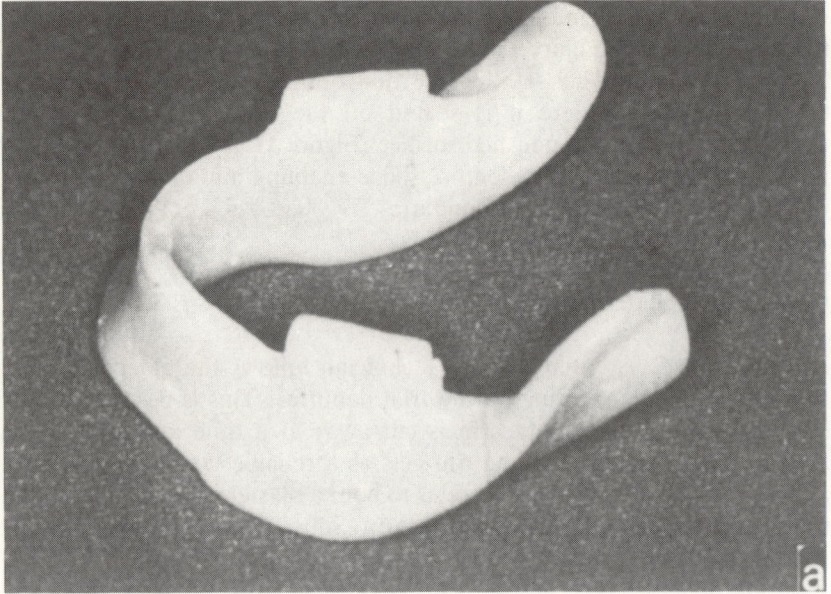

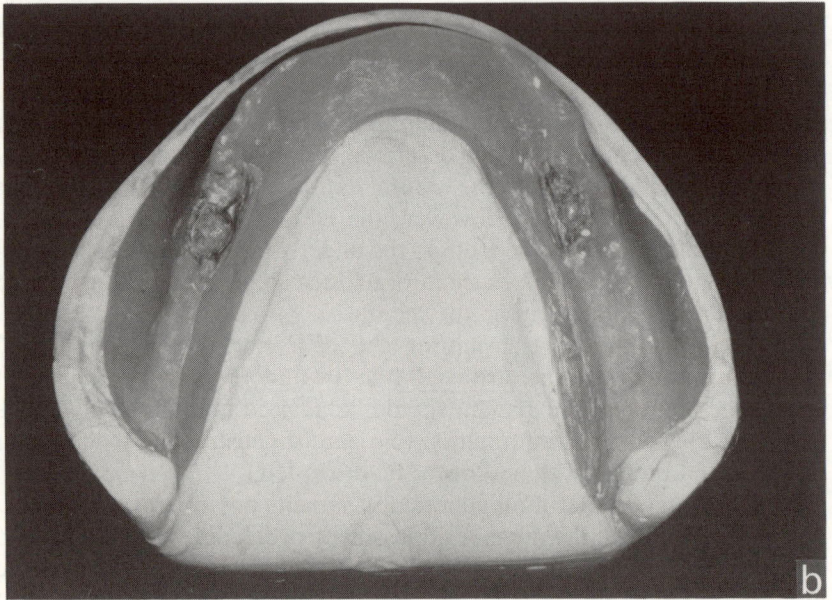

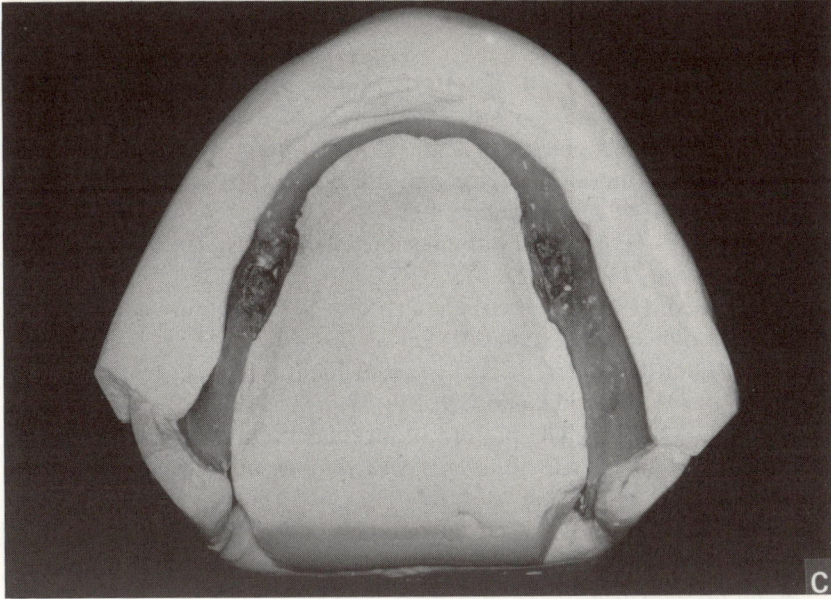

Figure 11.15 (a) Lower base for neutral zone impression. (b) Neutral zone impression which has been moulded by the muscles of the lips, cheeks and tongue. (c) Buccal and lingual indices in silicone putty

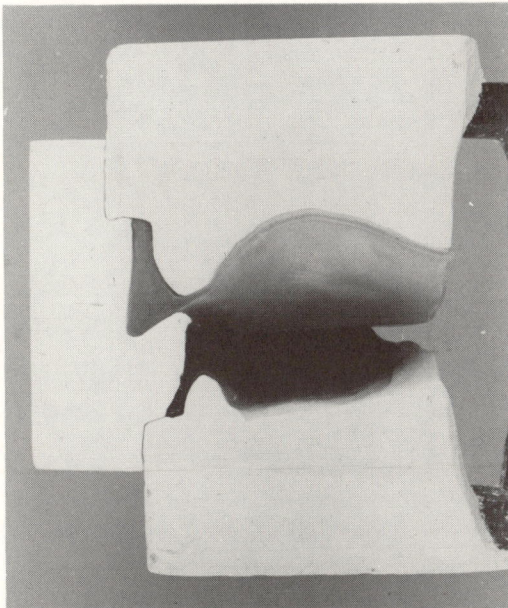

Figure 11.16 A plaster index poured over the record rims shown in Figure 11.14. This index guides the technician in placing the artificial teeth in their correct positions

BIBLIOGRAPHY

Berry, D. C. and Wilkie, J. K. (1964) Muscle activity in the edentulous mouth. *British Dental Journal*, **116**, 441–7.

Foster, T. D. and Walpole Day, A. J. (1974) A survey of malocclusion and the need for orthodontic treatment in a Shropshire school population. *British Journal of Orthodontics*, **1**, 73–8.

Liddelow, K. P. (1964) Oral muscular behaviour. *Dental Practitioner and Dental Record*, **15**, 109–13.

Murphy, W. M. (1964) Pre-extraction records in full denture construction. *British Dental Journal*, **116**, 391–5.

Neill, D. J. and Glaysher, J. K. L. (1982) Identifying the denture space. *Journal of Oral Rehabilitation*, **9**, 259–77.

Richardson, A. (1965) The pattern of alveolar bone resorption following extraction of anterior teeth. *Dental Practitioner and Dental Record*, **16**, 77–80.

Tallgren, A. (1963) An electromyographic study of the behaviour of certain facial and jaw muscles in long-term complete denture wearers. *Odontologisk Tidskrift*, **71**, 425–44.

Tulley, W. J. (1969) A critical appraisal of tongue-thrusting. *American Journal of Orthodontics*, **55**, 640–50.

12 Try-in Procedures

Trial dentures are constructed by setting up teeth on shellac or acrylic resin bases. These dentures are assessed in the mouth so that any errors can be identified and corrected before the dentures are finished. In addition to allowing the dentist to check all previous recordings, this stage also permits the patient to express an opinion on the appearance of the dentures so that modifications can be carried out where necessary.

The trial dentures should be examined first on the articulator and then in the mouth.

ASSESSMENT ON THE ARTICULATOR

A more orderly examination is assured if the operator inspects each of the denture surfaces in turn.

Impression Surface

If shellac bases have been used, the dentist should check that they are closely adapted to the casts. The border regions of the dentures should be shaped to conform to the depth and width of the sulcus on the cast. In the upper jaw, the base should be extended posteriorly to the post-dam cut in the cast and in the lower jaw half-way up the retromolar pads.

Polished Surface

If there are gross discrepancies on the lower cast between the position of the teeth and the crest of the ridge (Figure 12.1), one may suspect that the teeth are not in the neutral zone, and therefore may be the cause of instability in the mouth. This is not invariably the case however, so final judgement on this aspect must be delayed until the dentures have been examined in the mouth. If a biometric approach is being adopted in the

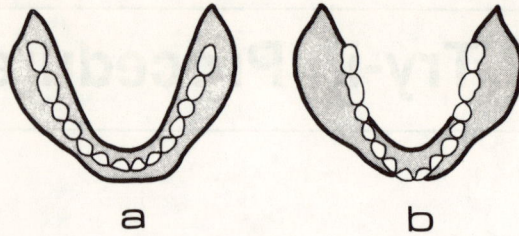

a   b

Figure 12.1   Occlusal view of two lower dentures: (a) the teeth follow the crest of
the ridge; (b) marked discrepancies between the position of the teeth and the crest
of the ridge are present suggesting that the teeth will not be in the neutral zone

design of the upper denture (Figure 9.4), the position of the teeth and
polished surfaces should be checked in relation to the palatal gingival
vestige and incisive papilla. The buccal and lingual aspects of the polished
surface should converge occlusally so that pressure from the soft tissues
contributes to retention. The exception to this rule is found in the upper
anterior region where the labial surface of the flange often faces upwards
and outwards.

If the patient already has dentures, they should be compared with the
trial dentures to see whether any planned similarities or differences, such
as arch shape or arrangement of the anterior teeth, have been produced
correctly.

Occlusal Surface

A check should be made that there is even occlusal contact and, unless a
simple hinge articulator has been used, that there is also balanced
articulation.

ASSESSMENT IN THE MOUTH

The dentures should first be assessed individually for physical retention,
base extension and relationship to the neutral zone, and then together for
occlusion, freeway space and appearance.

A bowl of cold water should be available so that frequent chilling of the
trial dentures can be carried out. If the dentures are left in the mouth for
more than a few minutes at a time, softening and distortion of the wax will
occur.

Physical Retention

An arbitrary test of physical retention is to attempt to dislodge the denture away from the tissues by exerting a vertical pull on the anterior teeth. If the retention is good, dislodgement may be extremely difficult or even impossible. This test is only really of any value when applied to the upper denture which would normally be expected to have good physical retention. In the case of the lower denture, retention is often poor because of the relatively small denture-bearing area and the difficulty in obtaining an efficient border seal. If the physical retention of an upper trial denture is not as good as one would expect from the anatomical conditions existing in a particular patient, the cause should be identified and, if found to be a fault in the denture, must be corrected. Contributory factors may include absence of a border seal resulting from underextension or inadequate width of flange, an ineffective seal at the posterior border or a poor fit of the denture base.

Base Extension

The accuracy with which the denture borders conform to the depth and width of the sulci must be determined. The posterior extension of the dentures over the retromolar pads in the lower jaw and to the junction of the hard and soft palate in the upper jaw must also be checked.

If marked overextension of the denture flanges is present, stretching of the sulcus tissues will occur when the denture is inserted into the mouth and their subsequent elastic recoil will cause dislodgement of the denture. Therefore, if the denture is displaced immediately after being seated, overextension should be suspected. A small degree of overextension may cause dislodgement of the denture when the dentist gently manipulates the lips and cheeks or when the patient raises the tongue. The exact location of such an error can only be determined by carrying out a careful examination inside the mouth; when overextension is present in areas where the visibility is good, displacement of the sulcus tissues will be seen as the denture is seated. However, in the lingual pouches, visibility is poor, so the dentist will have to make an assessment based on the behaviour of the lower denture as the tongue is moved. Correction of overextension is by reducing the depth of the offending flange. If this is not carried out, the finished dentures will traumatise the mucosa in that area and will be unstable because of the large displacing forces exerted by the soft tissues.

The presence of underextension is determined primarily by intra-oral examination, when the depth of the sulcus will be seen to be greater than that of the denture flange. In the case of the upper denture, however, a preliminary indication of underextension will be given by the existence of poor physical retention. Correction of any underextension will usually entail taking a new impression. Failure to do this will result in reduced physical retention of the finished dentures and inadequate distribution of load to the tissues.

Neutral Zone

The positioning of teeth in the neutral zone is of particular importance in the case of the lower denture because the physical retention is relatively weak. It may be difficult, however, to identify the neutral zone with any degree of certainty at the chairside. When the lower denture is inserted, it should remain in place when the mouth is half open and a limited range of tongue movements carried out. A useful 'rule of thumb' is that the lower denture will usually be stable if narrow teeth are used and are placed as far buccally, or labially, as possible without displacing the cheek and lip tissues. By this means, maximum tongue room is provided within the limits dictated by the lips and cheeks (Figure 12.2).

If, however, displacement of the denture does occur, the cause must be identified and the denture modified to correct the instability. An area where this difficulty commonly arises is the lower anterior region where the lip may exert excessive pressure, causing the denture to move upwards and distally. Correction of this type of fault should be carried out at the chairside so that the effect of the alterations can be assessed in the patient's mouth. The offending teeth may be reset in the correct relationship to the soft tissues or they may be removed and replaced with a wax rim which is

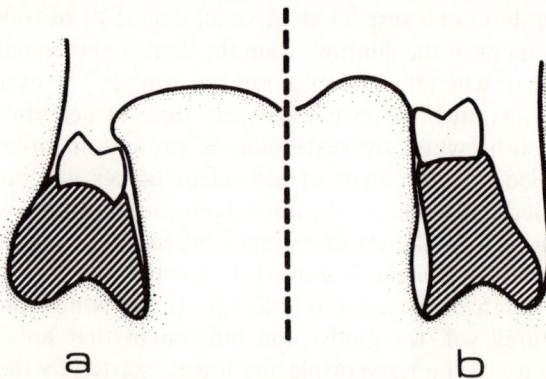

a   b

Figure 12.2 The relationship of the lower posterior teeth to the cheeks and tongue: (a) correct – buccal surfaces of the teeth are in close proximity to the buccal mucosa; the level of the occlusal plane allows the tongue to rest on the occlusal surfaces; (b) incorrect

shaped with a wax knife until a stable denture is produced. The technician should then be asked to reset the teeth in the position indicated by the rim.

If the dentures being constructed are replacements for dentures which have given good service in the past, it may usually be assumed that the relationship of the old denture to the cheeks, lips and tongue is satisfactory and that consequently this relationship should be copied in the trial dentures. Both old and new dentures should therefore be compared in the mouth to see whether this relationship has been faithfully reproduced.

While assessing the position of the lower teeth relative to the soft tissues, the height of the occlusal plane in relation to the tongue should be noted. When the tongue is relaxed, it should be able to rest on the occlusal surfaces of the teeth – a situation which favours retention of the lower denture (Figure 12.2).

Occlusion

The occlusion should be checked with the mandible in the retruded contact position. The patient closes slowly with the mandible retruded and the dentist carefully observes the *initial* occlusal contact. The final occlusal relationship can be misleading, as an uneven occlusion may have been masked by compression of the mucosa beneath the denture, tipping of the denture or posturing of the mandible. In patients where anatomical factors are unfavourable and a shellac base has been used, looseness of the upper trial denture may make it impossible to carry out an accurate assessment of the occlusion. In these circumstances, application of a denture fixative to the impression surface will overcome the problem.

If a relatively large occlusal discrepancy is present, it will be seen by the dentist without any difficulty. The existence of smaller faults however may be deduced from evidence such as slight tipping or lateral movement of the dentures as they occlude, and by asking the patient if the dentures are contacting evenly. Many patients are able to detect occlusal unevenness which is so slight that it could be overlooked by the dentist. Very small occlusal faults may be left until the finished dentures are fitted, when the necessary adjustment will be carried out; others however must be corrected at the trial stage.

Both vertical and horizontal discrepancies in the occlusion may occur. A vertical occlusal discrepancy may take the form of a unilateral, anterior or posterior open occlusion. If this type of fault is present, the retruded position should be re-recorded after modifying one or both of the dentures to produce an even occlusion at the correct occlusal vertical dimension. There are several ways in which this may be achieved, the choice of method depending on the occlusal vertical dimension of the trial dentures (Figure 12.3). Before carrying out the modifications, the dentist should

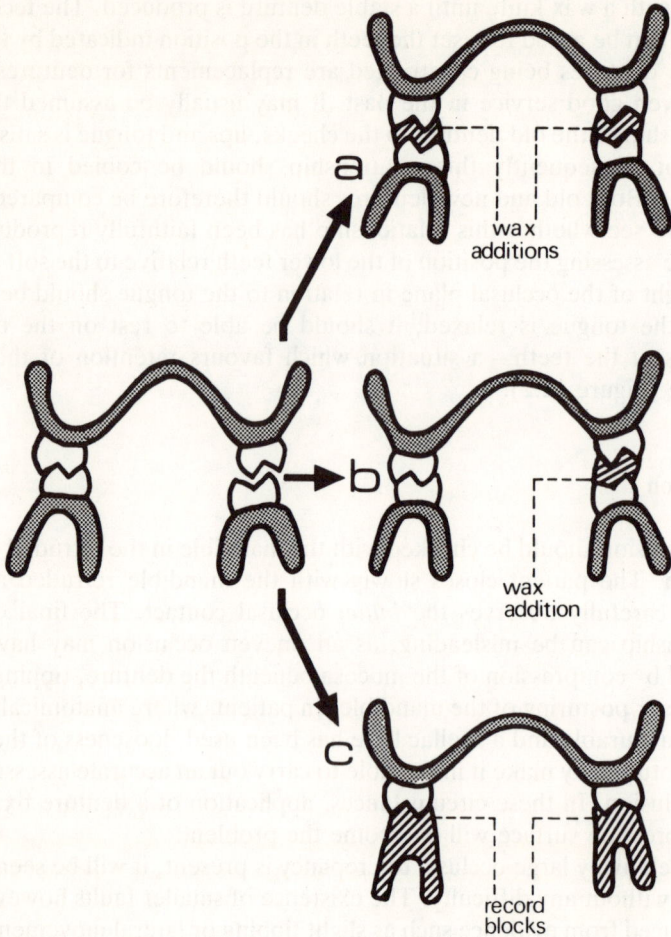

Figure 12.3   Methods of correcting a unilateral open occlusion at the try-in stage:
(a) if the occlusal vertical dimension is too small, an appropriate thickness of wax is
added to the upper or lower denture on both sides of the dental arch; (b) if the
occlusal vertical dimension is correct, wax is added to the side with the open
occlusion to produce even bilateral occlusal contact; (c) if the occlusal vertical
dimension is too large, the teeth on one of the dentures are removed and replaced
with a wax rim reduced in height by an appropriate amount. Final recording of the
retruded contact position may be made in each case using a suitable registration
material placed on both sides of the arch

determine whether or not the occlusal plane of the upper denture is
correct; if it is, the alterations will be carried out on the lower denture. If
the plane is not correct, the upper denture will also have to be modified by
resetting the anterior teeth or replacing the teeth with a wax rim to indicate
to the technician the required position of the occlusal plane.

An occlusal discrepancy in the horizontal plane may be detected by observing that the upper and lower centre lines are not coincident, that the posterior tooth relationship is not symmetrical, or that the horizontal overlap is not the same in the mouth as it is on the articulator. A new recording of the retruded contact position should be obtained after the teeth from one of the dentures have been removed and replaced with a wax rim. If the teeth are not removed, there is a danger that the cusps will guide the mandible back into the incorrect intercuspal position.

Freeway Space

The lower trial denture should be inserted and the rest vertical dimension measured. Then, after reinserting the upper denture and measuring the occlusal vertical dimension, an initial impression can be gained of the adequacy or otherwise of the freeway space.

This initial impression should be backed up by an assessment of the patient's appearance and speech. If the patient's facial proportions and lip relations appear to be appropriate when the teeth are occluded, it suggests that the occlusal vertical dimension is correct. This assessment can be broadened by asking the patient to occlude and then relax the mandible several times while the dentist assesses the freeway space by observing the amount of mandibular movement. Changes in facial proportions, lip posture and jaw relations during these movements will also help the observer to decide whether the occlusal vertical dimension is acceptable.

Finally, the patient should be asked to speak while wearing the trial dentures. The teeth do not normally contact during speech but approach most closely when the 'S' sound is made. The separation is known as the smallest speaking space and is usually about 1 mm. If the occlusal vertical dimension of the trial dentures is excessive, the space may be absent; correspondingly, it will be increased if the occlusal vertical dimension is too small. This assessment can be made by asking the patient to count out loud from 'sixty' to 'seventy'.

If the freeway space is too large, it is corrected by adding the appropriate thickness of wax to the occlusal surfaces of the posterior teeth on one of the dentures, adjusting the wax to produce an even occlusion at the desired occlusal vertical dimension and then recording the jaw relationship in the retruded contact position. If the freeway space is too small, or absent altogether, teeth will have to be removed from one of the dentures and be replaced with a wax rim before the new recording can be made. It is often sufficient to remove just the posterior teeth for this purpose but it may also be necessary to remove the anterior teeth where the horizontal overlap is such that further closure would be prevented by anterior tooth contact.

Appearance

At the try-in stage, the dentist must:

(a) reassess the information concerning the appearance of the dentures acquired when recording the occlusion. This includes the shade, mould and size of the teeth, the orientation and level of the occlusal plane, the position of the centre line and the degree of lip support;
(b) have a full discussion of the appearance of the dentures with the patient;
(c) create the final appearance by detailed arrangement of the anterior teeth, shaping of the gingival margins and, where necessary, grinding the incisal edges.

A check on basic aspects of the set-up, such as orientation of the occlusal plane and position of the centre line, can best be made if the upper lip is reflected so that a clear view of the maxillary teeth is obtained. However, this method of examination is not appropriate when assessing the overall aesthetic effect of the trial dentures. To make this judgement, the teeth should be observed during function by the operator engaging the patient in conversation and, if possible, introducing an excuse for the patient to smile naturally. This functional assessment is important because dentures which have a pleasant appearance in repose may suddenly become glaringly unsuitable as soon as the patient's lips move in speech.

If the position of the anterior teeth requires correction, the modifications should be carried out at the chairside so that the altered dentures can be tried in the mouth and the effectiveness of the modifications assessed by both the dentist and the patient.

When finalising the appearance, the dentist should attempt to create the illusion of natural teeth. In order to carry out this visual deception successfully, the appearance of the dentures should be appropriate for the patient in question and also appropriate for the population from which the patient comes. If these requirements are fulfilled, the teeth will appear to 'belong' to the patient and the deception will be complete.

In the UK, the prevalence of crowding is so high that a 'perfect' even arrangement of natural anterior teeth is rarely, if ever, seen. If, therefore, dentures are constructed with this type of arrangement, the risk of the resulting appearance seeming artificial is considerable. As a general rule, imperfection in the anterior tooth arrangement is a basic requirement in creating the illusion of natural teeth; complete symmetry should be avoided – the anterior teeth should not be placed so that the incisal edges are all at the same level. Some form of crowding should usually be incorporated into the anterior tooth arrangement; this crowding may vary in degree from minimal irregularity to marked overlapping of the teeth. When producing irregularity of the anterior teeth, care should be taken to ensure that a general impression of balance is maintained even though the two sides of the dental arch may not be completely symmetrical. For example, if the centre line between the central incisors is some distance from the mid-line of the face, or if the incisal level is not horizontal, a sense of imbalance will result and the appearance will be poor. The vertical axes of the anterior teeth can be varied but if the inclination of these axes on one side of the mouth does not approximately balance that on the other, an unsatisfactory appearance will result (Figure 12.4).

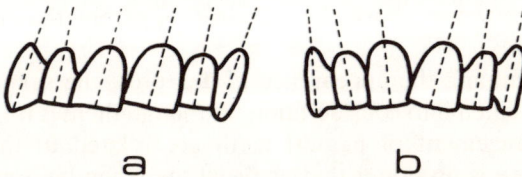

a   b

Figure 12.4   (a) Imbalance produced by inclining the vertical axes of the anterior teeth in the same direction. (b) The improvement in appearance produced by counterbalancing the inclination of the axes on one side of the mouth with those on the other

Restorations in anterior teeth are not uncommon. If composite materials of the correct shade have been used, these restorations should not normally be visible. However, there may occasionally be a slight discrepancy between the shade of restoration and the tooth; this feature of natural dentitions can be utilised in the construction of dentures to help create the impression that the patient still has natural teeth. Interstitial or cervical cavities may be cut in one or more of the artificial anterior teeth and then filled with composite or cold-curing acrylic resin of a shade which differs slightly from that of the tooth itself. It has been argued that this procedure is simply mimicking bad dentistry and is therefore not justified. There is an element of truth in this but the technique is a powerful weapon in the dentist's armoury of devices for creating the illusion of natural teeth. It can be brought out occasionally and used with considerable effect as the concept of restorations is so foreign to that of dentures that the patient's acquaintances may be deceived by this device alone.

Factors which are peculiar to a particular patient and which affect the appearance of natural anterior teeth are the skeletal relationship and age. These factors should therefore be borne in mind when constructing dentures.

The method of determining an incisal position which is appropriate for an edentulous patient's skeletal relationship has been discussed in Chapter

11. If a patient is provided with dentures which have an inappropriate incisal relationship, for example, a Class I incisal relationship on a marked skeletal Class II base, there is a risk that in addition to problems with stability, the dentures will appear incongruous and the aesthetic result will be poor.

Changes in the shape of the crowns of natural teeth commonly occur as a result of increasing age. These alterations in crown form are produced by incisal wear and gingival recession. Anterior teeth on dentures can therefore be given a definitely youthful, or aged, appearance by incisal grinding where appropriate and correct shaping of the gingival margins (Figure 12.5). If a 'young' dental appearance is provided for an elderly patient, or vice versa, it will be only too apparent that the patient is wearing dentures.

When determining the appearance of dentures, the sex of the patient should also be taken into consideration. Although there is no evidence that form and arrangement of natural teeth are related to the sex of the individual, there is no doubt that artificial teeth can be arranged to give either a 'feminine' or 'masculine' appearance to dentures (Figure 12.6). Masculinity can be suggested by increasing the irregularity of the arrangement and by using squarish moulds with obvious surface character while, conversely, a more even arrangement of rounded, smooth-surfaced anterior teeth will impart a feminine quality to the appearance. Rotation of the incisors in a vertical plane may also help to 'sex' the dentures; moving the distal margins labially will increase the vigour and masculinity of the appearance and vice versa (Figure 12.7). Features which help to determine the 'sex' of dentures can be summarised as follows:

Male	Female
Large teeth	Small teeth
Square moulds	Rounded moulds
Characterised labial surface	Smooth surface
Irregularity	Even arrangement
Distal margins labially	Distal margins palatally
Marked wear of incisal edges	Minimal wear of incisal edges
Diastemas	Closed contact points
Prominent canines	Canines not prominent

Once the upper anterior teeth have been adjusted, consideration should be given to the lower teeth. These, in most patients, will not make such an important contribution to the appearance; nevertheless, they should not be ignored completely. In a few patients, they may be displayed more during function than the upper teeth and therefore may be a dominant factor in determining the patient's dental appearance. Again, one should apply the same general rules regarding perfection and evenness of tooth arrangement which have been discussed previously.

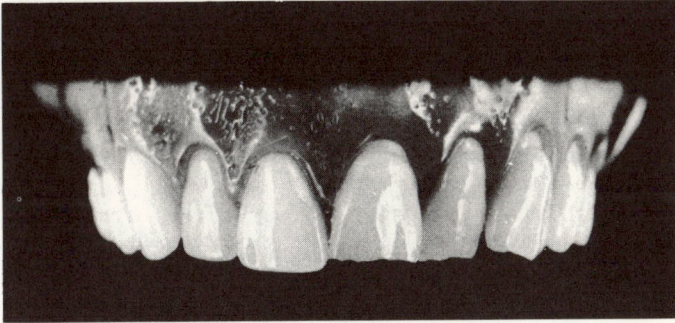

Figure 12.5 Use of incisal grinding and gingival contouring to convert a youthful appearance 3–1 to an aged one 1–3

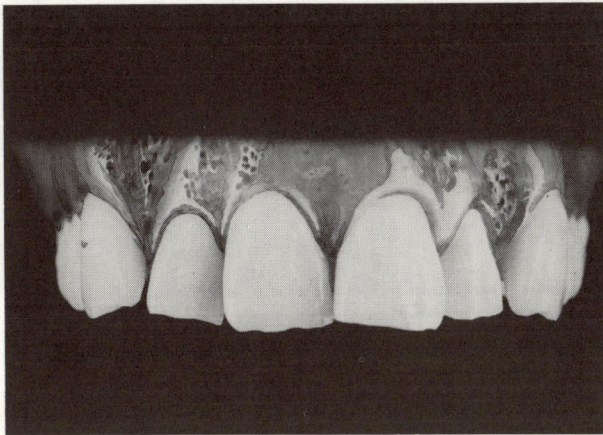

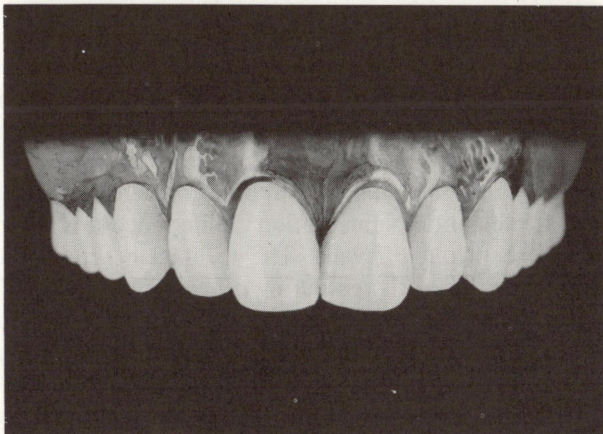

Figure 12.6 *Top*: An example of a 'masculine' anterior tooth arrangement. *Bottom*: An example of a 'feminine' anterior tooth arrangement

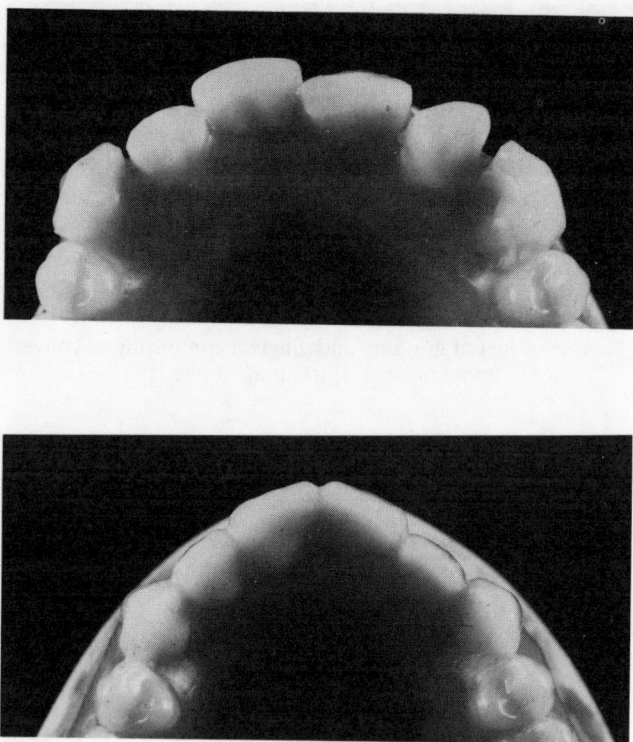

Figure 12.7   *Top*: Distal margins of incisors moved labially to increase the vigour of the appearance. *Bottom*: Distal margins of incisors moved palatally to impart a more feminine appearance (these are occlusal views of the set-ups shown in Figure 12.6)

In some patients, the upper labial flange will be visible during speech and smiling. If this is the case, a natural appearance will only be achieved if the acrylic flange is contoured to resemble natural gum, and if the surface of the flange is slightly irregular or stippled to break up any reflections (Figure 12.5). If melanotic pigmentation of the mucosa is present, a pale pink flange will seem out of place. The technician should therefore be requested to tint the labial flange during processing.

It is, of course, essential that the patient's requirements regarding the appearance of the dentures should have been discussed fully, not only at the try-in stage but also during the preceding stages of the course of treatment. The dentist's role in these discussions should be that of an adviser who ensures that the patient is in possession of all the information required to make a sensible decision regarding appearance. For example, some patients will request that their dentures have anterior teeth which are small, white and even – a combination which will almost guarantee that the dentition is easily recognised as being an artificial one. However, these patients will often change their minds if given the opportunity at the try-in stage of seeing the improvement that even a small amount of irregularity can make.

If a patient has strongly held views about how the dentures should look, the dentist should take great care not to persuade the patient to accept an arrangement of anterior teeth which conflicts with these views. If this happens, the patient may be dissatisfied with the finished dentures and could, with complete justification, request that they be remade. It is difficult for a patient to form a clear opinion regarding the appearance of the dentures in the short time available at the try-in stage and in the relatively strange surroundings of the dental surgery. If a friend or relative is available to offer an opinion, this can be of considerable help to the patient, particularly if the dentist leaves the room so that they are able to discuss the appearance in an uninhibited manner. In the absence of a friend, discussing the appearance with the dental surgery assistant may be beneficial. It is preferable for the patient to assess the appearance of the dentures by looking at them in a wall mirror at a normal viewing distance, rather than using a hand mirror which may be held too close to the face and give an unrealistic view. In exceptional cases where there is particular difficulty in determining what is an acceptable appearance, it may even be necessary to permit the patient to take the trial dentures home for a short time.

If instructions to the technician regarding the elimination of unwanted undercuts or the addition of a palatal relief have not yet been given, this must be done before sending the dentures to be processed. It is also appropriate at this stage to consider whether some form of identification marker should be incorporated into the dentures.

DENTURE MARKING

Identification marks may be incorporated into dentures to serve a variety of purposes:

(a) To allow identification of dentures in dental laboratories where large numbers of dentures are being processed. This procedure is widely practised by technicians and does not require instructions from the dentist.

(b) To allow identification of dentures in institutions such as hospitals and old people's homes where elderly and confused patients commonly misplace their dentures. Such losses are particularly regrettable because the dentures may be virtually irreplaceable as a result of an elderly person's difficulty in adapting to new dentures of different design.

(c) To allow identification of patients following loss of consciousness, memory or life. For this system to be fully effective, the marker needs to be indestructible and to incorporate a code which is universally acceptable. As the latter requirement has not been fulfilled at the present time, such markers are not widely used in general dental practice. However, they are routinely used in the Armed Forces and in certain countries such as Scandinavia.

Identification marks fall into two broad categories, surface markers and inclusion markers.

Surface Markers

Marks may be produced on the impression surface of the denture by scribing the cast before processing the denture. The irregularities produced on the denture surface are clinically undesirable and should therefore be reserved for identifying dentures in laboratories after processing. The marks should be removed before inserting the denture.

Marks on a denture can be made by writing with either a spirit-based pen or with a fine pencil. Pencil marks, however, require protection with a polymer varnish. Both techniques offer relatively short-term benefits. Exposure of spirit pen marks to hypochlorite cleaners can result in rapid fading. Also, there can be a rapid loss of definition of both pencil and spirit pen marks if an abrasive cleaner is used. Thus, unless the marks are checked at regular intervals and renewed as necessary, the methods are perhaps suitable only for the identification of dentures belonging to patients admitted to hospital for a short stay.

Inclusion Markers

These markers may be metallic, such as stainless steel strip, or non-metallic, such as tissue paper or ceramic materials. They can either be incorporated into a denture at the time of processing or can be inserted into the processed denture by cutting a recess, inserting the marker and covering with clear cold-curing acrylic resin.

Inclusion markers should be placed posteriorly in the lingual or palatal areas of the dentures. In this position, the stresses induced by the markers are unlikely to cause significant weakening of the dentures. Furthermore, the markers are less likely to be destroyed in the event of the patient's death by burning.

If identification marks of the inclusion type are required, the appropriate request must be made to the technician when the trial dentures are sent for processing.

BIBLIOGRAPHY

De Van, M. M. (1957) The appearance phase of denture construction. *Dental Clinics of North America*, 255–68.

Deb, A. K. and Heath, M. R. (1979) Marking dentures in geriatric institutions – the relevance and appropriate methods. *British Dental Journal*, **146**, 282–4.

Frush, J. P. and Fisher, R. D. (1958) Dynesthetic interpretation of dentogenic concept. *Journal of Prosthetic Dentistry*, **8**, 558–81.

Harrison, A. (1986) A simple denture marking system. *British Dental Journal*, **160**, 89–91.

Heath, J. R. (1987) Denture identification – a simple approach. *Journal of Oral Rehabilitation*, **14**, 147–63.

Lombardi, R. E. (1973) The principles of visual perception and their clinical application to denture aesthetics. *Journal of Prosthetic Dentistry*, **29**, 358–82.

Oliver, B. (1989) A new inclusion denture marking system. *Quintessence International*, **20**, 21–5.

Schwarz, W. D. (1963) Improving full denture appearance. *Dental Practitioner and Dental Record*, **8**, 319–27.

Turner, C. H., Fletcher, A. M. and Ritchie, G. M. (1976) Denture marking and human identification. *British Dental Journal*, **141**, 114–17.

Wright, S. M. (1974) Prosthetic reproduction of gingival pigmentation. *British Dental Journal*, **136**, 367–72.

13 Fitting Complete Dentures

Although all features of design are checked carefully on the trial dentures, the processing procedure will alter the occlusal and impression surfaces of the finished dentures. Thus, the main objectives when fitting new dentures are:

(a) to adjust the impression surface to ensure comfort;
(b) to modify the occlusal surface to ensure even occlusal contact;
(c) to give advice on the wearing of dentures, to encourage rapid adaptation, efficient usage and the maintenance of oral health.

THE IMPRESSION SURFACE

Any cause of pain must obviously be eliminated, not only to ensure comfort but also to prevent pain impulses encouraging the adoption of abnormal paths of closure of the mandible which prevent occlusal contact causing pressure at the site of discomfort. The common causes of pain arising from the impression surface of a denture are shown in Figure 13.1. Acrylic nodules and sharp ridges are detected readily by observation and by passing a gauze napkin or cotton wool roll over the surface so that the threads catch on the acrylic projections. An undercut flange is likely to cause pain as the denture is inserted and removed; the area is located by direct observation and by the use of a disclosing material such as soft wax. In the latter instance, an even layer of the disclosing material is applied to the suspect area and the denture inserted and removed. The precise area of undercut producing the pain is shown up as an area of acrylic from which the wax has been removed.

THE OCCLUSAL SURFACE

Having reached the stage when each denture can be inserted and removed from the mouth without discomfort and when firm pressure can be applied

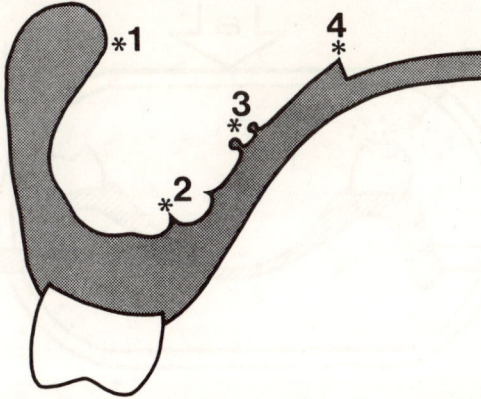

Figure 13.1 Common causes of pain arising from the impression surface of a denture are indicated by the asterisks: 1, overextension into bony undercut; 2, sharp projection associated with crease in mucosa; 3, acrylic pearls; 4, sharp edge of relief chamber

to the occlusal surface without eliciting pain, the occlusion is now checked. However, before discussing the methods of occlusal adjustment, it is necessary to appreciate the possible causes of occlusal error arising from the processing procedure.

Laboratory Causes of Occlusal Error

These are illustrated diagrammatically in Figure 13.2.

(a) If, during the packing procedure, the acrylic resin has reached an advanced dough stage and thus offers increased resistance to closure of the flask, excessive force will be needed to bring the two halves of the flask together. The excessive pressure may push the artificial teeth into the investing plaster. Similar tooth movement may result from rapid build-up in pressure if the two halves of the flask are closed too quickly.

(b) The layer of investing plaster may be weakened as a result of porosity in the mix, the use of an incorrect powder/water ratio or by an inadequate thickness of plaster between the walls of the flask and the denture. Normal packing pressure may break the investing plaster, resulting in movement of the teeth.

(c) If pressure on the flask is released during the curing cycle, the two halves may separate, thus increasing the height of the completed denture.

(d) The two halves of the flask may be separated by a layer of excess resin which should have been removed during trial closure of the

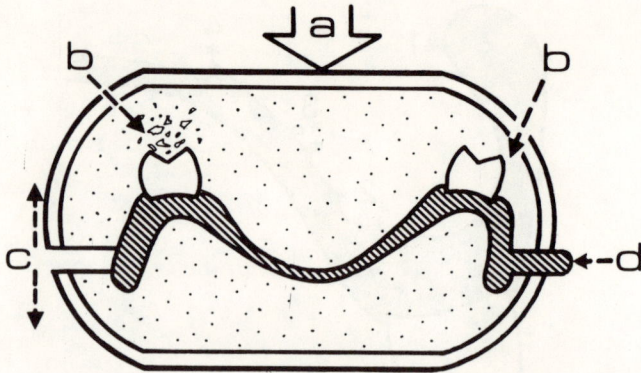

Figure 13.2   Laboratory causes of occlusal error (for a description of the causes, see the text)

flask. This 'flash' will result in an increased occlusal vertical dimension of the denture.

In spite of taking all due precautions to prevent the errors just described, small occlusal inaccuracies are bound to occur. It has been shown that a processed denture exhibits an average increase in height of 0.5 mm and a shift in tooth contact towards the posterior region. Such errors can be corrected in the laboratory if a split-cast mounting technique is used.

The basis of a split-cast mounting technique is to have a method of replacing the processed dentures, still on their casts, back on to the articulator in exactly the same jaw relationship as when the set-up was produced (Figures 13.3, 13.4 and 13.5). Any premature contacts, resulting from displacement of individual teeth, can then readily be seen. An overall increase in occlusal vertical dimension will be shown by the incisal pin failing to make contact with the incisal table.

Clinical Methods of Occlusal Adjustment

If all normal precautions have been taken while processing the dentures, any further occlusal error detected when the dentures are placed in the mouth is likely to be of clinical origin and to have passed undetected at the trial stage. Such an error can be corrected either at the chairside or by returning the dentures to an articulator using a check record procedure.

Chairside Adjustment

The reasons for recording the retruded contact position of the mandible, and not the muscular position, are discussed on page 74. The practical implications of the choice are considered in Chapter 10 and the case for

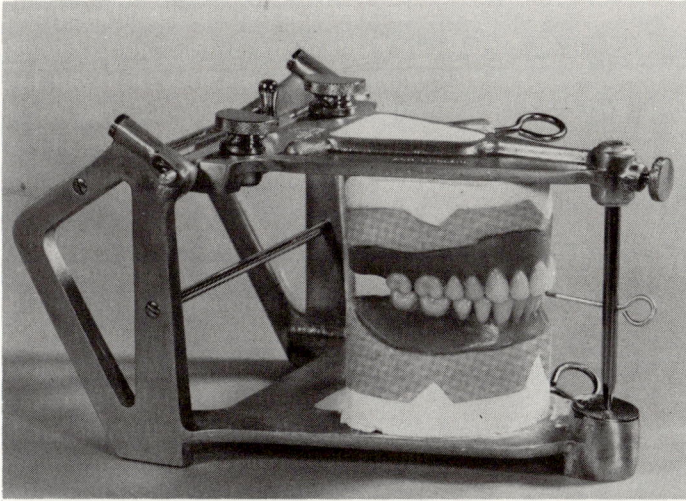

Figure 13.3   Split-cast mounting technique (a). The trial dentures have been mounted on an average-movement articulator. Before the casts are plastered to the articulator, 'V'-shaped location notches are cut into each cast. A film of petroleum jelly is applied to the location notches and to the peripheral areas of each cast; as a result, the master casts are readily detached from the topping plaster prior to processing

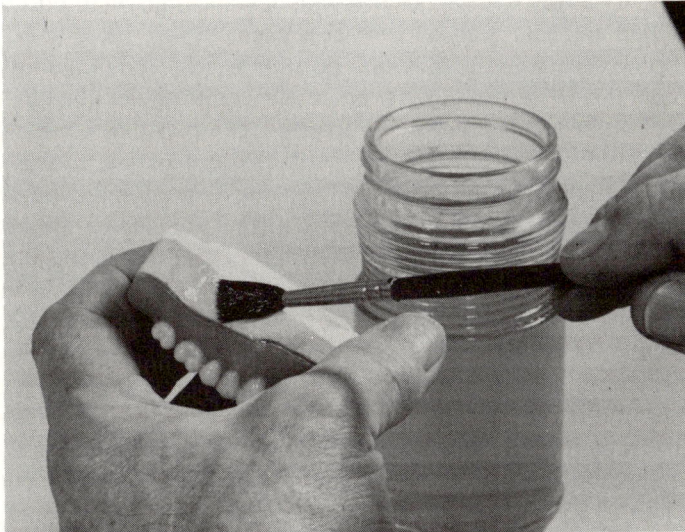

Figure 13.4   Split-cast mounting technique (b). A separating medium is applied to the cast before flasking. This allows the denture, still seated on the cast, to be removed from the investing plaster after processing

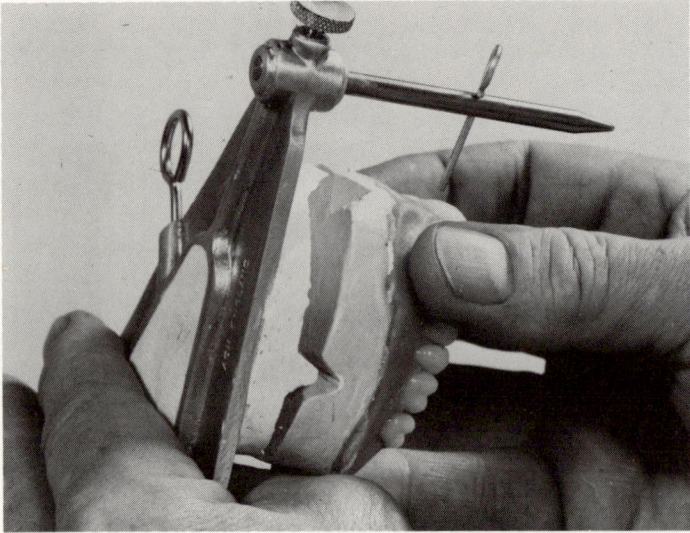

Figure 13.5 Split-cast mounting technique (c). The master cast is accurately relocated on the topping plaster and secured with either sticky wax or a cyano-acrylate adhesive

creating an area of free movement around the retruded contact position is presented at the end of that chapter (pages 186–93). The purpose of adjusting the occlusion on the finished dentures is to ensure that freedom of movement between the retruded contact and muscular positions is re-established and that occlusal contact is even.

Balanced occlusion in the muscular position is achieved in the following way. When the dentures have been made comfortable, the patient is encouraged to relax and is then instructed to open and close without making occlusal contact. In this way, the pattern of jaw movement is largely determined by sensory input from the temporomandibular joint receptors and from the muscle spindles in the muscles of mastication. Sensory input from the mechanoreceptors in the denture-bearing mucosa is then introduced by asking the patient to continue opening and closing in a relaxed manner but to make initial, light contact on the teeth and to report on the location of that contact. It is essential that the patient refrains from heavy contact; this ensures that the joint sensory input prevails and thus prevents alteration to the path of closure of the mandible. In addition, it should be remembered that heavy contact is likely to compress the underlying mucosa and so mask the presence of the premature contact.

The majority of patients are able to offer such comments as 'The dentures are meeting on the left side first of all' or 'I'm meeting on the back teeth only'. Such discrimination comes from stimulation of the mechano-receptors in the denture-bearing mucosa and it is the dentist's task to act on the evidence and eliminate the premature contacts. A piece of thin horseshoe-shaped articulating paper is inserted between the teeth and the patient asked to repeat the jaw movements. A single strip of articulating paper placed on only one side of the dental arch is likely to induce jaw movement to that side. Furthermore, instructions such as 'bite together' are likely to encourage protrusion of the mandible, whereas a request to 'close on your back teeth' will promote a normal closure pattern. Adjustment of the occlusal surfaces should be made only on those markings made by the articulating paper which coincide with the patient's comments. The process is repeated until the patient reports that the teeth meet evenly. Having established a balanced occlusion in muscular position, the dentist should normally check that there is an area of balanced articulation of 1–2 mm around this position.

The occlusal vertical dimension and occlusal balance in intercuspal and muscular position depend on contact between the palatal upper cusps and the buccal lower cusps of the posterior teeth (Figure 13.6(a)). These cusps are therefore known as *supporting cusps*. Having established even occlusal contact in muscular position, further adjustment of these cusps should be avoided wherever possible. Thus, if, in a lateral occlusal position, a premature contact is detected on the working side between a buccal upper and buccal lower cusp, it is the buccal upper cusp (BU) that should be reduced; similarly, if interference is observed on the working side in lateral occlusion between a palatal upper and lingual lower cusp, it is the lingual lower cusp (LL) that should be reduced (Figures 13.6(b) and (c)). This approach to correcting the occlusion on the working side is known as the BULL rule. This rule cannot be applied to the correction of premature contacts on the balancing side, however, because here both upper and lower supporting cusps are in opposition (Figure 13.6(d)). It is usually possible in this situation to reduce the *interfering* contact without eliminating the *supporting* contact. If this is not possible, it is necessary to adjust one of the offending cusps and to accept loss of supporting contact in this area. Overall balance in muscular position will not be lost as a result.

Check Record
Adjusting an occlusal discrepancy which is visible clinically is frequently a time-consuming exercise if carried out in the manner just described. This is especially so if the error produces an anteroposterior or lateral slide after the initial occlusal contact. There is, in fact, evidence to suggest that a check record should be undertaken as a routine procedure on the grounds that its use results in fewer post-insertion complaints of discomfort. If the dentures are rearticulated by means of a check record, much of the initial work can be carried out in the laboratory before the final adjustments are made in the mouth.

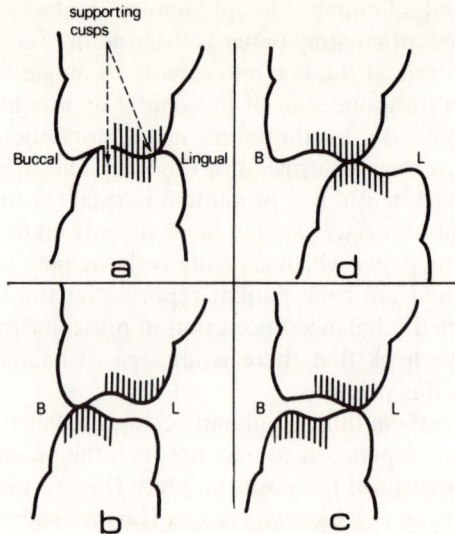

Figure 13.6 (a) Contact between supporting cusps maintains the occlusal vertical dimension and occlusal balance in tooth position. (b) Premature contact between buccal cusps on the working side in lateral occlusion is corrected by grinding the buccal upper cusp. (c) Premature contact between lingual cusps on the working side in lateral occlusion is corrected by grinding the lingual lower cusps. (d) Premature contact on the balancing side is corrected by reducing the interfering contact on one or other of the supporting cusps

After the denture bases have been made comfortable, a recording is made of the jaw relationship with the mandible in the retruded position and with the dentures just out of occlusion. This procedure ensures that normal jaw closure and the relationship of the dentures to the supporting tissues are not influenced by abnormal dental contact. The inter-occlusal recording medium used for the check record should offer minimal resistance to jaw closure. A wax containing fine metal particles is useful in this respect. The softened wax is placed on the posterior teeth of one of the dentures, care being taken to confine it to the occlusal surface. If an excessive amount of material is used, sensory nerve endings in the tongue and cheek mucosa are stimulated and the sensory input may influence jaw movement adversely. After initial closure into the retruded position, the dentures are removed and the wax inspected to ensure that there has been no penetration of the wax by the artificial teeth. Once a satisfactory initial record has been obtained the wax is trimmed using a sharp blade to minimise the chance of distortion. Buccal excess is removed because it obscures the contact relationship of opposing teeth with the wax record, making a visual check on accuracy impossible. Occlusal excess is removed until only the indentations made by the tips of the opposing cusps are visible. This is necessary because deep occlusal indentations increase the likelihood of denture displacement and mandibular deviation. Once the excess wax has been removed, the accuracy of the record can be checked.

Accuracy is crucial to the success of the procedure and it is common practice therefore to verify the accuracy of the all-important record before committing oneself to the occlusal adjustment. This involves obtaining more than one record and then only proceeding with the adjustment if both agree.

One approach involves the production of a wax record as described previously and using this to articulate the dentures. A second wax record is then produced on the articulator by closing the dentures through a sheet of wax until initial tooth contact occurs. This second record is chilled and trimmed as before and then checked for accuracy in the mouth. If consistency is achieved, the operator has verified not only the accuracy of the original record but also the articulator mounting and the arc of closure of the articulator. Occlusal adjustment can then be carried out with confidence. If the second record is not found to be correct, the intra-oral registration must be repeated and one of the dentures rearticulated. When undertaking this procedure, it is helpful to be able to remove the dentures and replace them on the plaster mounting casts. This can be achieved by blocking out any undercuts on the impression surface of the dentures with soft wax or wet tissue paper before pouring the casts.

If the dentures are mounted on an average-movement articulator, the relationship of the upper denture to the axis of movement on the articulator will be similar to the relationship of the maxilla to the hinge axis passing through the heads of the condyles. However, a more precise record of the relationship of the upper denture to the condylar axis can be obtained using a face bow; the recording is subsequently transferred to a semi-adjustable articulator (page 187). The pure hinge movement of the articulator will be similar to the movement of the mandible in the retruded position, as the check record has been made on the path of retruded arc of closure (page 67). Before starting the occlusal adjustment, the inter-occlusal recording is removed, the incisal pin raised and the articulator closed until initial tooth contact is made. The occlusion is then adjusted until even occlusal contact is obtained. If there is a gross error in the jaw relationship, it may be necessary to remove the artificial teeth and set up new ones in the correct position. In such a situation, it is wise to repeat the trial stage. When the jaw relationship is at last correct, the new teeth can be attached to the denture base with cold-curing acrylic resin. Stages of the check record procedure are illustrated in Figure 13.7.

The time required to mount the dentures on the articulator may act as a disincentive to the use of the check record procedure, particularly if there is no dental technician on the premises. However, the process can be speeded up considerably if the laboratory is requested to return the finished dentures with the upper denture already on a plaster-holding cast

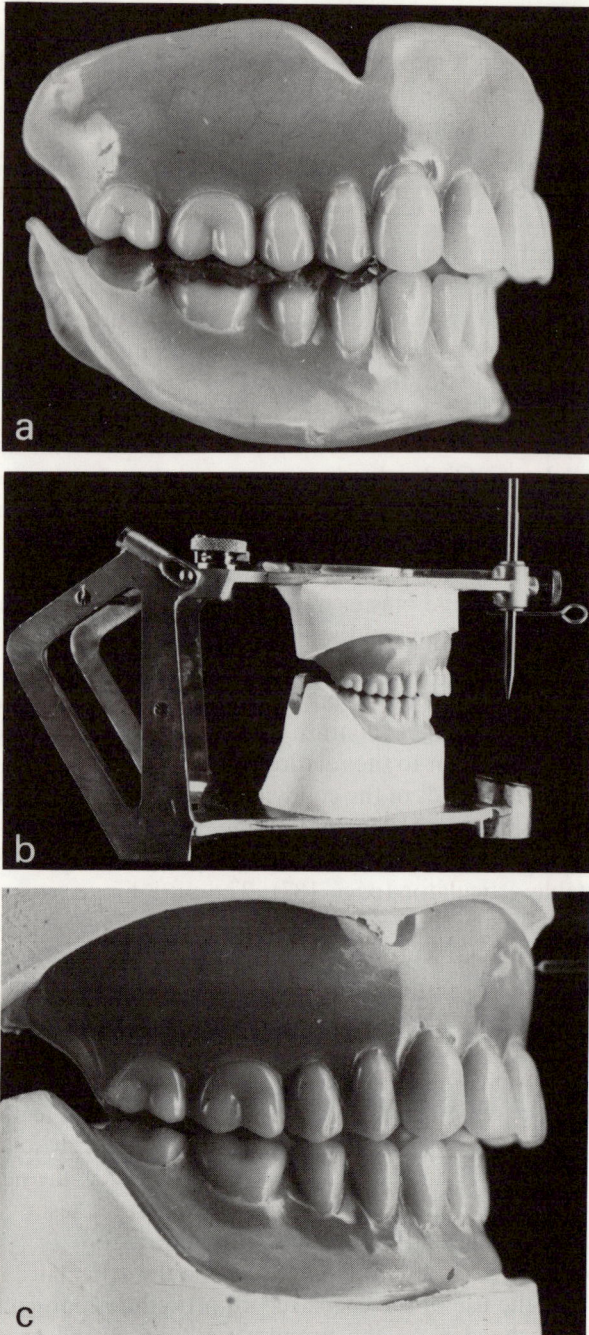

Figure 13.7 Stages of the check record procedure: (a) a recording of the retruded position with the dentures out of occlusion; (b) the dentures are articulated, the occlusal record removed, the incisal pin raised and occlusal contact made; (c) view of the dentures to show an occlusal error

on the articulator. It is then a quick and simple matter for the dentist to mount the lower denture against the upper when the check record has been obtained. This technique presupposes that the laboratory will return the articulator as a matter of routine. If not, or if one wishes to undertake a check record at some stage after the dentures have been fitted, a convenient chairside technique is as follows.

An articulator, kept in the surgery, has acrylic platforms fixed to the upper and lower arms (Figure 13.8); these platforms have small locating notches cut into their upper surfaces. Any undercuts on the impression surfaces of the dentures are blocked out. The dentures are then attached to the platform with impression plaster and the check record procedure is concluded in the normal manner. This technique is both rapid, convenient and accurate.

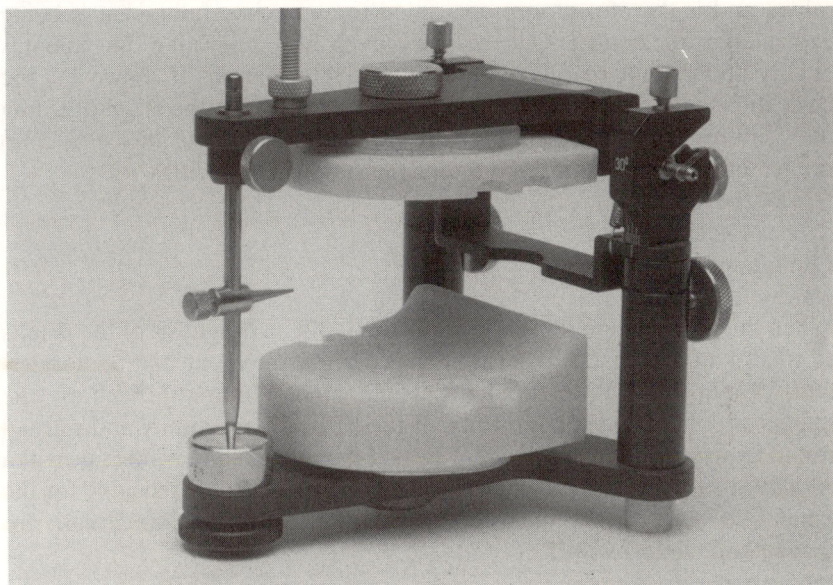

Figure 13.8   Acrylic mounting platforms attached to an average-movement articulator to allow a rapid check record procedure at the chairside

ADVICE TO THE PATIENT

The ultimate success of new dentures depends to a considerable extent upon the quality of advice offered by the dentist. Sensible advice put over in a clear manner gives confidence to the new denture wearer, and ensures that the patient starts off on the right footing. It is perhaps more effective to stress particular points by the spoken rather than the written word. Thus, the dentist should spend time in explaining the intricacies of denture wearing. In addition, it is useful to back this up with printed instructions which will act as a reminder. With regard to advice on denture cleaning, especially when given to elderly patients, it has been reported that verbal information alone is likely to result in no more than a short-term improvement. Long-term improvement in denture hygiene is likely to occur only if verbal information is reinforced by demonstration.

Although advice to the patient is considered in this chapter, it is most valuable to introduce the various topics during the earlier stages of treatment and reinforce at the trial stage. Information must be remembered and assimilated if it is to be effective. If new dentures have just been placed in the mouth, the patient is wondering how to control them, how to cope with the new sensation and what to do with the sudden outpouring of saliva, and is therefore too preoccupied to appreciate fully what is being explained by the dentist. This thought is even more relevant if the patient is elderly and cannot readily assimilate new information. If, however, the basic information has already been given, repetition at the stage of fitting the dentures can help to reinforce the earlier message. The advice given to the patient may be considered under the following headings.

Limitations of Dentures

When the patient's mouth was examined initially, a prognosis of the results of treatment was made. If, at that stage, it was apparent that anatomical and, perhaps, adaptive problems would create future difficulties, the patient should have been informed at the earliest opportunity and warned not to expect too much of the dentures. If the information is first given at a recall visit when complaints have been made, it is not unreasonable for the patient to believe that the valid explanation is, in fact, an excuse for inadequate clinical work.

Controlling Dentures

It should be explained to the patient that once the dentures have been fitted, new muscular behaviour must be developed in order to control them and that simple tasks should be mastered before advancing to more complex skills. Thus, the patient should be advised to take small mouthfuls of non-sticky food and to chew on both sides of the mouth at once during the initial stages. Such well-known phrases as 'learn to walk before you run' and 'practice makes perfect' convey the sense admirably. It is important to convey the impression that time is required to learn the muscular skills since it has been reported that although approximately 60 per cent of experienced denture wearers were able to eat and speak satisfactorily within a week of the replacement dentures being fitted, a further 20 per cent of these patients required up to one month to become proficient.

Appearance

If the new dentures make an obvious change to the appearance of the patient, as for example when restoring a loss of vertical dimension, it is very important to warn the patient in advance that friends and relatives may look twice and even pass a remark on a change in appearance. Unless this is done, there is a risk that the patient will interpret a chance remark or a second glance as realisation by the friend that new dentures have been provided. Whereas most people are more than happy that new clothes or new hair styles are admired, they may be particularly sensitive to new dentures being recognised. As there is a danger that such recognition may set the patient against the dentures, it is wise to remind him or her of the original aims of the treatment and that the much needed improvement in appearance may be noticed. The patient should be encouraged to appreciate that friends and relatives, as well as the patient, may require a period of adaptation to the new dentures.

Initial Sensations

It is wise to reassure the patient regarding the immediate changes that may be noticed when the dentures are inserted. For example, some inexperienced denture wearers salivate excessively and thus find it extremely difficult to speak. Reassurance that this outpouring usually settles down within several hours and that the strange sensations disappear within a few days helps to boost morale.

Wearing Dentures at Night

If dentures are worn at night for at least the first 10 days or so, continuous stimulation of the mechanoreceptors in the oral mucosa hastens adaptation.

Ideally, it is better if the dentures are left out at night following the initial period of adaptation because it has been shown that frequent tooth contacts are made during sleep with the possibility that the denture-bearing mucosa may be traumatised. Furthermore, continuous coverage of the denture-bearing mucosa prevents cleansing of the mucosa by the tongue and saliva and increases the exposure to denture plaque. If the dentures are not worn at night, the mucosa is allowed to recover from the day's activity. This is especially relevant for those patients with a thin atrophic mucosa and with a reduced ability to repair tissue, features commonly found in the elderly. However, the dentist's advice to leave the dentures out at night is frequently ignored because, as has been rightly said, 'To leave the dentures in a glass in the bathroom or at the bedside all night is an unattractive thought to most people, even if they sleep alone, or with partners whose capacity for simple domestic pleasures and skills has fallen off'. Advice to take dentures out just before sleep rather than leaving them out at night is a subtle variation which proves more acceptable to some patients.

Cleaning Dentures

Deposits such as microbial plaque, calculus and food debris on dentures may be responsible for a variety of problems including denture stomatitis, angular stomatitis, unpleasant tastes, odours, an unsightly appearance and the accelerated deterioration of some denture materials such as short-term resilient lining materials. The effective cleaning of dentures is therefore of considerable importance to the patient's general well-being and oral health.

When new dentures are fitted, the patient should be advised to brush them regularly and carefully using soap, water and a soft nylon brush small enough to reach into all areas of the denture surface. The importance of removing all deposits, not just the more obvious stains and food particles, should be emphasised. Disclosing solutions may be used by the patient at home as an indicator of when complete removal of denture plaque has been achieved. Food dyes, such as cochineal, are the cheapest and most readily available solutions suitable for this purpose. If the dentist needs to reinforce denture hygiene procedures at a later stage, 4 per cent Neutral Red is a suitable disclosing agent (Figure 13.9).

Conventional toothpastes and pastes designed specifically for dentures are used frequently by patients. There has always been a worry that these materials will abrade denture base resins. Recent studies have shown that pastes containing dicalcium phosphate are less abrasive than those containing calcium carbonate, but that the amount of wear that occurs even with the latter group of pastes is insignificant provided that the brushing load is not excessive. Pastes of high abrasivity are needed to remove tobacco stain.

In addition to brushing the dentures, regular use of an immersion cleaner is also advisable. Such a cleaner should remove any plaque left behind on the denture surface because of difficulty in brushing inaccessible

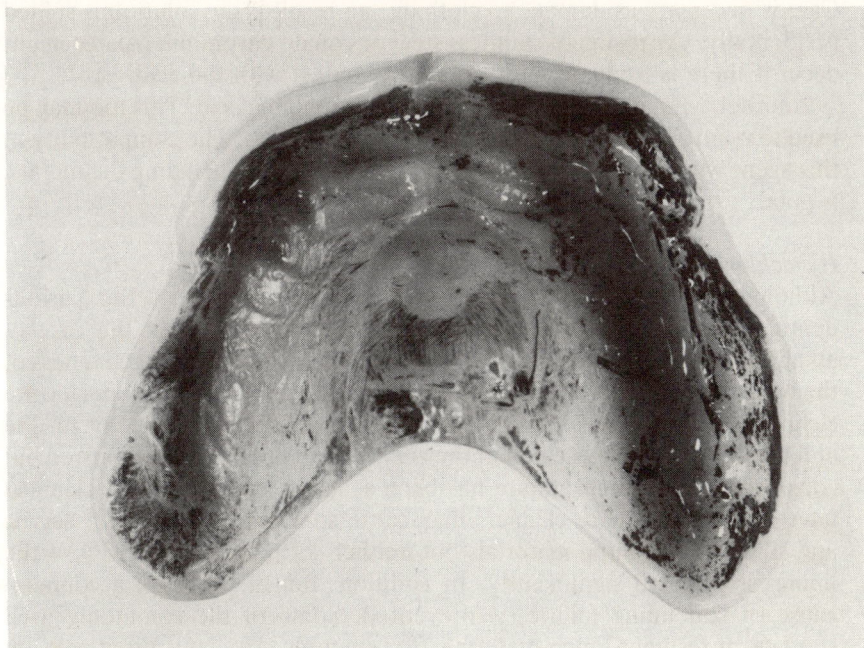

Figure 13.9 Microbial plaque stained by disclosing solution applied to the impression surface

areas or because of a patient's lack of manual dexterity. Immersion cleansers have been blamed for bleaching denture base resin. As a result of recent work, it has been shown that the products are innocent and that bleaching occurs because the manufacturer's recommendations for use have not been followed and hot water has been added to the cleaning agent. Such a cleaning regime will also reduce the flexural strength of the denture base.   *DENTURAL*

Alkaline Peroxide Cleaners
These are the most widely used type of immersion cleaner. Their cleaning action is largely due to the formation of small bubbles of oxygen which dislodge loosely attached material from the denture surface. They are safe, pleasant to use and do not damage acrylic resin or the metals used in denture construction. It has been demonstrated however that they are capable of causing rapid deterioration of certain short-term resilient lining materials. They are relatively ineffective cleaners and there is evidence that their ability to remove microbial plaque is severely limited.
                              STEREDENT

Acid Cleaners
One type of acid cleaner contains 5 per cent hydrochloric acid. It may be applied to dentures to soften calculus which is then removed by brushing.

Care is necessary as damage to clothing can result if the solution is spilled accidentally. Corrosion of stainless steel or cobalt–chromium palates might occur if there is frequent and prolonged contact with the acid.

Another type of acid cleaner consists of sulphamic acid. This too may be used to control the formation of calculus on dentures. The compatibility of this agent with the commonly used denture materials, including the metals, is good.

Hypochlorite Cleaners

Although investigations into the relative effectiveness of the various denture cleaners have produced some conflicting results in the case of alkaline peroxides, there is widespread agreement as to the effectiveness of the hypochlorite preparations. Immersion of the dentures in a hypochlorite cleaner for periods in excess of six hours will result in removal of plaque and heavy staining. Bleaching of the acrylic resin has not been reported but corrosion of cobalt–chromium has been seen when hypochlorite cleaners have been used. These cleaners may cause some loss of colour of acrylic and silicone soft lining materials but neither softness nor elasticity of the linings is affected significantly. In addition, fungal invasion, a common cause of soft lining failure, is prevented. Some of the commonly used short-term resilient lining materials (for example, De Trey Visco-gel) are compatible with hypochlorite cleaners; in fact, the regular use of such a cleaner can extend the useful life of a tissue conditioner from a few days to several months.

Recall Procedures

When the dentures are fitted, it should be stressed that a recall visit within the next few days is necessary and that, to reduce the risk of tissue damage or bone resorption, a check should be made every year. It is important that the patient is not under the mistaken belief that once the artificial substitute for the natural teeth has been provided there will be no further problems, and no need for further maintenance. Treatment carried out at subsequent visits is discussed in the next chapter.

BIBLIOGRAPHY

Altman, M. D., Yost, K. G. and Pitts, G. (1979) A spectrofluorometric protein assay of plaque on dentures and of denture cleaning efficiency. *Journal of Prosthetic Dentistry*, **42**, 502–6.

Ambjornsen, E. and Rise, J. (1985) The effect of verbal information and demonstration on denture hygiene in elderly people. *Acta Odontologica Scandinavica*, **43**, 19–24.

Bergman, B. and Carlsson, G. E. (1972) Review of 54 complete denture wearers. Patients' opinions 1 year after treatment. *Acta Odontologica Scandinavica*, **30**, 399–414.

Brill, N., Schübeler, S. and Tryde, G. (1962) Aspects of occlusal sense in natural and artificial teeth. *Journal of Prosthetic Dentistry*, **12**, 123–8.

Budtz-Jørgensen, E. (1979) Materials and methods for cleaning dentures. *Journal of Prosthetic Dentistry*, **42**, 619–23.

Crawford, C.-A., Lloyd, C. M., Newton, J. P. and Yemm, R. (1986) Denture bleaching: a laboratory simulation of patients' cleaning procedures. *Journal of Dentistry*, **14**, 258–61.

Davenport, J. C. (1972) The denture surface. *British Dental Journal*, **133**, 101–5.

Davenport, J. C., Wilson, H. J. and Basker, R. M. (1978) The compatibility of tissue conditioners with denture cleaners and chlorhexidine. *Journal of Dentistry*, **6**, 239–46.

Firtell, D. N., Finzen, F. C. and Holmes, J. B. (1987) The effect of clinical remount procedures on the comfort and success of complete dentures. *Journal of Prosthetic Dentistry*, **57**, 53–7.

Guckes, A. D., Smith, D. E. and Swoope, C. C. (1978) Counselling and related factors influencing satisfaction with dentures. *Journal of Prosthetic Dentistry*, **39**, 259–67.

Harrison, A., Basker, R. M. and Smith, I. (1989) The compatibility of temporary soft materials with immersion denture cleansers. *International Journal of Prosthodontics*, **2**, 254–8.

Harrison, A., Huggett, R. and Murphy, W. M. (1990) Complete denture construction in general dental practice: An update of the 1970 survey. *British Dental Journal*, **169**, 159–63.

Hutchins, D. W. and Parker, W. A. (1973) A clinical evaluation of the ability of denture cleaning solutions to remove dental plaque from prosthetic devices. *New York State Dental Journal*, **39**, 363–7.

MacCallum, M., Stafford, G. D., MacCulloch, W. T. and Combe, E. C. (1968) Which cleanser? A report on a survey of denture cleaning routine and the development of a new denture cleanser. *Dental Practitioner and Dental Record*, **19**, 83–9.

Murray, I. D., McCabe, J. F. and Storer, R. (1986) Abrasivity of denture cleaning pastes *in vitro* and *in situ*. *British Dental Journal*, **161**, 137–41.

Murray, I. D., McCabe, J. F. and Storer, R. (1986) The relationship between the abrasivity and cleaning power of the dentifrice-type denture cleaners. *British Dental Journal*, **161**, 205–8.

Neill, D. J. (1968) A study of materials and methods employed in cleaning dentures. *British Dental Journal*, **124**, 107–15.

Preiskel, H. W. (1967) Anteroposterior jaw relations in complete denture construction. *Dental Practitioner and Dental Record*, **18**, 39–44.

Robinson, J. G., McCabe, J. F. and Storer, R. (1987) Denture bases: the effects of various treatments on clarity, strength and structure. *Journal of Dentistry*, **15**, 159–65.

Wesley, R. C., Henderson, D., Frazier, Q. Z., Rayson, J. H., Ellinger, C. W., Lutes, M. R., Rahn, A. O. and Haley, J. V. (1973) Processing changes in complete dentures: Posterior tooth contacts and pin opening. *Journal of Prosthetic Dentistry*, **29**, 46–54.

14 Recall Procedures

It is essential to institute a programme of review appointments after fitting complete dentures to ensure that the tissues are not being damaged and that the dentures are functioning efficiently.

In the short term, modifications to the dentures may be required to *achieve* an acceptable level of function and comfort. As a result of subsequent changes in the tissues and in the dentures, modifications in the long term may be needed in order to *maintain* this level of function and comfort.

SHORT-TERM RECALL PROCEDURES

The first recall appointment should be no longer than one week after fitting the dentures. At this visit, it is necessary to obtain a careful history of any complaint such as pain or looseness of the dentures. Then, even if the patient expresses complete satisfaction and perfect comfort, it is essential to carry out a thorough examination. This is because it is not uncommon for mucosal injury, even frank ulceration, to be present without the patient apparently being aware of it. The absence of a complaint under such circumstances may be due to a high pain threshold or a desire to please. With the information gleaned from the history and an examination, a diagnosis of any problem should be established and appropriate treatment decided upon.

Problems with the dentures may be caused either by faults which passed unnoticed at the fit stage or by changes occurring in the mouth since that time. In addition, instability of the dentures may occur because the patient has not, as yet, learned to control the new shapes in the mouth.

With regard to changes in the mouth, it must be remembered that because new dentures are seated on a surface which is compressible and liable to change, the initial few days of function may have induced a slight alteration in the occlusion. It has been shown that patients attempt to adapt to an uneven occlusion by altering the normal pattern of mandibular movement. Such an attempt is liable to produce muscular disorders which, in the short term, may pass unnoticed by the patient. In an experimental group purposely provided with dentures which interdigitated maximally in a protrusive relationship, tenderness in one or more of the muscles of mastication was elicited by palpation in 60 per cent of the patients after only one week's wear.

Examples of injury to the mucosa which arise from faults with the impression surface include mucosal damage in the sulcus due to overextension and on the most bulbous part of a ridge where the denture base has been inadequately relieved from a bony undercut. Where there is a clear relationship between mucosal damage and the impression surface, appropriate correction of the denture should be undertaken. It is tempting to assume that all mucosal damage is directly related to faults in the impression surface. However, such a perception would be a fundamental error as damage may be due to faults in the occlusion causing movement of the denture or concentrations of occlusal pressure. It is important to appreciate that the occlusal error causing a problem may be some distance from the site of inflammation (Figure 14.1). It is also important to remember that an assessment of the occlusion must always be made and that the impression surface of the denture should never be adjusted in an empirical manner. Once any occlusal faults have been eliminated, a further check of the impression surface should be made using a pressure disclosing medium. If this sequence is not carried out, it would be difficult to judge whether an area of inflammation was due to an impression surface defect or occlusal error.

If the mucosal damage is localised, a material such as soft disclosing wax is applied to the impression surface of the denture in the appropriate area. The denture is then seated firmly for a few seconds and, on removal, any pressure points are indicated by the pink denture base showing through the wax. Adjustment of the impression surface can then be carried out in a relatively precise manner.

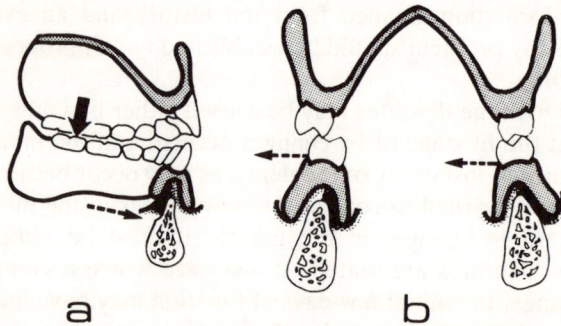

Figure 14.1   (a) A *posterior* premature contact, resulting in forward movement of the lower denture (dotted arrow), produces inflammation of the mucosa on the lingual aspect of the alveolar ridge in the *anterior* region. (b) Lateral displacement of the lower denture produces inflammation of the mucosa in areas closely related to the occlusal error

If the mucosal damage is more generalised, an alternative technique which is simple, quick and revealing is to obtain a wash impression over the whole of the impression surface using a low viscosity mix of alginate. The set impression gives a clear picture of pressure points and base extension, again allowing precise correction where necessary. If adhesive has not been applied to the denture beforehand, the alginate can be quickly and cleanly removed from the denture after the adjustments have been completed.

Treatment at the short-term recall stage might include occlusal correction and adjustment of the denture border and impression surface. Ways in which this treatment is undertaken have been described in Chapter 13.

In addition, a check must be made on the patient's progress in adapting to the new dentures. Bearing in mind that 20 per cent of experienced denture wearers require up to a month in which to become proficient with their new dentures, it is likely that a significant number of patients will benefit from the offer of further advice.

If necessary, a further appointment for short-term review should be made so that the dentist can ensure that any modification has been successful. The patient should be advised as to the importance of a yearly review for reasons that will become apparent in the next section of this chapter.

LONG-TERM RECALL PROCEDURES

The long-term changes in shape of the residual ridges and the consequent effect on dentures have been studied extensively. A continuing reduction in height of the alveolar ridges over a period of 25 years has been observed. There appears to be a marked reduction in the first year of denture wearing and in the next few years a continuing loss averaging 1 mm each year. Over periods of time, the loss in height of the anterior lower ridge is four times that of the upper. As the lower denture covers a much smaller area, the functional stress transmitted to the underlying tissues is greater; more bone is lost because of the increased likelihood of the physiological limit of these tissues being exceeded. The resorption of bone brings in its wake a loss of both occlusal vertical dimension and rest vertical dimension. The former dimension is reduced to a greater extent and thus the freeway space is increased.

The progressive deterioration in the fit of dentures also leads to a deterioration in occlusal balance, a change which may be apparent only six months after fitting the dentures. This occlusal deterioration will be aggravated by occlusal wear in the case of dentures with acrylic teeth.

The combination of loss of both fit and occlusal balance will encourage mucosal inflammation and further bone resorption, thus establishing a vicious cycle (Figure 14.2). It is clearly important, if oral health and function are to be maintained, that this cycle is broken by regular denture review and effective maintenance.

The progressive long-term deterioration of dentures which has been described is not invariably associated with a complaint by the patient. This is because adaptive changes can occur in the patient and a tolerance developed which allows the patient to continue wearing the dentures. Thus, a considerable amount of tissue damage can go unnoticed by the patient. Whereas successful adaptation to new dentures is a prerequisite for success, a patient who tolerates slowly developing faults will store up troubles for the future. In addition to the likelihood of tissue damage, reduction in rest vertical dimension and the adoption of abnormal mandibular postures create problems for both the dentist and the patient when replacement dentures are eventually made (Chapter 7).

If some loss of fit is detected at review but there is no complaint from the patient, nor any signs of tissue damage, the dentist is faced with the decision of whether or not to correct the deficiency. Certainly, in the absence of both signs and symptoms, it will often be foolhardy to tamper with well-accepted dentures just because the dentist considers that retention has been impaired slightly.

The deterioration in both the dentures and the health of the mouth is the result of patients not seeking regular denture maintenance. The size of the problem was highlighted by the first survey of Adult Dental Health in 1978 which reported that among those patients who wore their lower dentures all day, 26 per cent complained of looseness and 17 per cent experienced soreness. Yet only 20 per cent of this group planned to visit a dentist. In another study, it has been reported that more than 50 per cent of patients

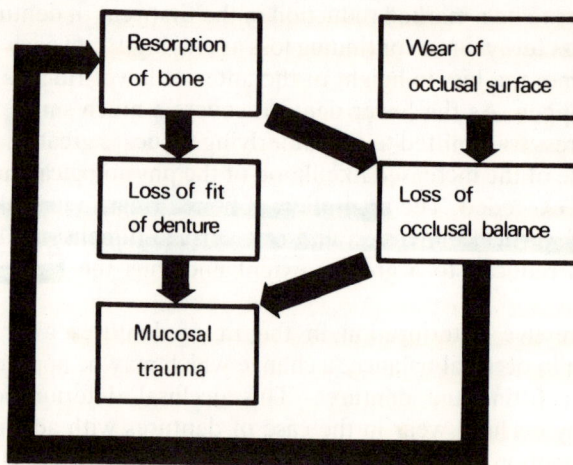

Figure 14.2   Cycle of tissue damage resulting from lack of denture maintenance

expected their dentures to last more than 10 years. Clearly, many patients do not have a realistic perception of what is required to maintain their dentures and mouth in good condition.

Another example of this kind of misconception is the not uncommon resort by patients to home denture reline kits, rather than seeking professional help when denture problems develop. Such ill-advised action can result in gross tissue destruction because the addition of such a liner can derange both the horizontal and vertical occlusal relationships.

The importance of the dentist convincing the patient of the need to seek regular denture maintenance is obvious in the light of this discussion. It should be explained that a recall appointment should be made no longer than a year after the dentures were first fitted. Thereafter, an appointment every two or three years is a realistic measure. Furthermore, the dentist should make the point that the dentures have a limited life and should advise the patient of the potential dangers of wearing dentures which have become inadequate.

Treatment required at recall visits will be one or a combination of the following:

(a) adjustment of impression surface or base extension,
(b) occlusal adjustment with or without a check record,
(c) construction of replacement dentures,
(d) reline or rebase of the dentures.

The first three items have already been considered in previous chapters.

Clinical Procedures for Relining or Rebasing

A reline procedure involves resurfacing the impression surface of the denture with new material. Rebasing entails the replacement of most of the original acrylic base of the denture. Technical details of the laboratory methods are described in standard texts on dental technology. In simple terms, a reline involves a straightforward substitution of the layer of impression material by a layer of new acrylic resin. Such a method is quite satisfactory for a lower denture but will increase the thickness of the palate of an upper denture, the degree of increase depending upon the impression material used. The more viscous zinc oxide–eugenol impression pastes are likely to produce an unacceptable thickness while minimal change will occur with the lighter-bodied silicone-perfecting pastes.

A rebasing technique does not suffer from the disadvantage just mentioned and is thus preferred by many for correcting the impression surface of an upper denture. Certainly, a rebase should be undertaken when the existing denture base material has deteriorated or when there is a history of previous fractures of the palate.

When a denture is relined, cold-curing acrylic resin should be used. As the original denture base material is still present, heat curing would release strains which had previously been locked within the structure of the old resin, and this would result in distortion of the material. As most of the original denture base is removed in a rebasing procedure, there is no danger of distortion due to strain release, and thus a heat-cure process can be used.

Whatever laboratory technique is requested, the basic principles of the clinical method remain the same. For simplicity, when describing clinical procedures, only the term 'reline' will be used.

It is apparent that as the reline alters the impression surface of a denture, it must be used only when a patient's complaint can be attributed to a defect in that surface. The common history a patient gives is one of recent looseness following a period of trouble-free denture wearing. If the complaint is the result of an unbalanced occlusion, it is quite useless to reline the denture and hope for an improvement. The uneven contact must be corrected either by occlusal adjustment or by constructing a new denture or dentures. Alternatively, the looseness may be caused by the once satisfactory denture no longer occupying the neutral zone. Relining a denture in this instance will, of course, be of little benefit to the patient; the appropriate treatment is to construct a new denture which is shaped to lie within that zone of muscular balance.

When an impression is taken within an existing denture, care must be taken to ensure that the jaw relationship in the horizontal plane is not altered. This is achieved by taking great care in seating the denture and checking the accuracy of this by asking the patient to occlude. Inevitably, the occlusal vertical dimension is increased slightly by the thickness of the impression material. As this increase should be kept to a minimum, it is usual to choose an impression material which is accurate in thin section. Low viscosity silicone elastomers and zinc oxide–eugenol impression pastes are good examples of materials which can be used. The more fluid silicone will produce the least change in occlusal vertical dimension.

When an impression is taken within a lower denture, excess material in the middle of the impression surface has only a short distance to travel before it escapes at the periphery. Thus, the force needed to extrude the material and seat the denture is small, and the risk of displacing the underlying tissues or of altering the occlusal relationship is minimal. The situation is obviously somewhat different in the upper jaw as the excess material has a longer and more circuitous route to follow (Figure 14.3). Greater force is needed to seat the upper denture, bringing with it the potential complication of undue displacement of the mucosa with consequent reduction in retention of the relined denture. Unless great care is taken, the denture may not be seated correctly in the anteroposterior plane; too much impression material may be left under the labial flange

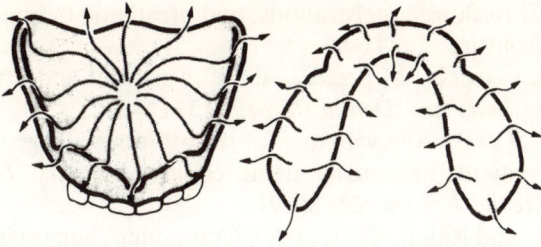

Figure 14.3   Escape routes for excess impression material

and as a result the relined denture is positioned more anteriorly, bringing with it inevitable occlusal and aesthetic complications.

Clinical Procedures for Reline Techniques

Three routine preparatory procedures are carried out whatever reline technique is followed.

(a) The occlusion must be balanced to ensure that, when the impression is taken, uneven contact does not bring about a bodily shift or tilt of the denture when the patient is asked to occlude.

(b) Any over- or underextension of the borders must be corrected.

(c) Undercuts within the acrylic impression surface must be eliminated so that the technician can remove the denture from the cast.

If a low viscosity silicone impression material is used, its setting characteristics are such that an excessive build-up of pressure beneath the upper denture is unlikely to occur. This danger is, however, more likely when using a zinc oxide–eugenol impression paste, but pressure in the palatal area can be reduced if small vent holes are drilled through the palatal acrylic before the impression is taken.

BIBLIOGRAPHY

Bergman, B. and Carlsson, G. E. (1972) Review of 54 complete denture wearers. Patients' opinions 1 year after treatment. *Acta Odontologica Scandinavica*, **30**, 399–414.

Bergman, B., Carlsson, G. E. and Ericson, S. (1971) Effect of differences in habitual use of complete dentures on underlying tissues. *Scandinavian Journal of Dental Research*, **79**, 449–60.

Bergman, B., Carlsson, G. E. and Hedegard, B. (1964) A longitudinal two-year study of a number of full denture cases. *Acta Odontologica Scandinavica*, **22**, 3–26.

Brill, N. (1957) Reflexes, registrations, and prosthetic therapy. *Journal of Prosthetic Dentistry*, **7**, 341–60.

Brill, N. (1962) Aspects of occlusal sense in natural and artificial teeth. *Dental Practitioner and Dental Record*, **13**, 114–21.

Ettinger, R. L. (1971) An evaluation of the attitudes of a group of elderly edentulous patients to dentists, dentures, and dentistry. *Dental Practitioner and Dental Record*, **22**, 85–91.

Jackson, R. A. and Ralph, W. J. (1980) Continuing changes in the contour of the maxillary residual alveolar ridge. *Journal of Oral Rehabilitation*, **7**, 245–8.

Osborne, J. (1952) Re-lining and re-basing. *British Dental Journal*, **92**, 149–53.

Shaffer, F. W. and Filler, W. H. (1971) Relining complete dentures with minimum occlusal error. *Journal of Prosthetic Dentistry*, **25**, 366–70.

Sheppard, I. M., Schwartz, L. R. and Sheppard, S. M. (1971) Oral status of edentulous and complete denture-wearing patients. *Journal of the American Dental Association*, **83**, 614–20.

Sheppard, I. M., Schwartz, L. R. and Sheppard, S. M. (1972) Survey of the oral status of complete denture patients. *Journal of Prosthetic Dentistry*, **28**, 121–6.

Stafford, G. D. (1973) Denture relining material for home use. Report of a case. *British Dental Journal*, **134**, 391–2.

Tallgren, A. (1957) Changes in adult face height due to ageing, wear and loss of teeth and prosthetic treatment. *Acta Odontologica Scandinavica*, **15**, 1–122 (Suppl. 24).

Tallgren, A. (1966) The reduction in face height of edentulous and partially edentulous subjects during long-term denture wear. *Acta Odontologica Scandinavica*, **24**, 195–239.

Tallgren, A. (1972) The continuing reduction of the residual alveolar ridges in complete denture wearers: a mixed-longitudinal study covering 25 years. *Journal of Prosthetic Dentistry*, **27**, 120–32.

Todd, J. E., Walker, A. M. and Dodd, P. (1982) *Adult Dental Health: Volume 2: United Kingdom 1978*. HMSO, London.

15 Some Complete-denture Problems

PAIN AND INSTABILITY

In this chapter, some specific complete-denture problems will be discussed and methods of treatment described. The most common problems associated with complete dentures are pain and instability. Many of the causes have been described in earlier chapters but to give a simplified picture they are summarised in Table 15.1. The most likely main complaint has been indicated in each case. It should be remembered however that there is considerable overlap between the two columns as any cause of instability may additionally give rise to a complaint of pain.

PERSISTENT PAIN UNDER DENTURES

It will occasionally be found that a patient continues to complain of pain under a denture which, in terms of design and construction, appears to be entirely satisfactory. This problem is usually seen in the lower jaw where the area available for distribution of the occlusal load is relatively small. There are several possible causes of this discomfort related to the tissues, namely mucosal atrophy, an irregular bony surface and pathology within the bone. Discomfort can also arise from overloading of the mucosa as a result of clenching or grinding the teeth. Such occlusal habits may be caused by increased activity of the masticatory muscles produced during stressful situations. In treating this parafunction, the patient must be made aware of the problem and should be told that it is normal for teeth to be free of occlusal contact for most of the time; certainly, dentures should be taken out at night.

Initial treatment should be directed towards reducing the size of the occlusal table; for example, the second molars can be removed and the buccolingual width of the teeth reduced. One effective way of providing a very narrow occlusal table is to use metal wedges which can be formed out of stainless steel sheet (Figure 15.1). Not only does this design reduce the

Table 15.1

Cause	Complaint (P = Pain L = Looseness)	
DENTURE FAULTS		
Impression Surface		
Inaccurate fit	P	L
Overextension	P	L
Underextension	P	L
Flange width inadequate for facial seal		L
Post-dam absent		L
Relief chamber absent but required	P	L
Roughness	P	
Cast damaged before processing	P	
Extension into bony undercuts	P	
Polished Surface		
Denture not in neutral zone		L
Shape unfavourable for muscle control		L
Occlusal Surface		
Occlusion unbalanced	P	L
Cuspal interference	P	L
Occlusal plane too high		L
Inadequate freeway space	P	
Occlusal table too wide	P	L
PATIENT FACTORS		
Bruxism/Parafunction	P	
Low Pain Tolerance	P	
Poor Neuromuscular Control		
Slow rate of adaptation (e.g., patient elderly)		L
Neuromuscular disorders (e.g., Parkinsonism)		L
Mucosa		
Flabby		L
Atrophic	P	
Bone		
Sharp spicules	P	
Prominences (mylohyoid ridges, tori, genial tubercles)	P	
Advanced resorption		L
Mental foramen near crest of ridge	P	
Pathology within the bone	P	
Saliva		
Deficient or absent		L
Systemic Disease		
e.g., iron-deficiency anaemia	P	

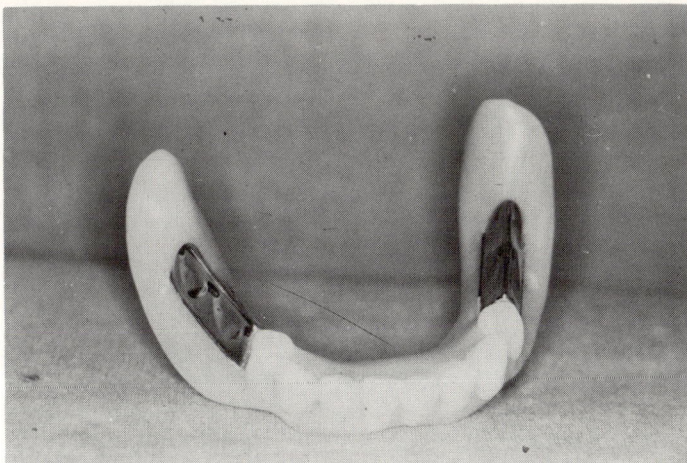

Figure 15.1   A lower denture with stainless steel wedges replacing the posterior teeth

occlusal load, but it also provides the maximum possible tongue space in cases where the size of the tongue, or the amount of tongue spread, has reduced the size of the neutral zone to an absolute minimum.

Soft Lining

Soft linings are also referred to as long-term resilient lining materials. This alternative terminology has value as it allows one to distinguish this group from the short-term materials which are often referred to as tissue conditioners (page 115).

If pain persists in spite of the measures described in the previous section, tolerance to a lower denture may be improved by using a soft lining material on the impression surface. This acts as a cushion, helping to reduce the trauma to the tissues. The soft lining must be at least 2 mm thick if its beneficial properties are to be fully effective. A corresponding reduction in the thickness of the hard acrylic resin of the denture base is necessary to make room for the lining. As this reduction weakens the denture, a strengthener in the form of a cobalt–chromium lingual plate may be added (Figure 15.2). Although the cushioning properties of a soft lining are valuable in appropriate circumstances, it is wise to avoid their use wherever possible because those which are currently available are not as serviceable as hard denture base material.

Soft linings can be applied to the denture either during its construction, at the flasking and packing stage, or can be added to an existing denture by means of a reline procedure.

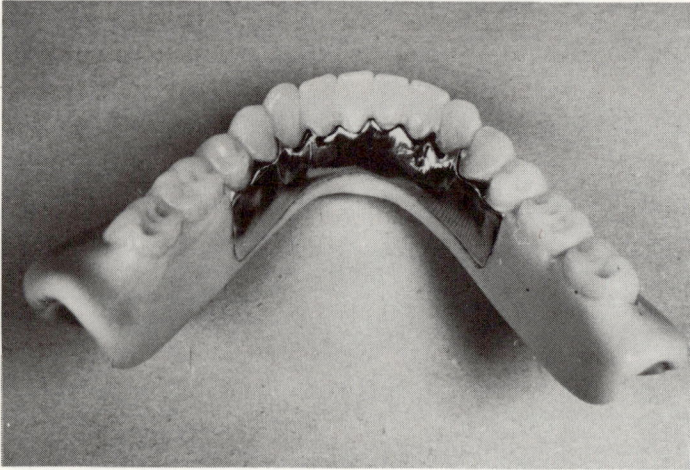

Figure 15.2   A lower denture with a cobalt–chromium lingual plate strengthener

An advantage of the former approach is that, with certain soft lining materials, a more reliable bond between the denture base and the soft lining can be achieved when the acrylic dough of the denture base and the soft lining are processed together. Also, if a heat-curing soft lining material is used, a single processing avoids the risk, present when reprocessing a denture, of stress release occurring within the original denture base.

The advantages of the reline approach are that it is often difficult to be certain at the treatment planning stage that a new denture made in rigid acrylic resin will not be entirely successful. Also, the compressibility of a soft lining in a finished denture can make it more difficult to detect premature occlusal contacts and therefore to carry out any occlusal adjustments that might be necessary.

The soft materials commonly available for lining dentures are the silicone rubbers and acrylic resins.

Cold-curing Silicone Rubber Materials

One of the most important variations in composition of available materials is the percentage of filler content. As the content increases, so does the level of water absorption with resultant worsening dimensional stability. The rupture properties of these materials are particularly poor; the soft lining is liable to tear and to become detached from the denture base. In isolated instances, the commonly used catalyst, dibutyltin dilaurate, has been found to be a mucosal irritant. The abrasion resistance of these materials is poor.

An advantage of this group of materials, shared with the heat-curing silicone rubbers, is an elastic recovery which is better than that exhibited by the soft acrylics.

Heat-curing Silicone Rubber Materials

In contrast to the cold-curing silicones, the water absorption of these materials is low. As a result, the dimensional stability is improved and accuracy of fit is little affected by the oral environment. Improvements in rupture properties and adhesion to the denture base complete the picture of superiority.

Published reports indicate that these materials can remain serviceable for five years or more. However, it is necessary for the patient to maintain a high level of plaque control in order to achieve this length of service. If the lining is not kept clean and disinfected regularly, microbial invasion of the lining occurs, resulting in its degradation and failure. Hypochlorite cleansers help to maintain the required level of plaque control and do not result in deterioration of the cushioning properties or bonding of the lining. However, these cleansers can cause loss of colour; the patient should be forewarned of this problem and reassured that it is of no clinical significance. If the denture has a cobalt–chromium lingual plate strengthener, hypochlorite cleaning solutions are contraindicated because of the possibility of corrosion.

The heat-curing silicone materials are relatively abrasion resistant, indeed so much so that adjustment of the lining can be difficult. However, the problem is not insurmountable provided the dentist uses stones and burs specifically designed for the purpose. *MOLLOPLAST B.*

Acrylic Resin Materials

Most of the materials use poly(ethylmethacrylate) as the basic polymer. The materials are heavily plasticised to create softness.

The advantages of soft acrylics over the silicone materials include better rupture properties and more effective adhesion to the remaining denture base. Their drawbacks include an inferior elastic recovery and a progressive loss of plasticiser to the oral environment; the latter factor results in a reduction in softness of the material and cracking of the surface.

COE SUPER SOFT.

THE FLABBY RIDGE

This condition is most frequently seen in the upper anterior region, classically under a complete denture opposed by natural anterior teeth. As a result of this fibrous tissue, the stability of a complete denture will be poor. In extreme cases, the entire ridge may be readily distorted.

The management of this condition is somewhat controversial, opinion falling broadly into two camps. In one, surgical removal of the fibrous tissue is favoured in every case where the health of the patient allows. This approach produces a firm ridge which is reduced in size. Advocates of the opposing view suggest that surgical removal should rarely, if ever, be carried out because the fibrous tissue may have a cushion effect which reduces trauma to the underlying bone. If the tissue is removed, it must be replaced by denture base material with consequent increase in the bulk and weight of the appliance. Furthermore, there will be considerable loss of sulcus depth. It is the opinion of the authors that in most cases a satisfactory denture can be made without surgery.

If the flabby ridge is retained, one is again faced with a clinical dilemma. Should the impression technique employed compress the flabby tissue in order to try and obtain maximum support from it, or should one use a mucostatic technique with the aim of achieving maximum retention? There is little firm evidence to support either view. However, it is the authors' opinion that it is more helpful to use an impression technique which does not displace this tissue. This is because, if the fibrous tissue is distorted during impression-taking, the denture will fit only when seated by occlusal pressure (Figure 15.3(a)). When the teeth are apart, elastic recoil of the displaced tissue forces the denture downwards (Figure 15.3(b)) and eliminates retention. In addition, intermittent occlusion of the teeth results in a pumping action of the denture which can traumatise the tissues.

If, however, the denture is constructed on a cast obtained from a mucostatic impression of the flabby ridge in its resting position, the denture maintains its contact with the tissues when the teeth are out of occlusion. Retention will therefore be optimal for the case in question. Support will be gained primarily from the hard palate and firm areas of the ridge rather than from the flabby tissue.

A suggested approach to the flabby-ridge problem is as follows. Preliminary impressions should be taken in a stock tray using an alginate of low viscosity. This material will cause less tissue displacement than if impression compound were used, with the result that less modification of the special tray will subsequently be required.

In many cases, it will be found that the denture-bearing mucosa is inflamed. Before the working impressions are taken, resolution of this inflammation should be achieved by leaving the dentures out for several days beforehand, or by appropriate modification of the existing dentures by occlusal adjustment or the application of a short-term resilient lining material to the impression surface (Chapter 7).

Where the degree of mucosal displacement is minimal, a satisfactory result may be achieved by taking a working impression in a spaced tray using an impression material of low viscosity. Suitable materials for this purpose are impression plaster, and low viscosity silicone impression material. In the case of alginate, pressure on the displaceable tissue can be further reduced by using a perforated tray.

Where the displacement is marked, it is usually better to use a two-part impression technique. A close-fitting tray is constructed in cold-curing acrylic resin and designed so that the flabby area of the ridge is uncovered

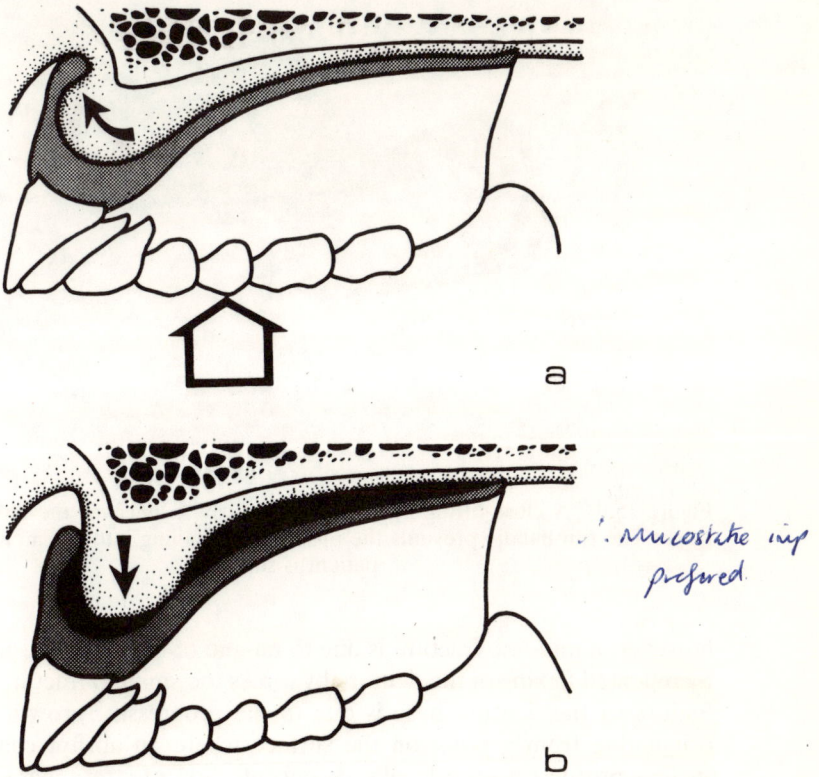

Figure 15.3 (a) Under occlusal pressure, the upper denture is seated and the flabby anterior ridge displaced. (b) When the teeth are apart, the flabby tissue recoils and displaces the denture downwards

(Figure 15.4). The tray is tried in the mouth and checked to make certain that it is not displacing the flabby tissue. The borders are corrected in the normal way and an impression is taken of the firm area using zinc oxide–eugenol paste. If this impression proves to be satisfactory, it is replaced in the mouth, the patient is tipped back into the supine position and an impression of the flabby tissue left uncovered by the tray is obtained by applying a thin mix of impression plaster using a spatula, brush or syringe.

MID-LINE FRACTURE

The mid-line fracture of an acrylic denture may occasionally result from careless handling by the patient; for example, accidental dropping of the denture while cleaning can cause an impact fracture. Characteristically,

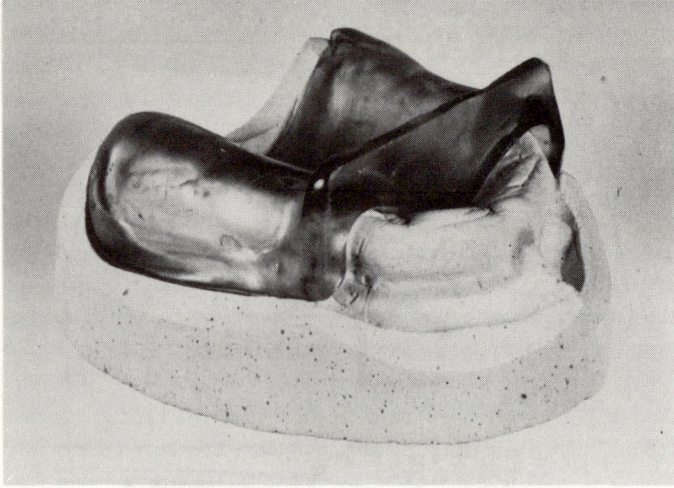

Figure 15.4   A close-fitting acrylic tray cut away to uncover the flabby anterior ridge. The rim handle prevents the unset plaster falling into the mouth when the patient is supine

however, a mid-line fracture is due to fatigue of the acrylic resin produced by repeated flexing of the denture by forces too small to fracture it directly. Failure of the denture base is due to the progressive growth of a crack originating from a point on the surface where an abrupt change in the surface profile causes a localised concentration of stress many times that applied to the bulk of the denture. The crack often starts palatally to the upper central incisors, grows slowly at first but undergoes an enormously increased rate of growth just before the denture fractures. A failure of this type most commonly occurs in dentures which are about three years old. Whenever possible, the cause of the fracture must be identified before the denture is repaired or replaced. Unless this is done and the cause corrected, the denture is likely to fracture again within a short period of time.

Causes of Mid-line Fracture – Denture Factors

Stress Concentrators
Changes in the surface profile of the denture acting as stress concentrators include scratches, a median diastema and a deep frenal notch. Inclusions within the denture base such as porosity, plaster, dust, nylon filaments and metal mesh so-called strengtheners may predispose to fracture and also contribute to the rapid growth of the crack. Stress concentration can also develop around the pins of the porcelain teeth.

Absence of a Labial Flange

An open-face denture is not as stiff as a flanged denture. Flexing will therefore be more marked and fatigue fracture more likely as a consequence. If this appears to be the primary cause of a fracture, and the anatomy of the anterior alveolus prevents the addition of a labial flange in the replacement denture, a metallic denture base is indicated.

Incomplete Polymerisation of the Acrylic Resin

If the curing cycle does not include a terminal heating period at 100 °C, the maximum degree of polymerisation is not attained and the strength of the denture base will be reduced.

Previous Repair

When a denture has fractured previously in the mid-line, and has been repaired using cold-curing acrylic resin, a further fracture may occur because the cold-curing material is more susceptible to fatigue than the heat-curing resin; in addition, the original denture base material on either side of the fracture line will already be fatigued.

Shape of the Teeth on the Denture

When acrylic posterior teeth are set up with a normal buccal overjet, they may wear and produce the situation shown in Figure 15.5, where a wedging action on the upper denture results from occlusion of the teeth. Locking of the occlusion also appears to predispose to mid-line fracture.

Poor Fit

When alveolar resorption has taken place beneath an upper denture, support will be provided only by the hard palate. As a result, flexing of the denture will occur when the teeth occlude. To correct this fault, the denture should be rebased after it has been repaired. By this process, the old highly stressed resin is replaced by stronger heat-curing resin.

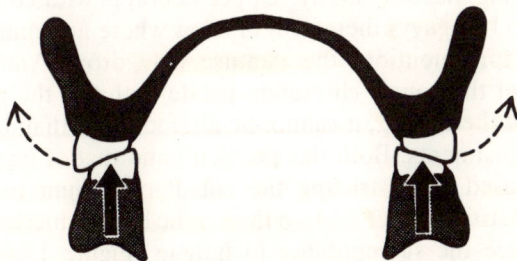

Figure 15.5   Wear of acrylic posterior teeth resulting in a wedge effect on the upper denture

If the two pieces of the denture can be located accurately and securely, possibly using a cyano-acrylate adhesive, it is possible to take a wash impression at the patient's first visit rather than waiting for the repaired denture to be returned for an impression to be taken at a subsequent appointment.

Lack of Adequate Relief

If the mucosa overlying the crest of the ridge is more compressible than that covering the centre of the hard palate, flexing of the denture will occur when the teeth occlude. To compensate for this variation in mucosal compressibility, and to prevent the flexing, a palatal relief chamber should be incorporated in the denture (page 179).

Causes of Mid-line Fracture – Patient Factors

Certain features of the patient may give rise to denture factors, already discussed, which predispose to fracture. For example, a prominent labial frenum will require a deep notch in the flange resulting in stress concentration in that area.

High Occlusal Loads

These may occur in patients with powerful muscles of mastication, in patients whose natural lower teeth are still present and in patients who are bruxists.

The replacement denture in this instance needs to be stronger than the old denture. Although increased strength may sometimes be achieved by altering the design of the denture, a stronger denture base material is often indicated. Materials which may be used for this purpose are described briefly below.

Cobalt–Chromium Alloy

This alloy is cast and therefore the impression surface follows the contour of the underlying mucosa closely. Upper dentures with cobalt–chromium palates tend to be heavy; therefore, in cases where anatomical factors are unfavourable for retention, the denture may drop. Another potential disadvantage of the cobalt–chromium palate is that if the post-dam is an integral part of the casting, it cannot be altered other than by carrying out very minor adjustments. Both this problem, and that of increased weight, can be minimised by restricting the cobalt–chromium to a horseshoe-shaped palatal strengthener set into the acrylic base to increase rigidity and therefore reduce the susceptibility to fatigue (Figure 15.6). This design ensures that the impression surface is made of acrylic and thus preserves the advantage of adjustability.

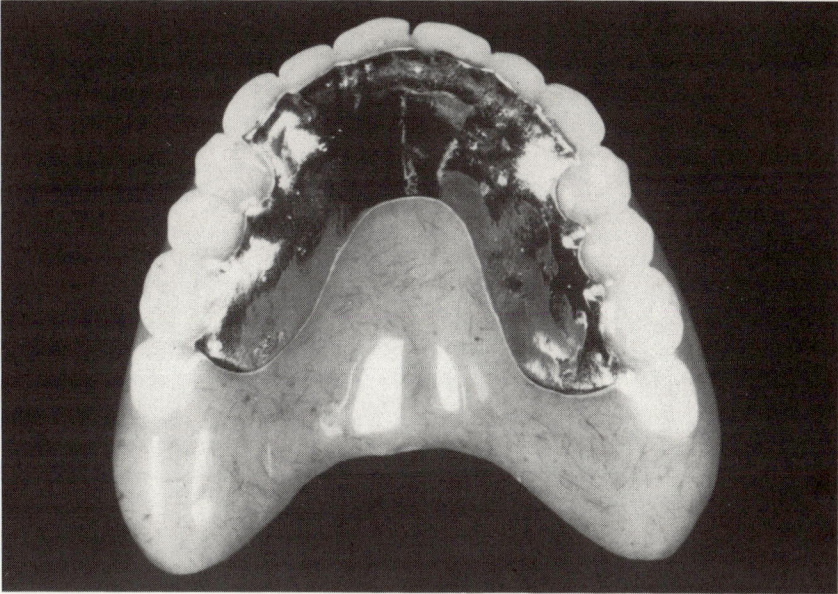

Figure 15.6   Upper denture with cobalt–chromium horseshoe-shaped strengthener

If it is judged that greater strength is required, a more extensive metal base can be used and still retain the advantage of an adjustable post-dam if the design shown in Figure 15.7 is employed. Acrylic resin, added to the mesh at the posterior border, becomes the material in contact with the mucosa; this material can be modified should the need arise. When constructing this type of denture base, the dental technician has to take great care to minimise the step between metal and acrylic at the finishing line.

Stainless Steel Palates
This material is swaged to the cast by slow-rate hydraulic pressure or by explosive-forming. It does not enter small clefts or pits in the cast and consequently the impression surface is relatively smooth; as a result, abrasion of the mucosa is less likely to occur as the denture moves in function. This material is therefore particularly useful in the treatment of patients with papillary hyperplasia (page 126). The smoothness of its surface also facilitates cleaning. Stainless steel palates can be fabricated in much thinner section than cobalt–chromium; therefore, although the density of the two materials is the same, the stainless steel denture is considerably lighter and in certain cases may be better tolerated by the patient. It may not be possible in a patient with a shallow palate to obtain sufficient rigidity to prevent the denture flexing if the occlusal loads are high. In these

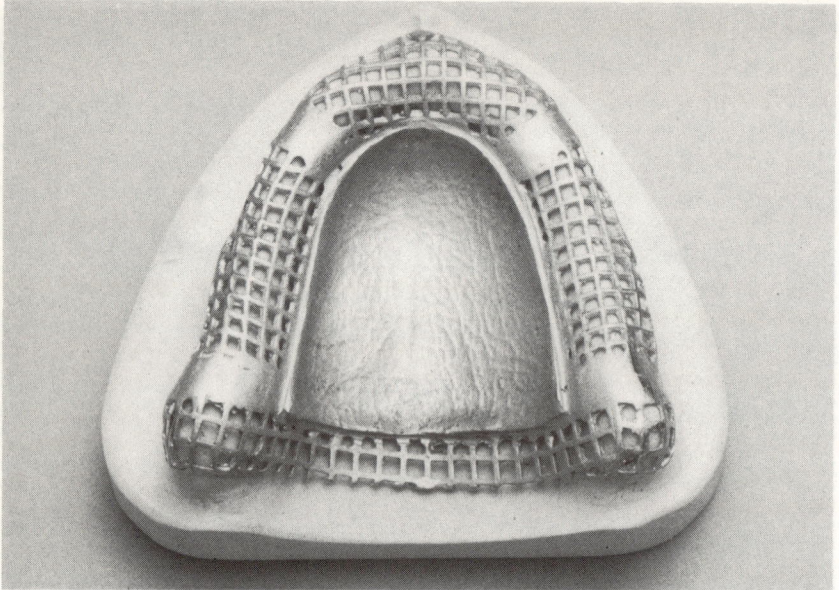

Figure 15.7   Cobalt–chromium palate with posterior mesh to which an acrylic post-dam will be attached

circumstances, although failure of the stainless steel palate is unlikely, fracture of the surrounding acrylic may occur.

Modified Polymeric Denture Base Materials
Vinyl copolymers and rubber–acrylic graft copolymers have better impact and fatigue strengths than poly(methylmethacrylate); crack propagation in the graft copolymers is slowed up by the rubber phase. Some of the vinyl copolymer materials require injection moulding and thus the production of dentures may be restricted to laboratories possessing the specialised equipment. However, the rubber–acrylic graft copolymers can be processed conventionally using a dough technique.

Techniques have been described by which conventional upper dentures are reinforced by the inclusion of carbon fibre inserts in the palate. This approach was reported to have reduced the incidence of fracture in a high-risk group of patients, but a disadvantage of the method is the black colour of the insert.

More recently, there have been reports of denture bases being reinforced with ultra-high-modulus polyethylene fibre. This material may be added either as a discrete insert in the palate or as chopped fibre incorporated in the polymer powder before the resin is mixed. The fibre is transparent and its inclusion in the polymer at a loading of 1 per cent has resulted in an increase in impact strength exceeding that of commercially available 'high impact' resins. At the time of writing, this technique is still at the experimental stage but it is mentioned in the text as a possible development for the future.

RETCHING

Retching is most commonly triggered by tactile stimulation of the soft palate, posterior third of the tongue and fauces. The stimulation may occur during prosthetic procedures such as impression-taking or result from the wearing of dentures. Other stimuli may also play a part; they may include the sight of impression material being mixed or the sound of another patient retching. Less frequently, the causative factor may be systemic disease, particularly conditions affecting other regions of the gastro-intestinal tract; for example, the link between retching and alcoholism may be related to the persistent gastritis found in such patients. Psychological factors are often important. The patient may, for example, be extremely apprehensive because of an unhappy first-hand experience of dental procedures or as a result of disturbing stories from friends. In rare instances, retching may be a manifestation of a psychological disturbance which is not primarily related to the patient's dental treatment.

Some patients begin to retch after new dentures are inserted. In most cases, this reflex disappears as the patients adapt to the dentures. It may persist however if the occlusal vertical dimension is excessive or if the dentures are stimulating the sensitive areas of the soft palate and tongue directly. This stimulation may be caused by palatal overextension, a posterior border which is too thick or poorly adapted, the teeth encroaching on tongue space or indeed by any factor producing denture instability. A denture whose posterior border does not go back as far as the junction of hard and soft palates can also cause retching for the following reasons. If the edge of the denture terminates on relatively incompressible mucosa, it is difficult to produce a satisfactory post-dam. This may result in poor retention which increases the apprehension of the patient. When this diagnosis is established, it requires a very careful explanation to convince the patient that to cure the problem it will be necessary to cover more of the palate.

Correction of these faults will usually eliminate the complaint. In a small minority of patients, conventional dentures cannot be tolerated at all; a palateless denture or a very thin stainless steel palate may provide the answer.

Retching is a serious problem in a minority of patients only, but in these cases it may be difficult, or impossible, for the dentist to carry out treatment procedures satisfactorily.

Patient Management

All but the most phlegmatic of individuals find impression-taking unplea-sant. However, retching can usually be prevented by the dentist having a confident chairside manner and careful technique. It is important to reassure the anxious patient and to encourage both physical and mental relaxation. In severe cases, sedation may be indicated; alternatively, relative analgesia will allow the dentist to obtain a satisfactory impression without causing the patient embarrassment. However, using either of these techniques will only put off the evil hour; although it may be possible to obtain a reasonable impression, ultimately the patient must meet the challenge of wearing a denture in an unsedated state.

When taking impressions, the dental chair should be adjusted so that the patient is sitting in the upright position. Impression trays should be well fitting. As close-fitting special trays are less bulky than spaced trays, they are better tolerated and should be used whenever possible. When trying trays in the mouth, firm, positive movements should be used. Most patients tolerate the lower impression better than the upper one, so if the lower impression is taken first, the success of the procedure is likely to reassure the patient. A saliva ejector should be used if copious amounts of saliva collect in the floor of the mouth. Instructing the patient to breathe through the nose is one of the most helpful methods of preventing retching; the soft palate remains stationary in its low position and the tongue in its 'guarding' position, protecting the nasopharynx from the threat of the foreign body in the mouth (Figure 15.8). If the patient breathes through the mouth, this protection is lost; movement of the soft palate results in intermittent contact with the setting impression material and increases the stimulation. The impression material should be mixed out of sight of the patient and the amount placed in the tray kept to the minimum necessary to record the relevant structures. It is during the insertion of the impression

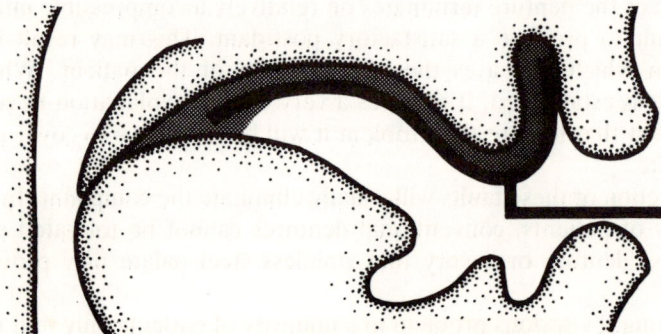

Figure 15.8 The tongue in its guarding position during the taking of an upper impression

and while the material is setting that it is particularly important to distract the patient's attention from what is going on. This may be achieved by insisting that the patient continues to breathe slowly and steadily through the nose. A refinement of this technique has been described in which the patient is instructed in a regime of controlled breathing which must be practised for one or two weeks prior to impression-taking. Breathing should be slow, deep and even; the required steady rhythm can be ensured by asking the patient to link it mentally to a well-known tune.

There are extreme cases where the retching reflex is so exaggerated that it is not possible to obtain accurate working impressions. In most instances, however, a stock tray impression using impression compound may be obtained, since the time required to mould the material is so brief that it is possible to remove the impression before retching occurs. In some of these cases, the patient may be conditioned to wearing dentures by constructing a thin acrylic baseplate on a cast from the composition impression. The fit of the baseplate may be poor but can be improved by peripheral adjustment and the addition of a tissue conditioner or cold-curing poly(butylmethacrylate) resin. The patient should attempt to wear the baseplate for increasing periods of time each day but not keep it in for so long that it actually causes retching. When the baseplate can be tolerated, conventional prosthetic treatment can be started. In addition, a lower baseplate can be constructed and teeth then gradually added to both bases. Initially, upper and lower anterior teeth are provided, and when the patient can tolerate this modification, posterior teeth are progressively added until the denture is complete.

When more orthodox techniques have been used to no avail, training bases may be of value when treating any patient with a long history of difficulties which suggest frank denture intolerance. The rationale for this approach is that new stimuli are introduced gradually, the patient has to cope with only one small step at a time and does not advance to the next stage in treatment until the previous stage has been mastered. The onus for making progress is therefore on the patient.

Having obtained the master casts, heat-cured bases are produced. To help stabilise the lower base, a spine of a poly(butylmethacrylate) resin may be added in the mouth; the muscles of the tongue and cheeks rest against this spine. As the patient accepts the basic shapes in the mouth, anterior teeth may be added and the patient told to wear the training bases at all times other than when eating (Figure 15.9). More additions may be made as progress dictates. If tolerance is increasingly successful, the final complete dentures are eventually developed. Because these dentures may look rather like a patchwork quilt, a copying technique may be used to produce the eventual replacement dentures.

The training base approach to complete denture treatment is inevitably a more complicated and drawn out affair. However, if all other more

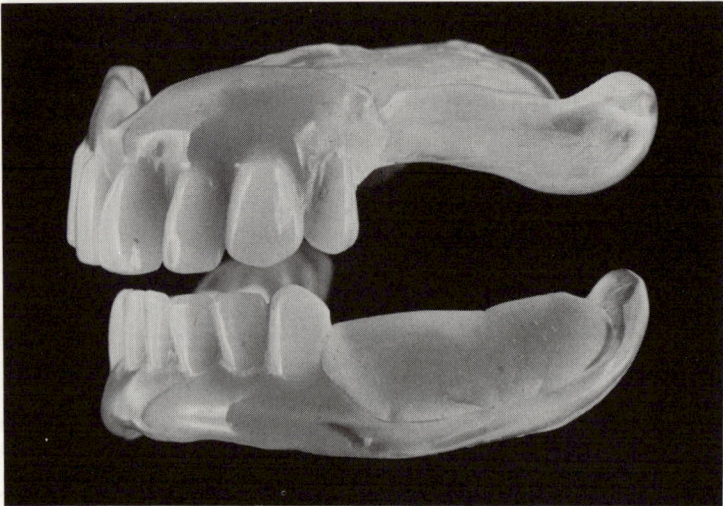

Figure 15.9   Training bases with the addition of anterior teeth and a spine of cold-curing poly(butylmethacrylate) resin

conventional techniques have been used, the approach may be the one remaining chance of providing a successful outcome.

THE BURNING MOUTH SYNDROME

This particular complaint can be very troublesome to the patient, presents problems of diagnosis and often involves prolonged treatment. It has been reported that the symptoms occur in up to 5 per cent of the adult population. Of those who seek treatment, there is a predominance of women with a mean age of approximately 60 years. The most common sites of the complaint are the tongue and the upper denture-bearing tissues. Rather less common are the lips and lower denture-bearing tissues.

Causative Factors

The many potential causative factors can be grouped conveniently under three broad headings (Table 15.2).

Local Irritation

Errors in denture design which cause a denture to move excessively over the mucosa, which increase the functional stress on the mucosa or which interfere with the freedom of movement of the surrounding muscles may

Table 15.2

Local irritation	Systemic	Psychogenic
Dentures	Iron deficiency	Anxiety
Design errors	Vitamin B complex deficiency	Depression
Residual monomer	Diabetes mellitus	Cancerophobia
Infection	Xerostomia	Parafunction
Smoking		
Mouthwashes		

initiate a complaint of burning rather than frank soreness (Figure 15.10). High levels of residual monomer in the denture base have been reported and the tissue damage produced is considered to be the result of chemical irritation rather than a true allergy (Figure 15.11). It is possible that the high levels of residual monomer, which have ranged from three to ten times the normal value, are due to errors inadvertently introduced into the short curing cycles which are currently popular. If the requisite curing temperature of 100 °C is not achieved in the relevant part of the short curing cycle, there is a marked increase in residual monomer content. This content can be measured by specialised analytical techniques such as gas chromatography and high pressure liquid chromatography.

The role of micro-organisms in burning mouth syndrome (BMS) is controversial and studies have not shown a link between the presence of

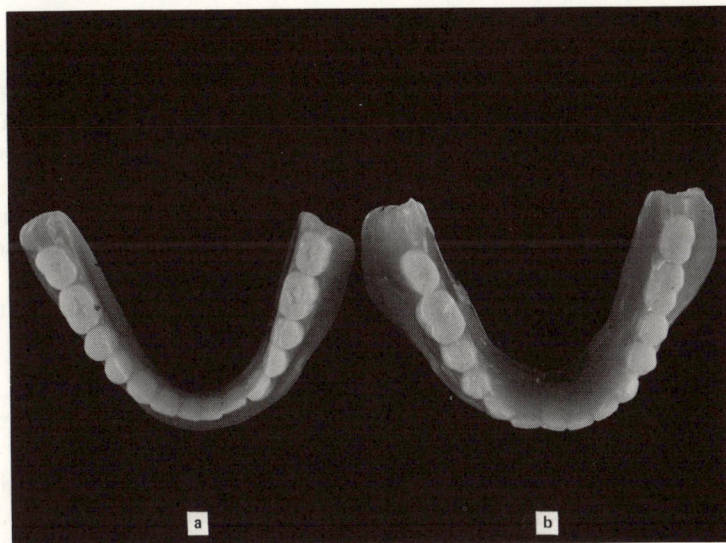

Figure 15.10   The restriction in tongue space produced by denture 'a' caused the patient to complain of a burning tongue. The complaint disappeared when denture 'b' was worn

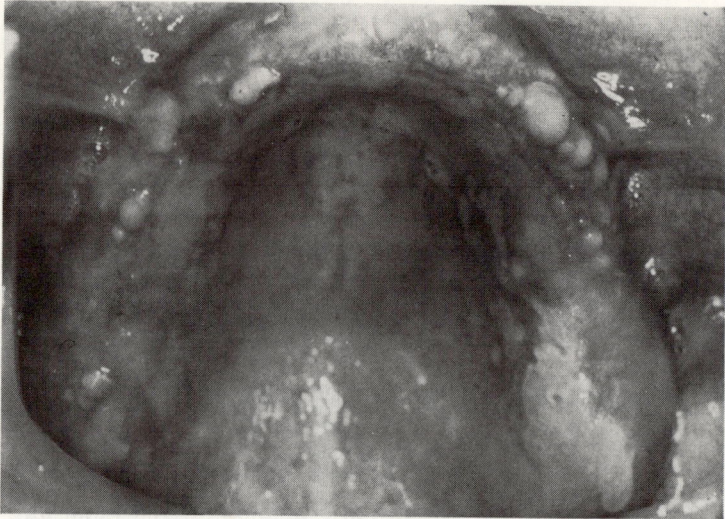

Figure 15.11   Severe blistering of the mucosa resulting from a residual monomer
content of 3.2 per cent

Candida albicans and the complaint. Finally, it should be recognised that the presence of a dry mouth is capable of accentuating the symptoms initiated by any of the causes of local irritation.

Systemic Causes

Contributions from nutritional deficiencies such as iron, vitamin B complex and folic acid should be highlighted. What is apparent is the relative unimportance of the climacteric as a causative factor, a modern viewpoint which is at variance with past clinical opinion. On rare occasions, the symptoms are found to be linked with an undiagnosed diabetes mellitus; treatment of the medical condition invariably results in complete resolution of BMS.

Xerostomia, frequently associated with BMS, has many causes. One that should be highlighted here is drug-induced xerostomia.

Psychogenic Causes

The more common disorders associated with BMS are anxiety, depression, cancerophobia and hyperchondriasis. Parafunctional activities such as bruxism and abnormal and excessive tongue movements are capable of inducing mucosal irritation.

Management

Faced with a multitude of causative factors, it will be recognised that the process of diagnosis and treatment is usually a time-consuming affair. It is beyond the scope of this book to discuss management in any detail, but the point should be made that establishing the diagnosis entails a very careful approach to history-taking and examination, and usually involves the need for a battery of special tests. Following the regime outlined below may well involve the establishment of a clinic dedicated to the purpose, as the services of dentist, doctor, psychiatrist, together with expert technical assistance, are frequently needed.

(a) Initial assessment (history/examination/special tests).
(b) Provisional diagnosis.
(c) Initial treatment (e.g., elimination of local irritants).
(d) Assessment of initial treatment.
(e) Definitive diagnosis.
(f) Definitive treatment (local/systemic correction/psychological therapy).
(g) Follow-up.

With regard to outcome, analysis of various investigations suggests that about two-thirds of BMS patients are either cured or improved to such an extent that the burning sensation is no longer an overwhelming problem. There remain a group of patients for whom the current state of knowledge can offer relatively little benefit. Some in this small group remain totally resistant to treatment.

DISTURBANCE OF SPEECH

The presence of complete dentures can modify speech by affecting articulation and by altering the degree of oral resonance. A number of sounds are articulated by contact of the tongue to the palate and occasionally to the teeth. Of special importance is the tongue tip to alveolar ridge contact which is required in the production of /s/, /z/, /t/, /d/ and /n/. Consequently, a change in the shape of these contact surfaces resulting from the fitting of new dentures will require a modification of tongue behaviour in order to produce sounds which are the same as before. In the vast majority of cases, the necessary modification occurs without any difficulty in a relatively short period of time. A change in speech which may be quite marked when the dentures are first inserted will usually disappear completely within a few days. However, if the changes in the contact surfaces require a modification of tongue behaviour which is beyond the adaptive capability of an individual patient, a speech defect will persist.

The sound most commonly affected in this way is /s/, a sound which is generally produced with the tongue tip behind the upper anterior teeth. A narrow channel remains in the centre of the palate through which air hisses (Figure 15.12). If the palate is too thick at this point, or if the incisors are positioned too far palatally, the /s/ may become a /th/. If the denture is shaped so that it is difficult for the tongue to adapt itself closely to the palate, a channel narrow enough to produce the /s/ sound will not be produced and a whistle or /sh/ sound may result. This is most likely to be the consequence of excessive palatal thickening laterally in the canine region (Figure 15.13).

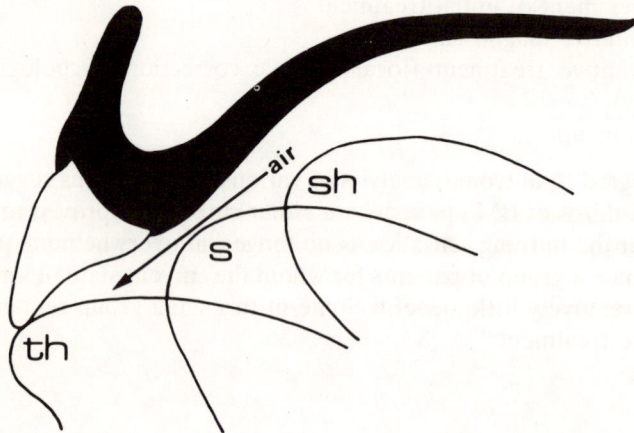

Figure 15.12   The position of the tongue for producing the sounds /th/, /s/ and /sh/

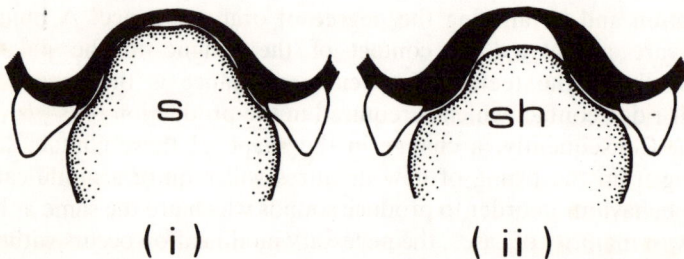

Figure 15.13   (i) The polished surface of the denture palatal to 3|3 is correctly shaped so that the tongue can form a narrow channel in the mid-line for producing the /s/ sound. (ii) Excessive thickening of the palate laterally prevents close adaptation of the tongue to the palate so that the /s/ becomes /sh/

A lateral seal between the tongue and posterior teeth is necessary to produce the English consonants, /th/, /t/, /d/, /n/, /s/, /z/, /sh/, /zh/ (as in measure), /ch/, /j/ and /r/ (as in red). Air is directed down this channel and may be modified by movement of the tongue against the teeth or anterior slope of the palate to produce the final sound. If the lateral seal can only be achieved with difficulty, movement of the tip of the tongue may be restricted with consequent impairment of speech. This difficulty arises if the posterior contact surfaces are too far from the resting position of the tongue as a result of the occlusal plane being too high, the occlusal vertical dimension too great or the posterior teeth placed too far buccally. In extreme cases, it may not be possible for the tongue to produce a complete lateral seal and so a lateral sigmatism develops.

The tongue of a patient who is wearing complete dentures has a dual function – to take part in speech articulation and to control the dentures. If the dentures are loose, the demands of this latter function may be so great that there is a general deterioration in the quality of speech.

The mandible moves closest to the maxilla during speech when the sounds /s/, /z/, /ch/ and /j/ are made. Normally, at this time, there will be a small space between the occlusal surfaces of the teeth. However, if the occlusal vertical dimension of the dentures is too great, the teeth may actually come into contact so that the patient complains that the teeth clatter. The labiodental sounds (f, v) are made by contact of the lower lip with the incisal edges of the upper anterior teeth. If these teeth are not placed correctly in the anteroposterior or vertical planes, difficulties with these sounds may be experienced.

BIBLIOGRAPHY

Austin, A. T. and Basker, R. M. (1980) The level of residual monomer in acrylic denture base material. *British Dental Journal*, **149**, 281–6.

Bahrani, A. S., Blair, G. A. S. and Crossland, B. (1965) Slow rate hydraulic forming of stainless steel dentures. *British Dental Journal*, **118**, 425–31.

Basker, R. M., Sturdee, D. W. and Davenport, J. C. (1978) Patients with burning mouths. *British Dental Journal*, **145**, 9–16.

Bates, J. F. and Smith, D. C. (1965) Evaluation of indirect resilient liners for dentures. *Journal of the American Dental Association*, **70**, 344–53.

Bearn, E. M. (1973) Effect of different occlusal profiles on the masticatory forces transmitted by complete dentures. *British Dental Journal*, **134**, 7–10.

Bjørlin, G., Glantz, P.-O. and Östlund, S. G. (1971) Silicone implants for reconstruction of flabby alveolar ridges. *Svensk Tandläkare Tidskrift*, **64**, 789–94.

Braden, M., Davey, K. W. M., Parker, S., Ladizesky, N. H. and Ward, I. (1988) Denture base poly(methyl methacrylate) reinforced with ultra-high modulus polyethylene fibres. *British Dental Journal*, **164**, 109–13.

Carr, L., Wolfaardt, J. F. and Haitas, G. P. (1985) Speech defects in prosthetic dentistry. Part II – Speech defects associated with removable prosthodontics. *Journal of the Dental Association of South Africa*, **40**, 387–90.

Davenport, J. C. (1970) An adverse reaction to a silicone rubber soft lining material. *British Dental Journal*, **128**, 545–6.

Davenport, J. C., Wilson, H. J. and Spence, D. (1986) The compatibility of soft lining materials and denture cleansers. *British Dental Journal*, **161**, 13–17.

Faigenblum, M. J. (1968) Retching, its causes and management in prosthetic practice. *British Dental Journal*, **125**, 485–90.

Fish, S. F. (1969) Adaptation and habituation to full dentures. *British Dental Journal*, **127**, 19–26.

Gutteridge, D. L. (1988) The effect of including ultra-high-modulus polyethylene fibre on the impact strength of acrylic resin. *British Dental Journal*, **164**, 177–80.

Hargreaves, A. S. (1975) Polymethyl methacrylate as denture base material in service. *Journal of Oral Rehabilitation*, **2**, 97–104.

Hoad-Reddick, G. (1986) Gagging: a chairside approach to control. *British Dental Journal*, **161**, 174–6.

Lamey, P.-J. and Lamb, A. B. (1988) Prospective study of aetiological factors in burning mouth syndrome. *British Medical Journal*, **296**, 1243–6.

Lawson, W. A. and Bond, E. K. (1968) Speech and its relation to dentistry. (i) Speech and speech defects. *Dental Practitioner and Dental Record*, **19**, 75–81. (ii) The influence of oral structures on speech. *Ibid.*, **19**, 113–18. (iii) The effects on speech of variations in the design of dentures. *Ibid.*, (1969) **19**, 150–6.

Liddelow, K. P. (1964) The prosthetic treatment of the elderly. *British Dental Journal*, **117**, 307–15.

McCabe, J. F. and Wilson, H. J. (1974) Polymers in dentistry. *Journal of Oral Rehabilitation*, **1**, 335–51.

Means, C. K. and Flenniken, I. E. (1970) Gagging – a problem in prosthetic dentistry. *Journal of Prosthetic Dentistry*, **23**, 614–20.

Murphy, W. M. (1979) A clinical survey of gagging patients. *Journal of Prosthetic Dentistry,* **42**, 145–8.

Osborne, J. (1960) The full lower denture. *British Dental Journal*, **109**, 481–97.

Osborne, J. (1964) Two impression methods for mobile fibrous ridges. *British Dental Journal*, **117**, 392–4.

Stafford, G. D. and Smith, D. C. (1970) Flexural fatigue tests of some denture base polymers. *British Dental Journal*, **128**, 442–5.

Thompson, J. C. (1971) The load factor in complete denture intolerance. *Journal of Prosthetic Dentistry*, **25**, 4–11.

Tomlinson, H. and Turner, C. H. (1984) A post-dam technique for metal based complete maxillary dentures. *Dental Update*, **11**, 655–7.

Tryde, G., Olsson, K., Jenson, A., Cantor, R., Tarsetano, J. and Brill, N. (1965) Dynamic impression methods. *Journal of Prosthetic Dentistry*, **15**, 1023–34.

van der Waal, I. (1990) *The Burning Mouth Syndrome*. Munksgaard, Copenhagen.

Vig, R. G. and Smith, R. C. (1972) Applied plaster impression for maxillary complete dentures. *Journal of Prosthetic Dentistry*, **27**, 586–90.

Wallenius, K. and Heyden, G. (1972) Histochemical studies of flabby ridges. *Odontologisk Revy.*, **23**, 169–80.

Watson, R. M. (1970) Impression technique for maxillary fibrous ridges. *British Dental Journal*, **128**, 552.

Wilson, H. J. and Tomlin, H. R. (1969) Soft lining materials: Some relevant properties and their determination. *Journal of Prosthetic Dentistry*, **21**, 244–50.

Wright, P. S. (1984) The success and failure of denture soft lining materials in clinical use. *Journal of Dentistry*, **12**, 319–27.

Wright, P. S. (1986) A three year longitudinal study of denture soft lining materials in clinical use. *Clinical Materials*, **1**, 281–9.

Wright, S. M. (1981) Oral awareness and oral motor proficiency in retchers. *Journal of Oral Rehabilitation*, **8**, 421–30.

Yemm, R. (1972) Stress-induced muscle activity: A possible etiologic factor in denture soreness. *Journal of Prosthetic Dentistry*, **28**, 133–40.

Index